Readers' Praise for

"This book is funnier than a leprechaun in a bag of Oreos."
~John

"Escaping from the hum-drum normality of the blogosphere like a shot of Hunter S. Thompson after a boring day, Vix could be the girl in the cubicle next door, and that's what makes her biting internal monologue and seductive wit all the more alluring. Come for the sexcapades and stay for the charming self-deprecation inside the mind of the chick we all want to share a bottle of bourbon with."
~ax

"From the second you start delving into the mind and tales of the Over-Educated Nympho, you will be taken by an avalanche of wit, adventure, sexual re-education and and plain entertainment. This book is many things: Shocking to some. Exciting. Arousing. And maybe an invitation to expand your personal sex life. But it is one thing for sure: A MUST READ!"
~Drago Schmidt

"When Googling "how to give a better blowjob," I came across something so much more powerful than a mere blowjob. I found someone else in this crazy world to identify with. Now I don't feel like such a freak while watching lesbo porn, eating an entire or two (no lie—it's insane) bag of Oreos, or letting the dark abyss of depression surround me. It's not just a nympho who writes a blog, it's a close personal friend of mine in Texas (Who I'm immensely jealous of for having not one amazing threesome… but two. Yes I'm bitter, I admit it freely)."
~beckster

"A paradox of wonder, fascination, and excitement, this book will leave you transfixed from beginning to end! Whether laughing at the exploits of the Triad or transfixed by her lack of the Bride Gene, this is one book you will not be able to put down!"
~Emmanuel A.

"If Dorothy Parker were writing today, this is what she would sound like. Vix has the nose-thumbing attitude of Parker, with the contemporary sexual frankness that would have gotten Parker arrested in the '20s. She offers instruction about giving blowjobs and reveals her own insecurities with equal deftness. She can make you laugh with her, and hurt with her, and feel what she feels. Her writing is honest, real and raw, and she can draw you into her head and let you see what she sees, the way she sees it in a way few writers can. If you know her work, there are favorites of yours in here. If you don't know her work, you will have favorites of your own in no time. Open up and enjoy."
~Tod Hunter

"I laughed, I cried, I tried to find the camera Vix has clearly planted in my bedroom. This book is an amusing romp through a world of contrasts between the smart, Catholic girl our parents wish us to be and the stripper that is hidden inside. More than a simple list of sexual tips and tricks, this book explores the hidden world of women who just happen to like sex...a lot."
~ Jessica

"...years later and I'm still getting complimented on the blowjob skills I learned from Vix! Her teaching has gotten me called everything from angel to goddess and has merited a few marriage proposals. Just this summer, an ex-lover mused on my impeccable skills with my mouth and eyes, calling it the best blowjob he ever had (sorry-not-sorry to his current girlfriend—maybe you could use Vix's book and learn a few things!)"
~ Brandinator

"Remember that blog you read several years back? The funny one with all the sex? Not that one...the good one! Yes! You found it by looking up blowjobs but stayed for the Oreos. Now you own it for yourself! Buy it and place it in your top drawer next to your bed. Next to your collection of special toys. You read OEN, I know you have that drawer (or drawers), you dirty girl."
~Barbie

RED WINE & OREOS

A collection of real-life misadventures adapted from the blog
www.theovereducatednympho.com

by

Vix

Over*Educated Nympho

AUTHOR'S NOTE
This book is a work of nonfiction. All names and identifying details have been changed to protect the not-so-innocent. Any similarity to a real person is strictly coincidence.

COPYRIGHT
© 2018 Vix the Over-Educated Nympho
All rights reserved. No part of this book may be used or reproduced in any matter whatsoever without the written permission of the Author.

www.redwineandoreos.com

© Ingrid Michaelson "Keep Breathing"

With sincerest thanks to Kelsey Wiseman of Wiseman Editing
www.wisemanediting.com

Questions? Comments? Email vix@redwineandoreos.com

To all the over-educated nymphos out there who are still scared to reveal themselves to the world.

Courage, my beloveds,
you have it in you, just as I did

It is not so much the example of others we imitate as the reflection of ourselves in their eyes and the echo of ourselves in their words.

Eric Hoffer

Contents

Foreword 12
Introduction 14

Part I

What If It Falls Off? 17
Knowing Sex, Being Sex 19
Forever Fifteen 21
Being a Meaty Chick 24
Nympho Statement 27
But My Medicine Cabinet Is Already Full 28
Naked *vs.* Raw 30
Assholes Need Not Apply 32
Real Romance Smells Like Sweaty Feet 36
Just Another Manic Monday 38
Sweet Smell of Comfort 42
Quiz: Are You a Nympho? 44
Necessary Lies 48
The Beginnings 52
The MOM 54
Quiz: Are You Over-Educated? 58
"O" Marks the Spot 60
The Story of the Russian 62
Speaking a Different Language 63
Smooth Hands & Gritty Memories 65
Overeducated and Unhappy 66
Wham, Bam, Thank Ya, SLAM 67
My First Threesome 70
How to Break Up in Fifty Words or Less 91
About Me: Raw, Ugly, Real 92
What You Think *vs.* What You Say During Sex 96
What I Miss About Being Single 99
Get That Thing Away From Me 101
My Tattoo 104
Preparations 108

Part II

Just Fucking Go For It 110
Red Wine & Oreos 112
My Story in Boxes 114
How To Get Your Coworkers Fired 118
Having a Girlfriend is Usually Considered a Cockblock 119
Am I Missing the Bride Gene? 123
Meet the Triad: The Pussy, My Brain & Me 126

Meeting Apartment #41 128
Douchebags at the Bar 131
How to End a Bad First Date 135
Dont' mind me it's the wine talking 137
The Rules of Fuck Buddies 138
The Triad: Abort, Abort, Abort! 141
The Pink Toothbrush Situation 145
My Future NYC Brownstone 147
Keeping the Mystery 150
187 Wrongs Do Make a Right 152
The One-Night Stand Contract 159
Fuck the Mystery 162
Bi-curious or Bisexual 163
The Triad Wants You to Take off Your Pants 164
Handsome & Pretty Twosome: A Proper Threesome Takes Nine Courses 170
I Could SO Be a Model. If You Squint. 191
TeXXXas Welcomes Porn Stars 193
Where Are You in the Blowjob Ring? 196
Blowjobs Are Not Icky 198
How to Give a Blowjob 201
Ducking the Family Guilt Stick 214
What I'm Really Thankful For 216
This Is Why I Don't Like Bars 219
How Do Guys Measure Up? 222
Are You Sure You Want to See My Place? 226
Hey Dumbass, I'm Trying to Flirt with You 230
Fuck Prince Charming, Where's My Frog? 236
Do Not Judge Me Based on My Impulse Purchases 238
Being Honest 241
Keep Your Happy Memories Away from My Soft Drink 244
My Careers Aren't Speaking to Each Other 246
Nympho Statement 249
My Boyfriend TiVo Broke Up with Me 250
Sometimes Love Isn't Enough 253
He Had Me at Hello... and Lost Me Anyway 255
Facing the Folks Again 259

Part III
Depression is a Big Fat Motherfucker of a Blessing 266
Perverts Perverts Everywhere 268
Revenge of the Cubicle Monkey 277
Does Your Cooch Smell Like Rose Petals Too? 279
One of Those Godforsaken Days 283
The Condom Aisle is Heckling Me 285
153 lbs, alcohol units 2, Oreos 62, calories approx. 9000 (v.g.) 287

Double Drama 290
Choosing to be Single, in Sickness and in Health 304
Cunt 307
I'm Mary Fucking Sunshine, Thanks for Asking 309
I Love Being Single, But 311
How to Talk Dirty 313
Look at Me Look at Me oh shit THEY'RE LOOKING AT ME 319
How to Answer 'If You're So Great, Why Are You Still Single?' 323
Is It Enough to Keep Breathing? 325
163 lbs, alcohol 2 4, bowls of Cinnamon Toast Crunch 3, calories 7 328
I Have Tits Too, You Know 331
More Than a Blowjob Queen 333
My First Time Sparkled 337
Waking Up Next to Hairy Man Ass 339
You Know You Need to Get Laid When 341
Who's on Track? 343
It's My Cooch, Not a Venus Fly Trap 345
Because I Love Cock 350
162 lbs (5 pending) Thin Mints 127, calories zero don't count on N.S.A.D 352

Part IV
Jazz Man, Meet Awkward. Awkward, Meet Jazz Man 356
The Cubicle Monkey Escapes 359
The Rhythm of Jazz Man 360
First Mission with the Marine 364
Base Camp One 368
Loving Pussy 371
You'll Shoot Your Eye Out 373
Because I Believe 376
But I'm Straight. -ish. 380
Farting in the Face of Sex 381
What No One Tells You About Losing Your Virginity 384
Wondering About Him 392
Why We Got the King-Size Bed 394
Slipping By 397

Recommended Reading 399
Afterword 401

Excerpt from the Next Book 402

Foreword

Why did I sleep around so much in my twenties? Was I insecure? Did I want to be liked? Was I recovering from sexual abuse? Did I want a place I belonged? Did I like being chosen?

Nah. That's all bullshit.

I just like sex. It's that simple. I like how having a cock inside me feels. Not how it feels emotionally, but how it feels physically, which is fucking awesome.

I love cock. It's that simple.

I'm not filling a hole in my heart, having daddy issues, or wanting someone to like me, even if only for one night.

I. Love. Cock.

I love a hard, veiny cock in my hand or pressed against my miniskirt. I love a hard cock released from a pair of blue jeans, eager to go where it belongs. I love a hard cock, period.

Because I love sex, many readers called me a slut. Because I love sex, some friends thought I was a slut, but were too nice to say anything. Because I was a slut, some of these same friends encouraged me to have casual sex, because they liked the stories I brought them. It's the nature of loving sex, that others will try to shame you. And you just have to deal with that. Ignoring them is usually the best option, or cutting ties. One so-called best friend broke up with me because she couldn't deal with my swinger lifestyle (see book two). I wasn't going to stop being who I was, so I let her go. I had already been censoring myself for her, which wasn't fair to myself.

I don't give a fuck what your father, boyfriend, or best friend tells you—*it's okay to love sex.* It doesn't make you a slut; it just makes you human.

You have to be true to yourself in everything you do, whether that's making art, going to culinary school, being a square, writing poetry, or only having friends who waited until marriage. Maybe you're reading this book because you love tales of salacious sex, even if you've only had a couple partners. That's fine.

Don't give in to pressure no matter which way it's pushing you. We're all just trying to be happy, after all, and that means something different to each of us.

What makes me happy is having a hard cock inside me. Oh my, am I even allowed to say that as a well-raised, privately-educated independent woman? I'm not saying it's the *only* thing that makes me happy, but it's definitely top five, along with writing, reading, making people laugh, and being with my family. I can be a well-rounded person and still love sex. I don't think our era gets that quite yet. Maybe our children's era will get it. Maybe girls will stop slut-shaming each other, but instead, bask in their sexuality and how much fun it can be, as long as they don't prey on anyone's feelings.

Maybe one day, sex can be just sex, without the word "slut" being thrown around at those of us who stand out from the crowd.

Go forth, girls and women, and have sex. Dare to love sex. Have fun and be safe.

Vix
October 27, 2018

Introduction

What the hell is an over-educated nympho, anyway?

I had meant to ask her that earlier in the evening. But later, it seemed a dumb question to raise while said nympho was kissing and undressing my girlfriend.

It's hard now to recall exactly the long, winding road that started with casual chats and ended between Vix's legs, but images remain. Oh, the images. So many. (Excuse me.) But thankfully, there's the full post, page 170.

I wish I could approach everything in life with the same hubris and intent that I approached my threesome with Vix and my girlfriend. Years ago, my girlfriend had admitted experimenting with women and that she was open to exploring such experiences again. Fortune favored me: I soon met a sex blogger through a friend. I was curious and charmed. And I was focused — focused on introducing this cheeky Vixen to my girlfriend. I persuaded, negotiated, and in no time, there was a fateful dinner meeting. We three ate, drank, laughed, and retired to my home. There was kissing and undressing. Lots of giggling.

The rest ended up on her blog. Page 170 to be exact.

What a blog. It's a bit surreal to read about yourself, learning about you through the eyes and fingers of a witty, sultry, and (over) educated writer. Sex brought us together, but Vix's intellect and stark honesty kept us together. She was generous, vulnerable, a lover, and a friend. The term "friends with benefits" never meant much to me, until I benefitted from this kind of friendship.

Sex is fun, yes, in that it's a liberating release and the culmination of wanton lust. But it's also exposure — literal and figurative. Vix exposes herself literally to a select few, but exposes herself figuratively to all. Her work is raw and real and sometimes uncomfortable. It's sometimes awkward, sometimes pure glee.

You know, like sex.

One of my great joys was mentioning her blog to various friends: I was shocked at the diverse audience. These were liberal, single professionals and conservative, married moms. They were young and old, gay and straight, prudes and freaks. Vix started her blog at a time when blogging was new. Sex writing was mostly in print. Her blog was quite the digital unifier.

I'm not surprised she's written a book; I'm surprised I'm writing the forward. Her work and her adventures (conquests?) have led her to many colorful, randy characters. They'd write a far better forward than I could muster.

Perhaps I'm writing the forward because I was so forward, long ago?

Enough about me. Welcome to the sultry, silly, sexy world of Vix. May you have the same joy that I did in devouring her every word when I first stumbled upon her.

And hell, after reading, may you one day have the chance to meet and devour her. I highly recommend it.

Handsome Twosome
December 1, 2018

Part I

One of the greatest moments in anybody's developing existence is
when he no longer tries to hide from himself but determines to get acquainted with
himself as he really is.

Norman Vincent Peale

What If It Falls Off?

The first time I masturbated I was six years old.

I didn't really understand what I had done, even years later in science class when we learned about masturbation, I didn't quite make the connection. Since it concerned "my private place" (what my mother called it), I understood it was something to keep to myself, to keep secret. I didn't see it as wrong or sinful, just ... well ... my secret. So I only did it at night when I was in bed waiting to fall asleep. I didn't tell anyone about it. I had just started a new school and didn't want to be known as the weirdo.

I first began noticing happy feelings when I would sit on one leg in class while waiting for my turn at the restroom. If I started rubbing myself on my leg, it would help ease the need to pee. If I rubbed a little differently, it felt nice. One day I put my little hand there and things felt *really* nice. From then on, if I was having trouble sleeping, I would rub myself until I sighed and I would fall asleep easily.

But I was worried.

What about Mom, when she did the laundry and saw my underpants, could she tell? Could she see anything that would suggest what I'd been doing? When I did it during the day and came to the kitchen for dinner, could anyone tell by my face? Could anyone at school tell I touched myself? Did I look naughty? Was it obvious?

As I got older I worried more and more. My friends didn't talk about it, my older cousins didn't talk about it and they even knew penis jokes, it wasn't on TV or in any of my books. What if what I was doing was bad? Was I doing it too often? Was I doing it too hard? What if I broke something? What if the next time I went to the doctor and he looked, and it looked wrong? Then what? "I've been rubbing myself for years, Doctor, I kept trying to stop because I worried it would fall off but it felt so good I started doing it every day?" Surely the doctor would tell Mom and she'd be mad because she'd have to buy me a new one for me and I knew she didn't like spending money.

I really did try to stop. I was more concerned about the thing itself and not so much morality. What if I like, used it up? How did it work? If you used it too much did it stop growing? If you did it too hard, would it get worn out and fall off? Why wasn't this mentioned anywhere, it seemed pretty important to me!

It was quite some time before I put together my sighs and masturbation. I only kinda got it during the reproduction unit in fourth grade science class, but the teacher avoided details because we were young and laughed every time she said "penis" or "vagina" (as I still do).

I didn't really get it until one of my old friends from came to visit when I was fourteen. Christopher was always getting into trouble, but I was friends with him anyway. We saw each other for the first time in eight years and he introduced me to Truth or Dare. He dared me to eat a dog biscuit (not as gross as I thought, just bland), I asked him if he had kissed a girl yet, he asked me if I masturbated. I paused on that one. I actually recall cocking my head to one side and thinking really hard.

"Don't you know what that means?" he asked.

"Yeah, I learned it in school."

"So . . . do you or don't you? Masturbate?"

I thought some more and finally said "Yes. I masturbate. Huh."

And I thought some more.

That's when everything started clicking together for me. I was already a horny little thing, but now things were processing much much faster. I started paying *much* more attention to boys as they went through puberty. They began to be taller than me, they got hard biceps, they got long lean legs, they started dressing better. I noticed it *all*. At night I'd go over my newest findings, a huge mental file cabinet of images of boys and some girls from school and what they looked like and what I wanted to do with them. I started talking to my friends and we pooled our information into a vast vat of knowledge over which we'd giggle and make fun of each other and say Ewwww to all the things we heard about from older kids, but secretly I wanted to find things out for myself.

And so it began.

Knowing Sex, Being Sex

It was different for a girl. So much harder. Nothing was nothing. Even a half-assed blowjob two years ago with a guy you maybe remember is something.

You had to keep all the boys a secret if you didn't want everyone talking about you and how easy your skirt pulls up and that you're thinking about getting your nipples pierced.

You had to make sure the nice boys didn't hear in case you ended up actually dating not just recreationally blowing one. You didn't want a nice boy at the time, but you knew you would eventually. So you had to be careful what you said and who you fucked. Just in case. Fuck the bad guys so you can save the nice ones for later, when you were ready.

It was always all about you. It was never about me, even when you talked about how much you liked gripping my firm ass and seeing the tattoo hidden there *No it doesn't mean anything I just like the way it looks* or how much you liked the sounds I make when you bit my neck a little bit hard like I liked it.

Even the baddest guy could flip to a good one in the time of one sentence. With his dick spent and still in your mouth he'd say something like *I could really marry a girl like you*. It would take all your good will not to bite down hard and demand he take it back. Maybe every guy wants to marry the whore after all.

Some days it was too much. You'd wear loose pants and flat shoes and keep your hair loose and wild and hope no one whistled at you or said *Hey baby* from a delivery truck or held your hand a second longer when handing back change. Some days you couldn't stand it, you wanted to detach yourself from your tits and legs and ass and all things that could lead to sex. It didn't matter though. They could still tell. Even the nice ones could tell. You wondered if it was your scent or something you couldn't cover up. You wondered if it was in your eyes. Like you can see Crazy in the eye of someone on the subway and just know to avoid eye contact. What could people see in your eyes that you couldn't see? You didn't think there was anything left to see except pupils.

I was good at sex. It was my thing, like some people are good at math or juggling or computers. The funny thing was that I was actually good at some things. Many things, really. Math, literature, writing, foreign languages. I was a very smart and talented child. I went to prep school. I learned prep school things like advanced calculus and how to ignore my inner bitch. I painted and filled out college applications and went to meetings of the National Honor Society where I sat in the back and read. I wasn't a whore in prep school. I wasn't anything, really. Just smart.

That's what I learned in college: smart means shit. I never got straight A's or made the Dean's List once I got to college. But I had something special when I started. I'd had a long-term high school boyfriend, which meant I knew sex. I knew sex better than anyone in my class. But a long-term college boyfriend silenced that until my senior year, when I was told I started to ooze Sex. It was no longer high school sex or college sex, it was woman sex. It only took one guy to realize that I was in a whole other league, one where people devour each other and even the most violent fucking is a peaceful death.

I fucked men as if it were my mission to extinguish them. I fucked beautiful men twice my age and they thought I was a demon with unfair sexual powers. I wanted someone to put me in my place, to remind me that a smart nerd girl didn't belong on her knees. I told them before or afterwards or even during that I was a smart girl, that I could recite Ovid and Eliot and make teachers cry with my poetry. They would always look at me as if I were speaking another language. And then we would fuck. They could tell fucking was what I knew.

I wondered if they knew I was different. I didn't know how I was, but I knew there was something about me that made so many men and women stop to look at me twice. For the longest time I thought I was crazy or egotistical or self-involved. They kept looking. I wondered if they could tell when I had been fucked the night before. If it was in my gait or ass-wiggle or posture. If it was in my proud face.

Forever Fifteen

When I was fifteen years old, I wasn't popular. I didn't listen to the right music, I didn't flirt with the boys, and I didn't have the right friends. I didn't wear the right shoes or expensive jewelry to make up for the fact that otherwise we looked the same in our uniforms.

When I was fifteen, I tried to tell myself that I didn't care. I was too busy studying to go out to movies or concerts. I didn't care enough about my looks to wear make-up. Besides, all the cool guys at my school told me I had ugly legs (the very legs that now rock a short skirt and high heels like they were meant to be rocked). I told myself that I would never be pretty like any of the popular girls, so I should concentrate on doing well in school. This obviously did not help the popularity situation.

Then I got my first boyfriend. A hot boyfriend. No one believed me because he went to a rival school. After a lot of begging he came to see me play softball. My teammates all crowded together on the bench and whispered loud enough for me to hear, "Oh my god, Vix's boyfriend is HOT. Why is he dating *her*?"

That question always rings in my ear when I'm with a guy. *Why the hell is he dating me. Why the hell is he fucking me. Why the hell is he even* talking *to me?* I'm twenty-fucking-eight years old with a great education, great career, great tits, and *this* is what I have to say? Sure I manage to push those thoughts aside most of the time, but the point is they shouldn't be there in the first place.

When I told my boyfriend after practice what my teammates had said, he grinned. Not only did he look smug, but he did not say any of the reassuring things a good boyfriend is supposed to say. That hurt extra hard because I suspected that he already thought the same thing as my teammates.

Now I'm older and smarter about the ways of the world, allegedly. I know that popularity in high school is a big joke, and that being pretty does not mean someone will automatically have a dozen BFFs. I know this on a logical level after years of trying to get over my stupid self. However you can't always rationalize away the way you feel when the cool kids don't invite you to happy hour after work, or even so much as include you in the funny email forward that goes around the office. Because I am forever fifteen.

Today I saw four of the other twentysomethings in my department walk past my desk, talking about what restaurant to go to. I looked over, expecting one of them to say "Hey Vix, got any lunch plans?" Instead they kept walking. I sulked. Not because they didn't invite me, but because I still care that the cool kids don't want to hang out with me. It didn't help that they are the four most attractive people in my department, and they only talk to me enough to be polite. I felt like I was in high school all over again, watching the cool kids from behind the wall of a textbook.

Even though I'm not the ugly nerd girl I was in high school, I still feel her alive and kicking inside me. When I see a cute guy checking me out, I tell myself that I probably have a stain on my crotch, or that I look like his little sister's best friend. On the rare occasion a guy hits on me, I assume that I'm reading into the situation because why would he hit on me? I was never popular, and I was never pretty. I was the nerd girl with ugly glasses and an armload of books, and now I can't shake it.

A lot of readers out there are probably shaking this book and asking, BUT YOU'RE A FUCKING *NYMPHO*. WE HAVE SEEN THE PHOTOS OF THAT ASS. STOP BEING A DUMBFUCK.

No. That little fifteen-year-old Vix has always been there, looking for some much cuter girl behind me when a guy waves in my direction. To this day I'm still amazed when someone cool talks to me, let alone fucks me. There have been a couple of guys in my past that I fucked just because they reminded me of the guys in high school who never looked at me twice. I'm embarrassed to admit that. Hell, I'm embarrassed about this entire post.

I worry that I will feel this way for the rest of my life. Don't let the tight pencil skirt fool you. Sure I act confident and sexy on the outside, but that's basic self-defense. There isn't a lot of room to show insecurity when you spend most of the day around half-familiar acquaintances and strangers. Being a young female at the bottom of the corporate ladder leaves no room at all.

Why is it that at the established age of twenty-eight I still feel like the goofy adolescent girl who doesn't wear the right clothes, the right make-up, or say the right things? It's all so fucking stupid, and yet I still care. What is there to worry about if I have great friends who love me as I am? What am I trying to prove, especially if I'm the only one who seems to care?

What really concerns me is that if I still feel this way now, I may never get over it. I don't want to feel like I'm fifteen forever, always assuming all anyone can see is the ugly nerd girl inside.

Being A Meaty Chick

I have always been a meaty girl. I have a predominantly German ancestry, with the last four generations being of the strong/drunk farming sort. Which means we're big and surly if we don't eat red meat every day. It also means we're thick, muscular, and athletic. We know how to throw our weight around. Especially the women in my family. Let's just say the reign of the matriarchy goes way back.

I say this because I am proud of being meaty. Note: meaty is not a euphemism for "fat." I am not and never have been fat by anyone's opinion (except that one bully in the 10th grade whom I slammed against a wall and cursed out, but he changed his mind after that incident, oddly enough). When I tell people my weight or size they are always surprised because I do not look it. I am lean, have no tummy rolls, no cellulite except where I am supposed to. But I definitely have an athletic build. I am 5'-8", 160 lbs and a size 10. And apparently I'm not supposed to admit this so readily. I should be ashamed and silent because I *am* 160 lbs and a size 10 (oh dear me!). But I don't. I'm proud, and after I tell you why you'll never look at a size 2 chick* the same way again.

Being a thick and noticeable girl is something to be proud of. If I see another *healthy* chick call herself a fat ass and take the bread off her low-fat no-mayo turkey sandwich (hold the cheese), I'm going to scream and drag her sorry (and decidedly not fat) ass to my apartment for some mental re-conditioning. Which will probably include a rib-eye, a piercing, and some *fuck you* heels that will make her stand proud with her booty sticking out.

There are so many wonderful things that come with being meaty. I am strong. My legs are built for playing sports, for jogging, for lifting weights, for riding a guy's cock all night long, for sprinting up subway stairs in heels, for never standing down to a physical challenge that the super skinny chick might think twice about.

Guys out there: is there really any better feeling than grabbing onto a woman and just pounding the fuck out of her without worrying about breaking the poor thing? Especially for the big guys out there. Sometimes you don't know your own strength, and not all girls actively look for that in a guy like those of us with handcuffs hidden in our purses.

I am big. That means I am noticeable, commanding when I enter a room or am standing in a crowded bar. With three-inch heels on I'm eye level or taller than the average guy. I like to put them in their place. ("Um, *while you're down there*, why don't you make yourself useful . . . "). Many people don't want to admit it, but goddamnit it's true: being tall(er) helps with the typical male-female power battle. I stand above my boss, look down to his eye level, and say "I'm sorry, John, but I spoke to the consultants and that is just *not going to happen.*"

When I was single and sizing up guys, height was an issue. I was more likely to go home with the shorter guys who looked me in the eye over the taller guys who flinched and asked if I had to wear such tall shoes. Yes, I do, because that's part one of the "Do you get to fuck me" test, and *you just flunked, asshole.*

I know how to make the most of my body. I love seeing so much muscle on my body even though I haven't been to the gym in months. I love being able to match my male coworkers forkful for forkful at lunch. I love that if someone tries to push me aside, I don't budge. I love that I can throw several 2×4s over my shoulder–while wearing a skirt and heels–and walk out of Home Depot without needing any help. I love that so many past lovers have complimented me on my body—for being so thick, so solid, that they're not afraid to throw me around and really pound me because my body can take a beating and then ask for more.

I have not always felt this way. Ohhhh no. In high school I was ugly, nerdy, and quiet. Never mind I was getting laid five times a week by my hottie boyfriend, but he went to another school so no one knew to think otherwise of my outward bookworm appearance. All the popular guys in my grade (this was a small private school, mind you, so everyone knew everyone else) picked on me every day for having such thick "elephant" legs. They teased me for years and finally there was the aforementioned throwing-asshole-against-wall -and-holding-him-by-his-neck incident which improved things, but not by much.

My boyfriend telling me that he didn't like me playing so many sports because it made my quads and calves too big didn't help either. And, anyone knows, if you hear something often enough you begin to believe it. After years of this, I started to believe that my legs were too muscular, that I should never show my legs under a short skirt, that I would never be attractive.

Fast forward many years. I ran into two of these former prep school assholes when I lived in New York City. I went out for drinks with both of them. One apologized for being so mean and asked me out (guess what my answer was). The other one was very friendly and respectful and while on the way out of the bar told me that I "had grown up well." Mmmmmmm hmm. That's right, fuckers. You can make nice all you want but I'll never let you kiss this sweet ass of mine.

Let's just say that now my outfit of choice is a short skirt to show off my well-defined quads with a tiny camisole to expose the strong back and Jennifer Garner-esque triceps. I will never ever again make the mistake of letting someone convince me that I should apologize and cover up my meaty body. This body was made to eat, to run, to live life, to fuck, and most importantly–to stand up to people when I want them to get the fuck out of my way.

---

*Yes, I know that of course there are tons of women out there who are not meaty, who are short or petite and that doesn't stop them in any way. I have been friends with many girls who are just as badass as the meatiest of girls. All I'm saying is that being meaty helps, and that it's something to be proud of, fuck what the skitches (skinny/bitches) in all the magazines look like.

Nymphos are lovely and do not deserve to be stoned to death
aka the Original Nympho Statement

This issue is a huge pet peeve of mine because I see and hear it everywhere.

Guy wants girl who's nympho
Guy gets nympho
Guy has sex with nympho
Guy thinks nympho is whore
Guy no longer likes that girl is nympho
Guy brags to other guys that girl is nympho
Guy tells nympho "Not tonight honey, I have a headache"
Nympho beats the shit out of guy with a baseball bat

Ok, except for that last line, I get this bullshit all the time. Apparently *I* am a nympho. I never really thought of myself that way. Although looking back I can see it was kind of inevitable. When I was five I was the little girl on the playground chasing boys trying to get them to kiss me (They never did. Stupid boys.) When I was six I started masturbating. When I was thirteen I was so horny I didn't know what to do with myself so I just masturbated more. First blowjob at fifteen. Lost virginity at sixteen (and I was the one who pressured my boyfriend into it). For 21st birthday got hood of clit pierced. Between serious boyfriends at age of twenty-one, I became player. By that time, I'd gotten so much shit that I figured I might as well have the fun that goes with it.

My high school boyfriend told me I liked sex too much and that was skanky behavior.

My college boyfriend told me I liked sex too much and couldn't I make less of a deal of it?

My current boyfriend told me I like sex too much and why can't I get over it?

Most guys just can't handle a nympho.

But My Medicine Cabinet Is Already Full

Yesterday was my last day at my job. I saw my therapist, Dr. Fixer Upper, the day before that. They go hand in hand well. Work makes me sad. Dr. Fixer Upper makes me happy. Even though I'm quitting the job I hate, it still got to me. It still broke my spirit. And so I thought it would the perfect time to see my therapist.

That, and I needed more happy pills before my insurance got caught off.

Between having chronic depression and attention deficit disorder and some nauseating bouts of anxiety, I've tried tons of medications over the years. I can cluck off the names of anti-depressants like a child can name Santa's reindeer. *Prozac, Paxil, Zoloft, Celexa, Lexapro, Wellbutrin, Effexor, Serzone.* I've tried nearly every single one of them. Actually, no. As of this week I have tried every single one these, because my psychiatrist gave me some new samples to try. Then there's the ADD meds, which I've had much less success with. I'm still looking for The One that will complete me. I know it's out there, I just haven't found it yet.

My medicine cabinet is full. This is in addition to the overstock shelf in the bathroom's linen closet. One entire shelf is old prescription bottles at various stages of emptiness, depending on how long it took me to figure out that the medication of the month wasn't working.

Mom occasionally calls me up and asks if I have any old so-and-so because she ran out and it will be another week before she gets her prescription from Canada, the land of cheap online drugs, or because my brother lost his bottle of Ritalin, or because one of my cousins heard good things about Zoloft and she remembers I tried it a year or two ago. This is normal in my family.

Then there's Aussie, my live-in Australian boyfriend of a year, who has never so much as taken over-the-counter drugs for allergies. He might take Tylenol if he has a peculiarly bad hangover, but that's about it. He looks at my pill-popping world and he doesn't understand it. I look at his mentally sound world and I don't understand *that*. What craziness. Surely something is wrong with Aussie—he just doesn't know it yet.

When we first started dating, I was very protective of my depression because it had already been a silent and lethal beast in my last relationship. With Aussie I was upfront about having depression from the beginning, but I only revealed a little at a time, trying to gauge how much he could handle. Which was probably a mistake in hindsight, but I didn't want the medicine cabinet full of half-used prescription bottles to scare him away.

Then was it really any surprise that he didn't get how bad my depression could be? A long time ago he asked me if I really needed to take all the drugs because I didn't seem that bad.

One, it's because of the anti-depressants I don't seem so bad.

Two, I don't let you see me when I lose it.

Three, you've never been depressed, so you don't know what you're talking about.

But the thing is, when I'm not going through one of those depressed spells, I can't remember how bad it can get while in one. Even if I was like that just the day before. It's not so much "forgive and forget" as it is "I need to forget".

Depression can be very black and white. While in a depressed spell, you can't remember what it's like to be happy, to smile, to want to get out of bed, to want to do anything. You only feel the wretchedness of not wanting to be inside your own head. Then when you're your normal self, you clap your hand to your head and think "Oh silly me, I was just having a bad day! I won't let that happen again." It is never ever like that though. There's always another bad day. Or in my case, months.

Then one day you wake up and you're happy to be alive again, and you forget how bad it was just twelve hours earlier and you vow never to let it get to you like that again. And you keep making yourself that promise every time it happens, and you keep thinking, "Maybe this medication will be The One," every time you leave the doctor's office with another bag of samples.

Naked vs. Raw

Being naked has never bothered me. As a baby I screamed if fully clothed. In most photos of me before the age of five I'm in various stages of carefree undress.

As a teenager I got naked with my first boyfriend as soon as it no longer felt slutty to do so. I proceeded to continue getting naked with him as frequently as possible, enjoying walking around his bedroom buck-ass naked with his boner as the reward for such comfort in only my skin.

In my first one-bedroom apartment where I lived by myself in New York City, I frequently walked around naked, even on the coldest nights when I could feel the chill from the window.

I have always been all about the naked. It's natural. Easy. No *problemo* there.

It only occurred to me recently that maybe this great ease with physical nakedness serves as a distraction from how emotionally distanced I am. This *rawness*—I don't believe that it's becoming in person. At least not on me. In the anonymous blogosphere it's becoming, endearing even because I'm brutally honest, which is a nice change from the laugh-out-loud primetime sitcom. I never expect to see any of you, so I don't hold back. I don't care if I say something and a dozen of you lose interest and stop reading me. As much as you see it and empathize over a computer screen, it's so much more raw in the flesh, so much more ugly and messy to handle.

That's why in person I hold back a lot. It seems the older I get and the more relationships I'm in, the more I hold back. Especially with guys. Experience has taught me it's better to hold back the really raw parts of yourself, at least if you want someone to stick around. That is a horrible thing to believe. Sure, you can sing show tunes about how it's the faults that make you beautiful, but no. Faults don't make you beautiful. How you *deal* with those faults can make you beautiful, but not everyone wants to see you falling on your ass and sorting your way through the mess over and over.

Where does that leave me. Easy with the naked, unyielding with the raw. Too scared to let anyone see me past all the exposed flesh.

Assholes Need Not Apply

Every straight girl has a list of criteria for The Perfect Man. This list often reads like a personal ad: "must be smart, funny, Protestant, a stock broker in the Northeast. Romantic walks on beach a must. Bonus if like antiquing." Except when I was in high school and college, the lists of criteria were way more out there: must speak five languages and run marathons, be non-smoker but not mind if I smoke two packs a day, must be vegan and have been in military, prep school and Ivy-League education required, not be too caught up in himself. He's a mama's boy who knows how to treat a woman i.e. like a princess who only accepts presents that sparkle.

I will admit I've had some bizarre criteria myself—must aspire to be a famous B&W photographer, plans to travel to every famous foreign art museum, cooks large gourmet meals while singing Italian operettas in a perfect accent, doesn't mind my excessive and often creative cursing. I fully admit to my former dumbassness.

Then some of us grow up and develop more realistic expectations, others don't. They'll die old and wrinkly and lonely still waiting for Prince Fucking Charming to find them and whisk them off into the sunset when all those years they could have been seducing men half their age.

So where do these realistic criteria come from? What makes a Perfect Man? What makes my perfect man different from every other straight girl's perfect man? I don't want to compete with three million other horny bitches in my city. I want him to be *my* perfect man.

The way my criteria became more realistic was after dating two different guys in high school and college. The first boyfriend is now known to my friends as Asshole Boyfriend, because he was an emotionally abusive, selfish, narrow-minded, used-douchebag. The college boyfriend is known to my friends as Nice Boyfriend. (Although depending on context, I may also refer to him as Man-Boobies Boyfriend.) Here's a list based on one I wrote up at the time:

1. I don't like assholes.
2. I don't like man-boobies that are bigger than mine.
3. I like guys who are smart enough that I can have real conversations with them, but not so smart that I'm embarrassed to read my brain candy (i.e. *Glamour* magazine) in front of them.
4. I don't like religious guys. I'm an atheist. Atheism and religion have a way of expressing themselves in bed.
5. I like guys who are funny, witty, sarcastic, and ironic. I don't want to have to explain why *The Simpsons* is funny.
6. I don't like mama's boys. They are pansies and you will never be as good as his mama.
7. I like guys who shower every day.
8. I like guys who are open-minded, whether it be about food, people, or telling his guy friends that feminists are the girls to date because they're the most fun in bed.
9. I don't like guys who tell me what to do. At all. Quick story: Asshole Boyfriend thought I showed my body off too much (back then I didn't) and told me to wear looser tops and longer shorts etc. The first day I started college away from my hometown I ran naked all over campus screaming to make sure every possible person saw my naked ass. I broke up with him the next morning and proceeded to date Nice Boyfriend who loved running around campus naked just as much as I.
10. I don't like guys who don't pay attention to me. I'm not talking about the little stuff, but the big stuff, like what month my birthday is, why I don't think racist jokes are funny, and why I'm not calling him anymore.

There are many more things I learned about what I like in a guy, but this covers the basics.

At this time, I feel I must point out that, thus far, I have written about the criteria for a Perfect Man with regards to a boyfriend/husband. The criteria for a one-night stand are entirely different. Here is a comprehensive list:

1. Hot, as in a smokin' hot body you can't wait to jump on.
2. Someone you don't mind the possibility of never seeing again.
3. Open-minded enough to think that your clit piercing is sexy, not skanky.
4. Foreign accents are a plus. Personally, I like to ask foreigners to talk nasty to me in their native language. Wooooweeee, let me tell you, hearing Russian to this day makes me wet instantaneously.
5. Someone strong enough to hold you up while you fuck against a wall.

After a couple years of dating with criteria list number two, I was beginning to get a little bit pissy with my selection of hot foreign men. Sure a couple of them had taken my brusque behavior the wrong way and showed up at my door with flowers (which I felt really really bad about, but how hard is "this is just sex" to understand?!), but it's hard to transfer from being a one-night stand to a boyfriend.

At this time, having moved back to Texas to finish my final degree after a one-year internship in Manhattan, I decided I was ready for a boyfriend again. After all the hook-ups and fuck buddies I managed to revise list number one to be something realistic and obtainable:

1. Funny
2. Intelligent
3. Nice
4. Cute. Not necessarily hot, but hot is good too

Here comes the oh-so-not-fairy-tale way in which I met my current beloved, Aussie, in the most unlikely of places and the unlikeliest of ways.

After a month in Texas with no luck of boyfriend material, but already several more hot guys, I was losing hope (Hey, I'd just spent a year in New York Fucking City. My spirit was broken, OK?). An old fuck buddy of mine who I still hung out with called me up to meet him and his new friends at a bar. OK. I showed up and Guatemalan told me that he thought I'd probably like to hook up with his buddy, Aussie, who was foreign and my tendency to drool around foreigners is well known.

I met Aussie, who at first I thought was kinda boring because he wasn't talking much, but hey, he was pretty hot and I wanted to get me a big ol' piece of that. I went home with him, we hooked up, we stayed up late talking, and we ended up spending fortysomething straight hours together that weekend.

The first morning together we went for bagels and coffee and talked several more hours, we watched movies, we ate, we hung out with Guatemalan and friends again, we drank, we slept, we got to know each other. I saw that he was nice, sweet, considerate, romantic (although that has since disappeared, and this will surely be a future topic of discussion), very smart, funny, witty, entertaining, and utterly loveable.

That was just over a year ago. We had our anniversary recently. Aussie became Aussie the Boyfriend who as I type this is downstairs watching game seven of the NBA and hollering for me to hurry up and finish writing about him so I can watch the game with him.

So, I guess the happy little annoying moral of this story is that one-night stands can become something serious.

I mean, it was bound to happen. If you fuck enough guys, one of them is bound to grow on you.

Real Romance Smells Like Sweaty Feet

Let's be realistic. Roses and backrubs romance is only for teeny boppers and relationship newbies. For the rest of us, however, romance is a four-letter word. (And not the fun one you hope for on Valentine's Day.)

So, for the rest of us, where do we find romance? Does it even exist after you've been dating someone more than four months? Well . . . it does if you kinda sorta redefine romance to include not so sexy things—

1. He rubs your feet for you after a long day of work, and sweetly pretends there is no nasty sweaty foot smell making him throw up a little in his mouth.
2. He calls just to say he loves you . . . and that he paid the overdue electricity bill.
3. You give him a BBB: beer, blowjob, and baseball game, all at the same time. That means you can't get mad if he doesn't pay attention to you when there's a double-out on TV.
4. He brushes the hair out of your face and tells you with utmost sincerity, "That new anti-dandruff shampoo smells great, sweetie."
5. You eat sandwiches during sex. Hey, George Costanza wasn't totally dim-witted.
6. You share a secret and highly embarrassing indulgence together, like watching four consecutive episodes of *Gilmore Girls*.
7. You make spaghetti loaded with mushrooms (even though you would rather eat the rat fetus someone from Fear Factor threw up during the commercial break) just because he loves them, for some bizarre reason.
8. He asks you why you don't ever wear that really slutty skirt he likes so much anymore.
9. He TiVos your favorite show (while he's watching *Dark Angel* and downloading Jessica Alba photos, but still, it's the thought that counts, right?)

10. He doesn't hold it against you for taking a month longer to give him a drawer than he did for you. He didn't mind keeping his clothes on the floor. They just end up there anyway.

Just Another Manic Monday

    I know I'm not the only cubicle monkey out there who feels like I've been having a case of the Mondays since 1999. I am still a pee-on and have minimal responsibility. The few responsibilities I have I execute quickly and precisely so I can go back to the happy thoughts in my head, most of which are highly inappropriate and therefore fantastic fun. Blame it on the ADD. Or maybe that's just my pervy mind, but whatever. My normal day goes something like this:

1:03 Return from lunch
1:04 Get coffee from break room
1:06 Sit down to work, think about sex with Angelina Jolie instead
1:08 Pick at cuticles; wonder if Angelina Jolie's cuticles are sexy
1:09 Conclude *yes*
1:10 Wonder how much Angelina Jolie's sexy cuticles would go for on eBay
1:11 Decide why bother, couldn't afford them
1:14 Wonder if anyone in office is secretly an aspiring porn star
1:15 Michelle. Definitely Michelle.
1:18 Look at clock three times to see if the time has changed yet, finally put Post-it over screen
1:23 Wonder where the original TPS report came from
1:27 Get water, a ploy to check out cute guy in conference room by water fountain
1:29 Imagine sex with cute guy on conference room table
1:35 Stare at dead leaf on desk plant, willing it to drop off the branch and therefore prove telekinetic powers
1:38 Take a dump on billable time
1:58 Do Google search for "damn the man". Unimpressed with results.
2:02 Wish had a pillow under desk like George Costanza
2:04 Review George Costanza's many brilliant ideas. A sandwich during sex *would* be nice
2:09 Intentionally fart while standing next to an obnoxious coworker. Run away.
2:15 Talk to another coworker about weather, wonder what he looks like naked

2:19 No longer have interest in coworker because have imagined him naked

2:23 Throw self into work to get mental picture of naked coworker out of head

2:42 Wonder who thought up tampons

2:44 Bathroom: sit in stall for five minutes doing nothing but stare at shoes (so pretty!). Had no intention of peeing. Needed to leave desk where coworker was telling neighbor *again* how happy she is to be pregnant *again*.

2:53 Discover huge coffee stain on boob

2:54 Wonder how long huge coffee stain on boob has been there

2:55 Stare at huge coffee stain on boob. Clearly boob wants attention.

2:58 Color in letters in company logo printed on notepad. Color in so hard that tears through paper and stains desk

2:59 Cackle at sweet justice of it all

3:04 Get coffee, everyone stares at coffee stain on boob while walking to break room

3:12 Think about boinking all the guys in "hottie row" on second floor at same time

3:14 Consider masturbating in bathroom

3:15 Decide against masturbating in bathroom. Old lady who pees frequently also talks to herself, not ideal masturbation environment

3:18 Lean over large stack of papers with red pen in hand, trying to look like concentrating really hard while am really thinking about boinking all the hot guys on the second floor at the same time

3:22 Pick up highlighter. Now look like am *really* working hard, while actually am still thinking about boinking all the hot guys on the second floor—while the hot ones on the first floor watch

3:29 Stare at huge coffee stain on boob

3:35 Twirl in swivel desk chair while listening to Christina Aguilera's "Candyman"

3:36 Think about playing strip Candyland

3:37 Think about sex for next twenty minutes while working (and actually get a lot done—proves theory that sex clears the mind, at least for girls)

3:59 Wonder if mother still has Legos in attic

4:04 Hope Chelsea becomes the next Pussycat Doll

4:05 Daydream about watching *America's Next Top Model* and *The Search for the Next Pussycat Doll* with the Go Fug Yourself girls while eating tubs of ice cream and having Intern George massage our feet

4:09 Wish were a drag queen

4:11 Think about all drag queens have ever seen/met/been propositioned by (only two)

4:14 Add drag queens to mental Happy Place, along with midgets, the Dread Pirate Roberts (naked except for the mask, obviously), Oreoes, and Biggie O'Toole the leprechaun

4:26 Wonder who thought Keira Knightley would make a good bounty hunter

4:28 Think about a drag queen band of singing bounty hunters who sing in rhyming couplets and kill using only bejeweled jazz hands and/or "cleavage"

4:31 Draw a sketch of a Pez dispenser that holds Ritalin

4:32 Decide dispenser should resemble Wonder Woman

4:34 Draw sketch of a matching compact that holds condoms

4:46 Pretend to work when boss walks by

4:47 Resume daydream about showing McSteamy what steamy *really* is. Hope Addison joins in.

4:50 Walk around office at random. Need to get excess energy out of system

4:55 Walk by "hottie row" and feel smug when they all stare at huge coffee stain on boob

4:57 Wonder why good cheese smells so icky

5:01 Wish had a window

5:02 Think about splicing together a colored poster of Hawaiian sunset (charge all printing expenses to client) and hanging up on cubicle wall in futile attempt at escapism

5:03 Sit on toilet, contemplate existence. Take another shit

5:14 Look through purse for Xanax, find none

5:15 Get in staring contest with clock

5:14 Lose

5:17 Wonder who in office has naughty piercings

5:18 Imagine that all guys in hottie row have naughty piecings–and need to be punished for it

5:21 Consider buying subscription to *Juggs* and sending it to the virgin intern

5:24 Try wiggling nose like Samantha from *Bewitched*. Look like dumbass

5:28 Stare at huge coffee stain on boob. Overall, an eventful afternoon

Sweet Smell of Comfort

As a child, I would often slip into bed to read with Mom before going back to my room to sleep. I remember sitting up in my parents' bed with my book, looking around their room at all the items belonging to adulthood: Dad's shiny shoes, Mom's bras and lacy nightgowns, money and business magazines, luggage, scarves, red and maroon nail polish, thick hardback books, ceramic items I'd made in school, fancy purses saved for date night. I recall looking around the room, fascinated, waiting earnestly for the day I would own such adult things.

Of all the items surrounding me, none I wanted to possess more than the smell of my mother when I snuggled up to her, the book abandoned on my lap. Often, she would smile down at me and maybe laugh at something I'd said, then turn back to her magazine and flip a page. She never realized that while my head was on her chest, I'd tilt my head up to breathe in the smell of her, something sweet and clean that I had not found anywhere else, what I later learned was the face cream shipped in from an overseas friend of hers. Once I asked her to use it on me but she said, as I commonly heard from grown-ups, I was too young for it—what six year-old needed face cream?

Now when I visit Mom and Dad very few of these adult things remain in their room. Most no longer hold importance for them, having grown well into middle age. Now I go into my parents' room and it no longer smells wonderfully exotic, just old and settled. There's no perfume or glorious travel books or beautiful clothes with foreign colors. All that remain of the original adult glamour are the stacks of magazines on money and business, many covered in dust. Books and clothes cover the bed, which Mom often sleeps on because she's too tired to clear them off first. When I first noticed the disregarded energy of their room as a teenager I was saddened, even a little ashamed for them. Now that I'm older I understand, and I wonder how they maintained that level of energy for as long as they did.

While I was living in New York City, my parents booked a last-minute flight for me to visit home because I had called them crying so many times. That first night home, weeping and broken and disappointed in myself for being a failure at my first attempt at adulthood, I climbed into their bed where Mom was reading one of her magazines. She looked up in surprise, but quickly made her small customary motherly smile. She had been in a similar place many years ago. Although she has never told me her story, I've heard enough pieces to know that it was her shaky first step toward being the strong woman I have breathed in all my life. Here she lay next to me, having long outlasted the exotic makeup and pretty nightgowns that I used to think were signs of being a woman. Her smile was no longer full or glowing, but it was there, holding steady.

This time I didn't use the pretense of a book to crawl into bed with Mom like when I was younger. I wrapped my arms around her and started crying quietly. Throughout my childhood I'd hide in my bedroom closet when I cried because I was too proud to be seen vulnerable, even in front of my parents. But for the first time, I was too *empty* to be embarrassed. I let Mom pull me into her, her sweet soft neck smelling just like it always had.

Quiz: Are You a Nympho?

Sorry guys, this quiz is intended for ladies only. Ha. "Ladies."

Please note that "nymphomaniac" and "slut" are not the same. Nor is "kinky". Webster's definition of a nymphomaniac is "excessive sexual desire by a female", which I have issues with because of the whole "men want sex more than women so any woman who wants sex as much as a man is a slut and any woman who wants sex more than a man is just a fucking nymphomaniac freak-of-nature" bit. Which I will get to in a later post because as you may have noticed this issue royally pisses me off. I'm still trying to come up with my own definition of a nympho, which is a large part of the reason I'm writing this blog.

1. Did you masturbate before you actually knew what it was?
2. Did you keep masturbating when you found out it was wrong, no one would ever marry you and you'd go straight to hell?
3. Have you ever used something other than your hand/sex toy to get off?
4. Has anyone ever videotaped you and you loved it?
5. Has anyone ever told you that you have a porno face?
6. Do you enjoy giving blowjobs?
7. Have you ever seen a really well-hung horse, dog, etc., and gotten just a tiny bit horny?
8. Do you enjoy getting spanked?
9. Do you prefer to be the one who spanks?
10. Do you read sexual connotations/innuendos/puns/double meanings into anything possible?
11. Have you ever thrown someone up against a wall and demanded sex?
12. Have you ever scared someone with your unusual sexual appetite?
13. Can people tell within minutes of meeting you that you are a pervert with sex on the brain?
14. When someone refers to you as "a lady" do others crack up to the point of snorting?

15. Have you ever done anything in public with a pole?
16. Are you an exhibitionist? (i.e. you take your shirt off in a bar, never mind that you're dead fucking sober?)
17. Do you have a nipple or genital piercing?
18. Do you carry a mini-vibrator in your purse or work/school bag?
19. Have you ever hit on or been hit on by the person piercing or tattooing you?
20. Have you ever scared away a reputed player or kinky SOB because you were entirely too much for him to handle?
21. In bars do strangers point at you and whisper to each other with looks of admiration/lust/intimidation?
22. Do you turn down guys who are not on your playing field? Or even remotely close (this is a key difference between nympho and slut. OK, well there's more, that whole confidence thing, but this is just supposed to be a fun light-hearted quiz, so I'll save that post for a later time when I feel like going on a rant)?
23. In a bar fight could you totally take Angelina Jolie? And turn it into a make-out session?
24. Have straight girls hit on you because you're just so damn irresistible?
25. Do you not bother getting drunk when you go out because you don't have any inhibitions to lose in the first place?
26. Have coworkers or bosses ever told you "You have too much sex appeal. Please tone it down"? Even when you wear slacks and loose sweaters/blouses (i.e. normal office attire) to work?
27. Has anyone ever admitted that he's cheating on his girlfriend/wife with you (whom you did not know existed) because you're "just too hot to pass up"?
28. ... And this is the first time he's been unfaithful to the girlfriend/wife of x number of years?
29. Do you regularly get bitchy, pissy, agitated, aggressive, even mildly violent if going too long without sex?

30. Has anyone asked if you're a stripper and meant it?
31. Has anyone ever suggested you be a stripper?
32. Back in the day when you were a virgin, did people assume you'd lost it ages ago?
33. Do you think you should know how to go down on a woman just because "it seems like one of those things you should know how to do"?
34. Do friends come to you for sex advice (should I really talk dirty to him? Really?! Are you sure??), resources (i.e. which store has the best selection of vibrators), definitions (what is a dong?), explanations (why are guys so obsessed with anal sex?), and sympathy (why are boys so dumb?)?
35. Have friends told you that you should write a sex column because you're a better sexpert than the ones who do have columns?
36. For you is going without sex like a vampire going without blood?
37. Have you ever had orgasms numbering in the double-digits?
38. Do you have to keep a list so you remember what your Number is? Or did you just give up?
39. Has anyone told/accused you of dating or fucking like a guy?
40. Did your sex drawer turn into its own huge sex box?
41. You roll your eyes at the sex articles in *Cosmopolitan* and *Glamour* because you did all this stuff when you were, like, *seventeen.*
42. In a fit of frustration and self-consciousness, have you ever genuinely wondered, "What is wrong with me?"
43. ... And then said, fuck them, there's nothing wrong with me! I'm safe, classy, and confident, and those assholes can go fuck themselves?
44. Have you ever gone so long without sex that you started humping every lamp post you walked past?
45. ... And gotten off?
46. Does it ever feel like your Brain and Good Sense are at odds with your Pussy, but goddamnit Pussy always wins out?

47. Are you ever NOT in the mood? (Exceptions: visiting your parents, seeing another Pauly Shore commercial, visiting friends with a baby, hearing that Jennifer Garner is carrying Ben Affleck's spawn-child.)?
48. Do you still insist on having sex while you're sick?
49. On the day you went from being single to having a boyfriend, did the city cloud over, thunder roar, animals run to low ground, and the sun disappear?
50. Have you ever showed up late to work because you were masturbating? For an hour?

Scoring: Two points for every yes. Count on your fingers and toes if you need help keeping your score straight.

0-20: Um, you *have* had sex, right?

21-40: Eh. You're the cute Charlotte-type-character like on *Sex and the City*. But admit it, you're scared of the penis, aren't you? Oooh, watch out, HERE COMES ONE NOW!!! RUN!!!!

41-60: Not bad. You're definitely some fun in the bedroom. You won't have *too* difficult a time finding a husband. Unless he finds out you once took this quiz because you had *suspicions* that were a nympho. Think about how ashamed your children will be.

61-80: Congratulations! You don't mind putting icky things near your mouth. You're practically a ho!

81-100: Full-fledged nymphomaniac. Welcome to the club. You're fucked.

101+ Whooooa. OK, you're just a freak. Do you fuck leprechauns or something?

Necessary Lies

Sometimes for the sake of your relationship, you must lie. No big lies, no coordinating of alibis, none of that shit like you see on *The O.C*—just little lies . . . like that song, "tell me lies, tell me sweet little lies, tell me lies, tell me tell me lies . . ." from the eighties? Yeah? Well it's dead on. The most popular lie in relationships: *Do I look fat in this?* "No honey, you look beautiful. You're always beautiful."

This is the sort of lie I'm talking about. Now sometimes it's clear you're lying, in which case don't bother. (ex: if he asks you if you can tell he has man-boobs underneath this shirt and his tits are 40Ds, then don't bother lying. It's just hurting both of you.) But if there's a possibility you're telling the truth, both of you will accept the lie because it could *conceivably* be true.

For example: "Our kids won't be like that. They'll be different. They'll be well-behaved." But then again, you married/childed readers may know by now that's a big, fat, blatant kick-you-in-the-shins lie.

Here is a more detailed list of lies you should tell to protect your relationship. Especially if it's new, somewhat new, old, or fragile. Note: if the proper/false answer does not have the desired effect, proceed cautiously with either sex (i.e. pleasing the offended partner until he/she forgets what original topic was) or profuse apologizing. If apologizing occurs, this was not my fault for my scripted proper answers, it was your fault for not lying better.

For Her Sake:

Is this girl on the cover of Victoria's Secret prettier than me?
True answer: According to the dick-meter, she's SPANKIN' HOT, *whoooop whooooop*!
Proper answer: Eh. She's OK. Not my type. But *you*, sweetie, you're my type!

Does my butt look big in this?
True answer: Uh, well, J. Lo's big butt is in style now, right? 'Cause baby, you could booty-shake her off *any* stage.

Proper answer: Oh sweetie, your ass looks *wonderful.*

True answer: I'm dating you because of your big ass. With an ass like that I thought you would be all about the anal sex. Obviously I was wrong, which is why I hope you never find the four gigs of porn on my computer.

Wrong answer: I love your ass! So when are you going to let me hit that?

Does it bother you that I've been with so many other guys?

True answer: Excuse me? "*So many* other guys?!" Slut. Whore.

True answer: Every night after I make love to you, a part of me dies inside.

True answer: How dare you have slept with more people than me! *I'm* supposed to be The Man, not you!

Proper answer: Not at all! It's in the past. Besides, I'm the one who benefits from you being able to deep throat, sweetie.

Do you think my best friend is hot?

True answer: paSHAWWWWW! Mmm, I'd spank that shit SO HARD. Oooooh, THREESOME! I KNOW WHAT I WANT FOR MY BIRTHDAY OH PLEASE, OH PLEASE!

Proper answer: Who? Jennifer? Oh, don't be silly. Guys don't like girls with huge tits like that.

Do you think about other people while we're having sex?

True answer: Uh, *yeah.* Your sister, your best friend, the UPS chick, the sandwich chick, my boss in that skirt of hers, Jessica Rabbit, my third-grade math teacher, your mother, your other sister when she wears those leather pants . . .

Proper answer: Of course not. I'm thinking about you! I'm not attracted to anyone else.

Agh! Look at that girl, she's dressed like such a slut! Don't you think so?

True answer: –blood rushing to penis–

Proper answer: Agh! *Such* a slut.

True answer: Dirty dirty slut . . . I bet you talk dirty too, don't you, you dirty dirty slut . . .

For His Sake:
Do you wish I was big and muscular like Brad Pitt in the movie Troy?
True answer: Mmm . . . Brad Pitt in *Troy* . . . my nipples just got hard.
Proper answer: What, oh *him*? Eh. He's not my type. I don't like guys whose pecs are super defined like that.

Am I better in bed than your last boyfriend?
True answer: You mean Stan the Man? The boyfriend who made me cum so hard I blacked out and swore to name my first child after him?
Proper answer: Oh, don't be silly. Of course you are! You're so nice and . . . *gentle* . . . –sigh–

So what did you think of my best friend?
True answer: Dumbass. Who smelled. Like ass. Dying old man ass.
Proper answer: He's . . . nice! What an interesting scent he had . . . He's very.... *bohemian.*

Is my dick smaller than average? Tell me the truth.
True answer: No, it's not small. In comparison to the average 8- to 11- year-old boy.
Proper answer #1: Is that the phone I hear ringing? The office is supposed to call . . .
Proper answer #2: No. (As in, "No, I will not tell you the truth." It's all in the literal interpretation)
Proper answer #3: It's fine, honey! It's exactly as much as I need.
True answer: But then again, I'm 5'1" and have a freakishly shallow vagina, according to my gynecologist.

Do you think about other people while we're having sex?

True answer: Um, *yeah*. Brad Pitt, the lawn boy from *Desperate Housewives*, your brother, your imaginary twin brother (since it apparently would take two of you to get me off properly), my yoga instructor if he were straight, your other brother, my art professor, my last boss, the bank teller, that hot chick at the gym, Matthew McConaughnewhatshisname, the carpool dad who winked at me . . .

Proper answer: What? Did you say something?

Does it bother you that I have a third nipple?

True answer: It bothers me that you have it pierced.

Proper answer: Not at all! That huge hairy mole makes it barely noticeable!

Does it bother you that I don't go down on you very often?

True answer: Yes. Asshole. Why am I dating you again?

Proper answer: Yes. Asshole. Why am I dating you again?

. . . because there are times when you really need to be honest.

The Beginnings

I love to tell stories, I always have. When I was a child I loved to watch my father and uncles exchange stories on Grandpa's patio on the farm in deep North Texas. I was a lone girl in a company of men. They'd sit out there for hours telling stories of laughter, triumph, and a helluva lot of bullshit.

When it was hot they'd sit in a circle in patio chairs and drink from their bottomless beers that it were my duty to refill from the Kegerator. When it was cold they'd stand in a huddle, arms perched over the barbed wire fence with mugs of whiskey in hand. The stories came easily. They'd been gathering on that patio for so long that they often got caught in their bullshit stories, having told them differently before.

I don't know why they always let me sit with them. Not once did any of the men wave me off. They often forgot I was there, telling stories full of *motherfuckers* and *gotdamnsumbitches*. Over the years I learned there was an art to words, especially dirty ones. They taught me the fine nuances in saying *jackass*, depending on whether I was pissed, amused, or amazed. From them I saw when to pause while telling a story, how to change tone when talking as someone else, and to intentionally wait until someone was drinking his beer to spill the punchline.

It was at that young age I became fascinated with storytelling. I came home from school with stories I'd collected to tell my father, hoping to earn a loud hearty guffaw like the ones I often heard when he was among his brothers. My stories were cute, young, and, at best. received a chuckle.

I read constantly, trying to figure out what made a story worth hearing. What makes a laugh come from deep in the gut? What moves a grown man to tears? What makes a group of people fall silent in thought when they were laughing only moments earlier?

As I grew into a teenager, I never lost interest in the group of men out on the patio. Eventually they started letting me drink a beer of my own and later I grew brave enough to attempt sharing my own stories. My stories still fell short of the round of belly laughter I craved, but. Regardless. the men in my family looked at me with respect, proud that I was out there with them in the circle of lopsided chairs and dripping beers.

For a long time I only attempted funny stories, ones of dumbassery (others', not mine), embarrassment (mine), and smartassness (always, always mine), because that was what I knew. I grew up in a house where my parents' laughter woke me up in the mornings. Funny was what I saw every day.

Tales of set-backs and overcoming inner demons were not something I was so familiar with. When depression took me down at the age of twenty, my father turned his ear. Mom pulled me away and said he lived in a happy world, but not a realistic one. He could only hear laughter.

I grew silent. There was no room for stories of my kind out on the patio, or anywhere else.

Forfeiting my voice didn't keep me from trying to find the story inside the mess. Hours and hours I spent with a pen in my hand, trying to make sense of what was clouding my head. Doctors and books said it was mostly biochemical—something I had minimal control over—but I didn't believe it was nearly so simple. There were so many things that a pill couldn't explain, let alone fix.

Many of those first months were nothing but waves of senseless emotion on paper. The handwriting looked like it belonged to someone with a half-paralyzed hand, it was more erratic with each turn of the page. I wrote the same things over and over, waiting for the fog to clear just a tiny bit in hopes of giving me a glimpse of what was really there.

I wrote and wrote and one day things started to make sense. I kept writing. I needed to know that my voice existed, that my feelings were valid. I needed to know that my story was worth telling, worth hearing—but most importantly I needed to know that I wasn't going through everything for no reason at all.

The MOM

Mom just called.

She has her own special ring on my cell phone. For her cell phone, work phone, and home phone, they all have the shrill YOUR MOTHER'S CALLING ring. Whenever I hear it, even on someone else's phone, I automatically recoil in preparation of The MOM. In all her emails, she types normally until the signature where she always capitalizes MOM. Like she's a deity or a monster or arch-enemy. Which, she is. All of the above. No one intimidates me more than The MOM. None of the razor-blade-spitting bosses I've had have ever put the fear of death into me like The MOM.

I think she figured out the separate phone ring though (over the course of two years) and now calls me on Dad's cell phone because then I actually think it's Dad and pick up, only to hear, "Have you read my email?? I emailed you yesterday! When are you going to therapy again? Did you tell him you need to go every week? Did you tell him your pills aren't working?"

–sigh–

And she had the nerve to ask Aussie last weekend why I never pick up the phone. As if there were any question, really.

After two unanswered emails and three unanswered calls (and a bitchy blog entry), I decide it's time to pick up the phone so she doesn't call Aussie at work and demand to know "IS MY DAUGHTER DEAD OR JUST FAKING IT AGAIN?" Yes, she has actually done this. Despite what the all capital letters suggest, my mother does not scream or shout or even raise her voice. No. She's The MOM. She doesn't need to raise her voice. Her tone alone can make people drop to the ground as fast as cow shit.

"Are you going to see Dr Fixer Upper tomorrow?"

Yes, Mom.

"Are you going to ask to try new medication?"

Yes, Mom.

"Are you going to ask if you can have weekly therapy sessions?"

Yes, Mom.

"Are you going to haggle to see if he'll charge less for you?"

Yes, Mom.

"Are you going to tell him about how you're unproductive and can't send out your resume?"

Yes, Mom.

"Are you going to tell him about all the time you're spending in bed?"

Yes, Mom.

"Are you going to tell him that you *must* get his taken care of? Every day you lose to depression is a *day of your life you've lost.*"

Yes, Mom.

"Have you set up a separate therapy session?"

Yes, Mom.

"I read in the newspaper that some people just have bad genes. They get depression for life and never get over it, no matter what pills they try. Do you want me to send you the article?"

No, I want you to withhold any information that may make me start to cry. Like now. I'm about to cry.

"Oh honey, don't cry. You're just making yourself depressed all over again!"

No, you did.

"Don't you even think about going to that fridge and getting out the ice cream. I know how you are with that ice cream. I noticed you've gained weight."

Yes, Mom.

"Your aunt told me about this new surgery technique they're trying called transcranial something-or-other that is a procedure that fixes your brain so it releases the right hormones when it's supposed to so you don't get depressed. You should look it up. In a couple years maybe you can get it done."

You want me to get my brain probed?

"Not *probe*, sweetie, FIX. Look it up on the internet."

Yes, Mom.

"So I think you may have that bad gene I was just talking about where you're depressed for life and nothing can fix it, you're just like, *screwed* for life. I think that's you, because you're not doing as well as me or your brother or any of our other relatives on anti-depressants."

Thanks, Mom, that's your *gene that's screwed me up.*

"It could have come from your father, you know, I swear they're all depressed."

They're just alcoholics, Mom. Happy *alcoholics.*

"Don't you think that's caused by depression?"

No, I think mothers that send them depressing articles all the time are what cause depression. Then they drink so they lose brain cells and can't remember what they read in all these damn articles.

"Stop being negative, that's not going to get you anywhere."

Yes, Mom.

"You know, you should be so thankful you've got all these people around to help you with your depression."

Yes, Mom.

"Especially Aussie, he has to see you ALL THE TIME and that's not easy, especially for someone who's never been through depression himself."

Yes, Mom.

"You be careful, you can't let your depression get any worse or you'll scare him off."

Yes, Mom.

"That's why I'm nagging you to take care of this NOW, before you get worse."

Yes, Mom.

"Well, I'm glad we've talked. Call me tomorrow and let me know what new medication he suggested you try."

Yes, Mom.

"And since you're feeling better today, why don't you send out a couple resumes? You'll feel better once you get a job."

Yes, Mom.

"Bye, sweetie!"

CLICK.

I need to ask the psychiatrist for stronger Xanax tomorrow. This pissy little .5mg shit ain't holding up. I need a force stronger than The MOM. Like Xanax in the water filter and cheap vodka.

Quiz: Are You Over-Educated?

Do you, have you, are you, –insert proper grammar here–, etc.:

1. Ever speak only in anagrams, iambic pentameter, or Latin?
2. Get in a huge argument with your boyfriend about how to organize your combined book collection: alphabetically, by genre, by date of original publication, by undergrad/graduate/doctorate program?
3. Say "prep school" using the same innocent tone as "I assumed everyone read Rilke?"
4. Know what "meretricious" means (bonus points if you know the Latin root)?
5. Can name every "-ism" in modern European History in alphabetical or chronological order?
6. Refuse to use monosyllabic words for an entire day?
7. Were informed by the anesthesiologist that while she was putting you under you kept reciting bits of Chaucer?
8. Had sex with a nuclear physicist? (I actually did)
9. Read the authors whose main ideas are now commonly known as S&M? (bonus points if you own any of their works)?
10. Own anything from Dover Publications (example titles: *Life Histories of North American Marsh Birds*, *The Triumph of the Darwinian Method*, or *The Diary of an Early American Boy: Noah Blake, 1805*)?
11. Read all of *Moby Dick*, including the entire chapter on whale anatomy (without throwing the book against the wall)?
12. Take notes in books reading for recreation?
13. All your masturbation fantasies begin with you reading in a private library stocked with first-editions?
14. Understand Proust?
15. Get into heated arguments about Post-Modernism in American and European art—while drunk?
16. Could easily pursue three different careers with little additional training?
17. Own the same book in English, French, and German?

18. Have a one-night stand and use it as research for an article you're writing, "Third Wave Feminism and the New Generation of Fuck-Me Feminists"?
19. Won a middle school science fair for making a hydraulic pump to generate electricity using only your pet hamster and items found inside her cage?
20. Can't readily remember how many degrees you have?

The more *yes* answers you have, the more over-educated you are. I dunno, one of you engineering/math nerds can come up with some elaborate equation or something to illustrate just how too-educated for your own damn good you are. I'm going to go watch *Friends* to attempt compensation for the fact that I made up this entire list on my own in thirty minutes. And that I answered *No* only four times.

"O" Marks the Spot

I am a huge fan of the clit piercing. I got mine years ago for my twenty-first birthday. Best present to myself EVER.

Half the sex appeal of the clit ring is that it's a nice surprise the first time I'm with a guy. (Yes it is incredibly difficult keeping such a fun secret to myself.) Think about it: on the outside I'm a nice well-polished young woman, suitable for taking home to meet the parents. Then take my clothes off and there's tattoos and piercings galore. Well not really *galore*, I don't have a trashy number of body art—just enough to be sexy.

Then you can play it the other way and casually mention in conversation (it's surprisingly easy to drop in, "when I got my clit pierced—", I swear) around someone you like, or a friend of someone you like, and that thought will be burned into his head until he sees it up close and personal. Multiple times. What does it look like? A ring or a bar? What color? How does it work? Is it easier to get her off? How does it work with oral sex? So many questions with which to torture.

I want to dispel a few myths and fears.

The clit piercing is actually through the hood of the clitoris, not through the clit itself. It is *not painful*. At all. I've had my ears, cartilage, nose, and belly button pierced, and getting my clit pierced was as easy as getting the ear lobes done. I swear. Sure, I am known for having a freakishly high pain tolerance, but I can still tell you relative to other piercings and tattoos that the clit piercing does not hurt. Seriously. It felt the exact same as getting a shot at the doctor's office.

Having the piercing does not make me get off every two minutes or spontaneously just from wearing tight jeans—but *Yes, Mom.*

Yes, Mom.

it does make it significantly easier to get off. I have a ring with a ball through it, and I roll the ball down underneath the hood to rub directly against the clitoris. It's strategically awesome.

It's a dirty secret of indulgence. That's all there is to it. I love being so well polished and pressed from eight to five, knowing the entire time that I have naughty tattoos and happy piercings and *if only they knew*. It's fantastic fun having a secret identity. I don't need a shiny cape and tiara! I have bling of my own.

The Story of The Russian

A couple years ago was the only time I dated someone who didn't fit easily into the relationship or the casual sex category. I have been on exactly four second dates in my entire life. Three of them were with guys I entered long-term relationships with. The fourth one was with The Russian.

It was on my way to work the year I lived in New York City. I always stopped at Bergen Bagels in Park Slope before going on the 2-3 subway line into the city. That day I was wearing a long, pink bias-cut skirt that added extra sashay to my hips and extra confidence in my shoulders.

I pushed open the door *ring ding ding* and that stupid bell felt like it froze time for the next ten feet as I walked from the door to the back of the line, where a gorgeous man's man sort of guy stared at me with the sexiest combination of lust, bewilderment, and simple *awe*.

I will never forget those ten seconds. Before I even knew his name, he made me feel like the sexiest and most breath-taking woman ever to walk before him. He immediately started talking to me, and he had my phone number by the time we left the shop.

And those ten sexiest seconds of my life marked the downfall of the entire year I lived in New York City, with the one I could never figure out.

Speaking A Different Language

I looked over at The Russian lying next to me in bed. My wonderful bed, my heaven, my haven. I called it my princess bed because it was up so high (due to risers, so I could store as much as possible in my 300 square foot Manhattan studio apartment) and I had strung shimmery curtains from the ceiling all around my bed. I could pull those curtains closed around my bed and create a soft place for me and The Russian to sink into together for hours.

That particular night had been wonderful. For the first time since we'd met, we had gone out to eat a nice dinner. When we headed out of my apartment, The Russian pulled my arm down 1st Avenue to a Ukrainian restaurant he liked.

We drank fancy cocktails, fed each other food, talked for ages, and looked at each other with lover's eyes. It didn't matter we had nothing in common, that he often had to ask me to describe to him "Eh, whad does dis mean? Dis wohrd?" We always found something to enjoy in each other.

There was this one moment in particular at the restaurant I will always remember: we had just finished talking about something and the laughter gave way between us. His lips parted just a tiny bit like he was about to say something. For that split second, he looked at me like he cared and I looked at him like I was happy.

Later that night, drunk on wine-flavored denial, we started kissing and slowly pulling off each other's winter clothes. I could hear him murmuring things in my ear as he kissed my neck.

I leaned into his own ear and kissed it delicately before asking him, *Say something sexy to me in Russian.*
He had the tiniest hint of a smile on his face. "Why you want ta hear ma Russian? Do you not a like me in English, oh what?" I giggled and smacked him.

Please. I want to hear the way you really talk.
The Russian succumbed to the plea in my eyes. He resumed kissing my neck and rubbing his hands up and down my bare back. First, I felt the different pace of breath on my face and then I heard the words follow.

Hard, thick murky words came from The Russian's mouth. Russian is not a soft or lyrical language. It is rough, coarse—like the country itself, like the man beside me.

Only a sentence or two passed his lips. I moaned from deep inside and asked him what he had said.

He said nothing. Just shook his head and pulled me back down to him.

Smooth Hands & Gritty Memories

It was in the way he said my name. Long and breathy, thick. There was more to it than his murky Russian accent. He used the nickname that so few use. I loved hearing my name halt on his tongue and linger for a split second before returning to broken English.

His hands didn't show the years of subway construction work, the sixty-hour weeks of sweat and grit. I teased that he didn't really lift manhole covers but sat in at a desk all day and that's why he never had black under his fingernails. His small hands looked worn but durable. Artist's hands. Just watching them caress my bare stomach was enough to make me forget to breathe. I loved to take one of his thick, soft hands and hold it in my own. I'd turn it over and examine every knuckle, vein, and line, as if drumming my fingertips against his could reveal how they knew my body so well in such a short time.

He always tasted sweet, fresh. Even after he smoked a cigarette, the taste seemed to disappear as soon as the smoke left his mouth. Then he would kiss me on my lips, and he'd taste like me.

Afterwards I would look over at him lying on the bed next to me. Once his body's rhythm slowed to normal he'd place his hands behind his head, close his eyes, and smile. That was my favorite moment. Sometimes I would place my hand on his flexed bicep and gaze at the taut muscle. The male and female bodies are so different that I can't help but reach out and touch it. After all these years, there are still so many displays of masculinity that make me bite my lip.

A few times I woke up early in the morning to the touch of his knuckles trailing up the small of my back. I would smile to myself and enjoy it while it was there.

After he left in the morning I would go back to bed and drift in and out of the night's memories. I wanted to cover myself in the scent of our sex, our heat tangled in the sheets. The smell of his cologne on my pillow would keep me hovering there for hours while I wondered when—if—I would see him again.

Overeducated and Unhappy

From psychologytoday.com, Nov 22, 2006 By Colin Allen new research from Stanford School of Medicine.

Highly-educated Americans may earn more money, but they're also in for more misery, according to new research from the Stanford School of Medicine. The findings indicate that people with advanced degrees are at greater risk for mental health problems than the rest of the US. Employees at a Northern California office where 51 percent of works had a master's or doctoral degree were evaluated for their overall mental health status. The highly educated workforce scored well below the national average.

Overall, those with advanced degrees fell into the 32nd percentile, 18 points below the national average. Those who had recently completed their graduate programs were at greatest risk for mental health problems. The researchers attribute this to a lack of experience in coping with life's hardships.

Well, fuck me and my three degrees.

Wham, Bam, Thank Ya, SLAM

I just had fantastic sex. The hot sweaty slap-me-harder kind of sex that can be hard to find in long-term relationships.

The only trouble is that this great fuck was my boyfriend, and now I wish I could gracefully wash my face, kiss him on the cheek, and walk out the door before he remembers to ask for my phone number.

I don't want to cuddle with my boyfriend on the couch while the dogs wrestle to get in-between us and Aussie tries to sweet talk me into fetching him a beer while I'm too busy trying to discreetly release a fart.

While we're at it, let's throw into the equation any of normal daily occurrences: stepping in a puddle of puppy piss or erupting in a huge sigh instead of screaming, "DON'T YOU DARE YELL AT ME ABOUT THE PLANTS DYING WHEN WAS THE LAST FUCKING TIME YOU WATERED THE FUCKING PLANTS I DIDN'T EVEN WANT ALL THESE PLANTS ALL I WANTED WAS SOME FUCKING BASIL TO COOK WITH AND DO YOU SEE ANY GODDAMN BASIL IN THIS APARTMENT???" or jumping out of bed in the morning to be the first in the shower and thereby leaving the other to walk the dogs in the cold or seeing skid marks again in the fucking laundry in spite of asking him ever so nicely to please, kindly wipe his ass thoroughly before you forsake the institution of marriage and join a lesbian commune.

What I want after a hot fuck is to be left alone so I can enjoy the afterglow and raw pussy muscles without hearing him talk back to a Geico commercial.

I want to go to bed while my skin is still damp from sweat, sex, and heat so I can savor the memory of GREAT sex. I want to close my eyes, feel the cool fan on my face, burrow down into the cool covers and play over in my head all the hot fantasgasmic things that my body just experienced—that first pull and tensing as I lower myself on his cock, the first rock of our bodies together and then against each other, the hovering and teasing of muscles, the heavy, heavenly sigh breathed in my ear, the instant my mind blanks out from anything except heat and quivering, the pride in my body for being capable of such things over and over.

What I don't want is for my boyfriend, still flushed from fucking, to ask me if his work shirts are clean.

This is why the hot, one-night stand is entirely underrated. It's a win-win situation. Either you have sex and it's great and you leave shortly after with a lovely time under your belt or you have sex and it sucks and you let the air out of his tires on your way out and tell the story to your friends who laugh so hard they piss themselves. Either way, you get to *leave*. Leaving is key to an enjoyable evening.

Now, don't get me wrong, I love cuddling as much as a bug as snug in a rug, but save that for pillow talk about what to name your children. When I have sweet sex of the making-love variety, of course I want to snuggle and whisper sweet nothings and dream about having a million of his babies. When I have hot, nasty, porn star sex, it's right up there with drinking down a couple Xanax: sweet escapist indulgence, best enjoyed alone and asleep.

Nothing can ruin a good fuck like reality. Seeing her in the morning with racoon eyes and bedhead, smelling a serious Number Two coming from your bathroom, hearing your mother on the answering machine reminding you to get "that rash *down there* checked out", seeing him in good lighting, or, god forbid, finding out he's a virgin and "this was so special."

Reality is to be avoided whenever possible, especially if an orgasm is involved. Which is why hot sex and relationships (specifically: once you've gotten to know each other enough that you read before going to sleep instead of fucking) just don't happen that often. Living together, being around each other constantly, being married, having children, it's amazing anyone manages to continue having sex, let alone *good* sex, once they've been together a long time. I am impressed when it happens. Quite frankly, reality makes you lose your hard-on. Assuming you had the energy to get it up in the first place.

This brings us back to why random sex is a wonderful thing to be enjoyed and appreciated while the having is there. After sex, you get to kick him out. You get to be alone. You get to enjoy the wonderful intimacy of sex without the possibility of a Dutch oven, a request for another beer, or him asking for a list of things he could improve on. In other words, the afterglow of good sex is best enjoyed *alone*.

My First Threesome

After reviewing the notes from my old journal to prepare for this, I only managed to write one paragraph before the overcoming whirlwind of sexual memories knocked me on my ass and forced a vibrator into each hand. *Okay?* Want to know the secret to masturbating for two and a half hours, without any reading/viewing material? Real-life memories like this.

It was me and two guys. Two *hot* guys. Like hottie, hot, McHottie, *hot*. And to top it off, they were from the country. I tell you, it's like it was right out of *Penthouse*. Except way better because it happened to *me* and before then I thought things like that only happened in porn.

This is the sexcapade that was mentioned in my interview in *Maxim*. The crazy sexcapade which I somehow forgot to mention to my ex-boyfriend, according to him. Hmm. Quandary.

Note: this is my ONLY story that starts "So I was at this bar . . ." (At this point in my life, it was true). I'm not into the bar scene (because normally I bomb out and run out of dignity before I run out of cash), which makes this night all the more triumphant.

So, I was at a neighborhood bar with two friends for happy hour on a random Tuesday night. I had told Cool Friend and Shy Friend I was looking to get laid and I had dressed appropriately for it: tight booty jeans, four-inch tall stiletto boots, and a slinky black top that was full in the front and fully exposed in the back with only two tiny strings keeping it tied on. Cool Friend had a boyfriend, so she offered to play wing(wo)man. Shy Friend was, well, shy, and seemed flustered with the whole idea of picking up a guy and using him for sex.

But sex wasn't my only reason to be there. Cool Friend and Shy Friend were both about to move to the other side of the country, so we were spending as much time together as possible before they left. We shared an order of onion rings, drank our three dollar margaritas, and shot the shit. Cool Friend started egging me on to hit on some guys already.

Fine. I blatantly looked around the bar for some guys worth looking at. I was being really obvious. Like half-propping myself up on the bar with one arm so I could stand and lean over for a better look obvious. Let's not forget the 180-degree turn-around-and-check-out. Yeah, I've got that one down so that it's funny and endearing rather than utterly lame. At least that's what I like to think.

It was during one of these blatant stares that I noticed a guy at the pool table blatantly staring back. This guy was *hot*. He was working a plain cotton T-shirt in that sexy and rare way that makes for instant wet between my legs, and he was staring in my direction with such interest that I was sure he was looking at some super-hot blonde standing behind me. I turned around to look for her. I shit you not, I *turned around* because I honestly expected him to be staring at someone else. I was not used to getting stares like that from anyone other than the creepy maintenance guy.

There was no one behind me other than tables of guys chugging two-dollar beers. Now, I am so lame, I have to warn you, I actually pointed my finger to my chest and mouthed "Me?" –putting head in hands– I can't believe I did that. I can't believe he didn't change his mind after such a dumbfuck move. But I did, and he smiled and nodded. I hesitated. He motioned for me to come over. I got up and then looked at my friends, who had stopped talking to watch me be a first class dumbass. I pointed to them. He motioned for all of us to come over.
SCORE.

I wasted no time walking around the bar to the pool table, where I saw another hot guy come out of the shadows.
DOUBLE SCORE.

I introduced myself to them and asked if they minded us joining them for a game of pool. They grinned and said sure thing as we made introductions all around.

The first guy was Army Cowboy. He was mid-twenties, strawberry blond hair, warm smile, tall, in the army, and looked like he had quite the ripped body underneath all those clothes. Thin tight T-shirt, jeans, brown leather boots (the kind of work boots country boys wear, not cowboy boots). And to top it off, he was as sweet as could be. Very easy to talk to, if I gave him shit he gave it right back—my kind of guy.

As soon as he spoke, and a sexy-slow Texas accent came out, I asked him exactly where he was from. Army Cowboy said the name of a small town about an hour and a half away. I teased him for wandering off a long way from home and he said that he and his best friend Dark Cowboy had just come to the city for a night of fun before he shipped out that weekend.

Mmmmm hmmmmm. I know what *that* means.

Dark Cowboy was also sweet, fun, and easy to talk to. And hot. Oh, so very hot. He wasn't quite as beautiful as Army Cowboy, but *shit*, that's like comparing Katherine Heigl to Elle MacPhereson. Like his best friend, he was tall, thick body, handsome—and a devilish gleam in the eye. Oh, how I love it when the eyes are asking to get into trouble. And, of course, by trouble I mean me.

I suggest playing pool girls against guys, but Army Cowboy vetoed that and said it wouldn't be fair. He said we should be on one team and Dark Cowboy and my two friends would be on the other team. We played a couple rounds, having great fun teasing each other and flirting shamelessly. Army Cowboy was clearly into me and it looked like Dark Cowboy was into Cool Friend. She had a boyfriend, however, and was politely side-stepping all flirtations. I whispered this in his ear as encouragement to switch his preference to Shy Friend. But Shy Friend was, duh, shy. The beer helped her to loosen up and flirt some, but Dark Cowboy wasn't quite into her like he was Cool Friend. However, being the Southern Gentleman, he kept buying rounds for everyone nonetheless.

By the end of the last round, Army Cowboy's hand had made it onto the top of my hip a couple times and I kept playfully touching his arm (stroking, whatever), which is classic guy-girl TOUCH ME MORE behavior. Neither of us wanted to make the next move though, so for the rest of the night this was the extent of our physical flirtations.

We moved on from bar to bar, enjoying a pitcher of beer at each. Cool Friend went home to the safety of her boyfriend, leaving me and Army Cowboy paired up and Shy Friend and Dark Cowboy awkwardly attempting to talk. The booze helped, but it can only do so much. If the chemistry isn't there, it's not going to magically appear from a tabletop sticky with beer. None of us drank so much that we got drunk, thanks to the slow waitstaff.

Finally a bartender announced last call. It was now or never, and I wanted my hot country boy RIGHT NOW.

The two guys were talking to each other when I put my hand on Army Cowboy's knee. He didn't move or give me anything to go on. *Shit.* I moved the hand up. A tiny grin. *Excellent.* Let the teasing begin.

Shy Friend got up for the restroom. My hand was inside his thigh. I started making slow circles with my finger. The grin is still there. I start lightly running my fingertips up and down the upper part of his thigh. Dark Cowboy got up to pay the tab. Immediately I felt Army Cowboy's hand pulling mine onto the bulge in his pants. *HELLS YEAH!* NOW THAT'S WHAT I'M TALKING ABOUT.

Without even thinking I found myself pushing back the table and straddling his lap. My lips were on his, his tongue was in my mouth, my hands were all over his shoulders and arms, his hands were on my ass—

"A-HEM. LAST CALL. THAT MEANS *LEAVE*."

Army Cowboy pulled back in embarrassment at having the bartender catch us. I looked around for our friends. I saw neither, and the bartender walked away. Still straddling him, I leaned in to whisper, "Do you want to come back to my place?"

"*Fuck yeah,*" he exhaled, and I started biting lightly on his neck.

Then our friends came back. As we walked out of the bar Shy Friend pulled me aside and said she thought it was cool if I wanted to go home with my guy, but she had never done that before and didn't want to go home with hers. I said that was fine with me, I'd get them to drop me off at my place.

I got in the car with the two guys and wondered what the fuck to do with Dark Cowboy. They had driven into town in one car. Shit, shit, *shit*. Maybe he could fall asleep on the couch… or watch a movie? In the living room? *Aw shit,* I had no idea. OK, yes, I did, but that would only happen on a cold day in Hell.

I wasn't the only one thinking that. From the back seat Dark Cowboy stuck his head between us and said "So, uh, what are we going to do next?" We all looked at each other.

"Well, I'm going to have wild hard sex with your best friend... although I don't really know what to do with you . . . Um, I have movies. . . ?"

Silence. *Shit.*

Then I laughed and added, "Unless if you're really open-minded..." Pause. He cocked his head to the side. "I'm okay with that."

No fucking way . . .

They looked at each other. I watched them visually talking it out. After a few seconds, Army Cowboy looked at his friend and said, "I guess that's okay."

"Are you sure? Because I'm serious."

I placed my left hand inside Dark Cowboy's thigh to help him think.

"Yeah . . . "

". . . Yeah"

YESSSSSSSSSSSSSSSSSSSSSS!!!!!!!!

We all looked at each other in a completely different *WTF?!* way and then busted out laughing.

"Shit, we've been friends since kindergarten, but I never expected this!" said Army Cowboy.

"Are we really going through with this?" asked Dark Cowboy. Mmm, such a sexy southern drawl.

I looked at both of them and said "*Fuck yeah.*"

Army Cowboy drove the three of us back to my apartment, which was only a couple minutes away from the bar.

I'd like to say I was all suave as we walked from the parking lot to my apartment, but in my head I was totally doing a full-on booty shake, complete with twirls. *I got two boooys, I got two boooys, I am so cool, I am so coool*! It's a good thing people can't read my mind, otherwise there's no fucking way I'd ever get laid. But I was chill. I can hide the goofy girl inside when there's an orgasm or six on the line.

They followed me into my one-bedroom apartment (This situation right here is exactly why I do not have a roommate. Roommates generally don't like naked boys roaming the apartment in the middle of the night, and if they do like it then you'd have to share one of the boys and I DON'T LIKE SHARING MY THINGS).

"I'd, uh, like to take a shower, if that's alright? I smell like bar smoke," said Army Cowboy.

"Oh yeah, no problem. Let me get you a towel . . ." I went into the bathroom. Thank god it was clean. Nothing turns you off from sex like a nasty bathroom.

Dark Cowboy quickly added he'd like one too. Plenty of towels, no problem. Thank you, my dear mother, for teaching me to always have plenty of clean towels.

"Hmm . . . that's a good idea . . . that way I can get a little one-on-one time with each of you first . . ." Oooh I'm such a smoothie. Devilish grin.

Army Cowboy headed toward the bathroom as he took off his shirt. Naked back. Thick, manly, naked back. The door closed. I looked at Dark Cowboy. I grinned and came up behind him to pull off his shirt. Naked back number two. Ohhhh, how I like this already.

Even in my four-inch heels he was taller than me. As much as I may feel naturally drawn to foreigners (I have no idea why . . . I like traveling? The accents? The trilling the foreign tongues can do? *Mmmm,* yes, that must be it), I love my Texas boys. Everything IS bigger in Texas, babe. I'll raise my beer to that any day.

Dark Cowboy looked a little nervous. I knew how to take care of that. I put my hands on his bare chest and not-so-gently pushed him down onto the couch. With his blue jeans-clad legs spread (is there anything hotter than a bare-chested guy in a nice-fitting pair of jeans? Oh, there is: *two* bare-chested guys in jeans. *Mmmmm,* can I get a HELLS

YEAH?), I stepped between his legs and towered over him. Making eyes at him the whole time, slowly I bent down so that my face was level to his. His hands reached out for my hips and pulled me down so that I was straddling his open lap.

His face lifted toward me. My hands cupped his neck and pulled his face into mine. Dark Cowboy's hands started at my hips then wrapped around to my ass and up my back, which was bare because of the style of the delicate top I was wearing. The kissing was hot as hell. It felt like we were devouring each other—and we still had most of our clothes on.

I've got quite the exhibitionist side when it comes to sex. I love the idea of someone watching me with someone else and getting off on it. So, when I heard Army Cowboy in the bathroom, I really started putting on a show. I bit Dark Cowboy's neck—not lightly—and started grinding into him. I felt the moans in his throat as I bit harder.

"Hey."

We looked up.

Army Cowboy stood there with a white towel loosely wrapped around his waist. I felt my grin grow three sizes like a greedy Grinch.

"Your turn for the shower, buddy. I did my best to leave some hot water for you."

I stood up so Dark Cowboy could get up from the couch. His hard-on was noticeable through the jeans. His best friend snickered and then closed his eyes in embarrassment—I assume because he realized he was going to be seeing a hell of a lot more than that.

Dark Cowboy closed the bathroom door behind him. I walked over to Army Cowboy. Daaamn, he looked fine in a towel. To this day I can say he's one of the three hottest guys I've ever had the honor of fucking. Perfect toned body, thick shoulders, not too lean and not too thick. The gorgeous eyes and smile weren't too shabby either. But enough of that. I WANT TO SEE THE GOODS, BOY.

I walked over to Army Cowboy. He had such a big shit-eating grin and that wasn't the only thing I wanted to make bigger. Without a word I pulled his towel off and dragged him toward the couch. He sat down with his legs spread. *Mmm,* I know what *that* means.

We had already kissed heavily in the bar. I thought it was acceptable to dive right in for the good stuff. I figured Army Cowboy wouldn't mind. He didn't. Let me just say, I hadn't seen the good stuff beforehand. *This* was the good stuff. Just the right length (too long makes anal sex a bit difficult) and *thick*. Large girth doesn't get nearly enough credit. Under normal circumstances I love giving head anyway, but this? This was FUCKING AWESOME. I sucked on his hard cock in a slightly teasing way. Every once in a while, I looked up at him so he could see my eyes, which hopefully he could tell were saying *I can't wait to mount you and ride you like the big strong cowboy you are.*

Army Cowboy was writhing below me. I saw his hand digging into the couch cushion, which set me off. He looks like he's going to be some serious bitchslapping fun.

We heard Dark Cowboy turn off the shower. I could tell Army Cowboy was close, so I went all out. Within fifteen seconds he came, all over my top. My *dry clean only* top, asshole. Okay, *that* I did not like. But if a fancy top is the price of fucking two hot guys at the same time? Fuck it.

Dark Cowboy came out and went straight into the bedroom. My turn for a shower, but first I had to get all my silly clothes off.

I walked into the bedroom after Dark Cowboy, where he was sitting nervously on the bed. His best friend followed me in, a towel on now. A single lamp in the corner was on. I leaned into Dark Cowboy to kiss him. *Mmmm,* there's nothing I love more than a hot guy fresh out of the shower. Except *TWO* hot guys fresh out of the shower.

As I was kissing one guy, I felt the other come up from behind and press himself into me. Instinctively, I pushed back against him and ground my hips in a circle. I heard moans come from both directions. OH MY GOD, THIS IS *AWESOME*. And I'm still wearing clothes. Why the fuck am I still wearing clothes. The clothes are getting in the way of more AWESOMENESS.

Coyly I broke loose and asked one of them to untie my top, which was held on by two thin strands, one around my neck and the other across my back. Dark Cowboy jumped to attention. His large hands fumbled at the small ties. I could tell he was nervous. He untied one and I did the other. You'd really think guys would be better at getting a girl out of her clothes.

I pulled the strands apart and dropped the top to the floor. As I turned around one of them audibly gasped. Wow, and I still have my jeans on. I'd done more with Army Cowboy so I figured it was Dark Cowboy's turn for some action. He was sitting on the bed, at the perfect height. I walked into his open legs and felt them close around me. His arms went around my waist as he pulled me into him so he could suck on my nipples. I sensed Army Cowboy stir behind me.

Abruptly I broke away from Dark Cowboy and walked right past Army Cowboy toward the door. Slowly I unzipped my jeans and pulled them down, revealing a black thong and a small tattoo on my ass cheek. Without a word I walked into the bathroom and started the shower.

While I was in the shower soaping up and shaving at the same time (less time in here means MORE TIME OUT THERE), I was getting a tad nervous. I admit it, I wondered *am I really going through with this? Am I really going to fuck two guys at the same time? Isn't that kind of slutty?* Then: *WHO GIVES A SHIT IF IT'S SLUTTY. I'M FUCKING TWO HOT GUYS AT THE SAME TIME. GO ME!!* I turned off the shower and dried off. I stood naked in front of the mirror. Pep talk time. *I am going to fuck two guys at the same time. Two* hot *guys. I am not nervous! I don't always think I'm attractive, but they obviously do. GO WITH IT. I AM AS HOT AS THEY THINK I AM. I AM A SEX KITTEN. NO, I AM A SEX LIONESS! RAWWWR!* –snicker– Okay, start over. Get serious, Vix. *I AM GOING TO DO THIS. I AM SO NOT NERVOUS. I AM IN CONTROL. I DO CRAZY SEX STUFF LIKE THIS ALL THE TIME. IN THEORY. I WILL BE THE POWER-SEX GODDESS THEY SEEM TO THINK I AM. I WILL ROCK THEIR WORLD SO HARD THEY CAN'T SEE STRAIGHT FOR TWO DAYS.*

Okay. Ready to go. I wrap the towel around my body and open the bathroom door.

They're still there. *PHEW*. Part of me worried they'd freak and take off while I was in the shower. Another part of me worried they'd rip off my TV and I'd come out of the bathroom seeing the TV cord being dragged out the door. Nope. Two guys still here, TV still here. AWESOME.

Army Cowboy and Dark Cowboy had moved back to the living room. I guess they didn't like the idea of being together in a bedroom without a girl. Understandable.

They were both naked. And laughing. Hmm. Fascinating behavior.

"Yeah . . . we figured we were going to be seeing everything in the next couple hours, so might as well look at each other's dicks and get used to it," said Army Cowboy, laughing.

Dark Cowboy chuckled a little, but looked out of it. His friend came up to me and whisperered, "I think he's chickening out. You may want to, uh, *persuade* him." We looked at each other. I nodded. He went to the bedroom to wait.
Dark Cowboy looked up at me. He was nervous as hell. I dropped my towel to the ground.

"You a little nervous, babe? You know I can make you feel a lot better . . ." I knelt down on the floor between his legs. Instantly his dick started to harden. *Mmmm. I like you too.* I placed my hands on his knees and then fanned out my fingers as I caressed the length of his thighs. His head fell back. My hands ran down the inside of his thighs, intentionally bypassing his cock.

I lowered my head down between his legs. I breathed heavily on the tip of his rock-hard cock, jumped up to kiss him hard on the lips, bit him lightly on the neck, then trailed my fingernails down his bare chest back to his cock. I took it in my left hand. Hard pump twice, fast pump a couple times, then I dove in with my mouth to do what I do best.

A couple minutes later I felt Dark Cowboy squirm. I looked over with my mouth still full. Army Cowboy was peeking at us from around the corner. I locked back down on Dark Cowboy's cock and smiled at his best friend with my eyes. This just got twice as hot.

"Hello? I'm getting lonely in here!" laughed Army Cowboy.

I looked up at Dark Cowboy. He shuffled around like he was preparing to get up. Reluctantly I gave up his cock so we could both stand up.

There we were. Two guys—best friends since childhood, mind you—standing buck-ass naked in my living room with matching boners. And me, naked in the middle.

CAN I GET A BIG FAT MOTHERFUCKING *HELLS YEAH*?

They looked at each other and shrugged. Good. We're cool. YOU TWO BITCHES READY TO FUCK ME HARD? LET'S GO!

I grabbed Dark Cowboy by the dick and led him toward the bedroom. Hey, he needs to know who calls the shots here.

All three of us walked into the bedroom. They fell back and waited for me to lead the way. I climbed up on the bed and turned around to face the two ripped naked bodies in front of me.

Seriously. Is there anything hotter than *two* boners on *two* hot guys waiting their turn to have their dirty way with you? If there is, I WANT TO KNOW WHAT IT IS AND GO HIT THAT. –gasp– *Three* boners on *three* hot guys at the same time. –eyes get wide– *Oooooooh*. Must add that to my list of "Guys to Do."

"So . . ." said Army Cowboy, the more ripped and slightly hotter one. *Oh I can't wait to get on that. I want to devour him.* "I noticed you had quite a collection of toys over there," and he pointed at the bookshelf next to my bed, which held my collection of sex toys. He picked up the massive ten-inch pink jelly dong and held it up to me. "Should we be worried here?" he laughed.

I looked down at Army Cowboy with a sly grin. This guy was hung. He had some serious girth going on. To this day, it is one of the three most beautiful cocks I've ever had the honor of sucking off.

"Um, NO. You do not need to be worried." I reached out for him. Army Cowboy came to me, knowing exactly what I wanted. He leaned down and started sucking on my nipples. It only took Dark Cowboy a second before he jumped up on the bed. He started kissing on my neck from behind me.

YESSSSSSSSSSSSSSSSSSSSSSSSSSSS! I AM TOTALLY PULLING THIS OFF!! I RULE SO HARD!!!

I was already moaning. How could I not be when this shit is so fucking hot?

Army Cowboy's hands started roaming all over my body. They started at my breasts, then down over my belly button ring, down to my hips—all the while he's still sucking on one of my nipples, *hard* like I like it—then his hands continued to my thighs and all the way down the inside of my calves. At this time, I still spent two hours a day at the gym so my entire body was nice and firm.

Meanwhile Dark Cowboy was working his magic behind me. He alternated between kissing my neck and running his hands down the length of my back. I could tell he was antsy to get his turn at my breasts but as long as his best friend was anywhere close, he was staying away.

That's how it would be for the rest of the night. Being very heterosexual—and from the freaking *country*—Army Cowboy and Dark Cowboy were very aware of where the other was at all times—and staying *away*. One was always south of the equator, the other north. It was kinda funny, actually. But I'll give them props, because there was never any accidental *touching* of any kind. Chandler and Joey would have been proud.

Poor Dark Cowboy was getting impatient. Army Cowboy had been working his way toward my pussy anyway, so time to adjust position. I shifted and lay back into Dark Cowboy's lap. Immediately he went for my breasts. Army Cowboy went down on his knees between my legs.

Oh, wow, this just keeps getting better and better.

Army Cowboy wasted no time going for my pussy. He started with full-on tongue. Outside, inside, all around, inside—that boy was digging for gold. Or rather, platinum. He ate me inside out like he could not get enough. It doesn't get much hotter than that.

Oh, except that it does. Because while Army Cowboy was tending to me between my legs, his best friend was keeping me occupied everywhere else.

Every girl should experience this at least once—being worshipped from head to toe by two guys at the same time. To this day this is my favorite memory for masturbating. I've done some crazy shit in my time (whips, blood, fire, library basement, in a church copy room), but this beats them all, hands down.

Dark Cowboy had scooted back on the bed so that I was now lying flat on my back. He hovered over me, sucking on my nipples and rubbing his hands all over the top half of my body (like I said earlier, they stayed to their respective halves the entire time). At one point he was kneeling over me, directly behind my head, so we did the reverse Spiderman-style kissing. Odd, but fun all the same. I did my best to reach around and stroke his cock to keep it hard, not that it looked like it needed much help.

Army Cowboy was audibly lapping me up. *Daaaamn. You can stay down there as long as you want, sweetie.* I started to squirm. I wanted an orgasm, and I wanted one RIGHT FUCKING NOW. I'm all for girls who can get off with only the clit, but I'm not like that. I need some good hard, deep penetration. Fingers are a *start*. With nearly every single guy I go through the same process of whispering *harder . . . harder . . .* until finally I'm demanding *I said HARDER!* and then grabbing them by the hand and shoving their fingers in so deep they're choking. I'm no fucking delicate flower. "This is some *Amazon* pussy," as one guy had described it a few weeks earlier.

Yeah. So, fuck me accordingly.

Army Cowboy started off better than most. I only had to tell him *harder* once before he got it. Within seconds I was losing my mind. Having guys at both ends will do that.

Dark Cowboy moved in closer to get a good look look at my pussy and his friend's fingers having their dirty way with me. That really got me going. I'm a total exhibitionist (in case that wasn't shamefully obvious), so having one guy watching his best friend get me off—well, that's making me wet as can be writing about it now years later. Imagine how fucking hot it was to *be* there. *Mmmmmm.* – shudders–

Needless to say, it only took a few seconds after that for me to cum, and I came *hard*. When that happens, I have no control of my body—it shudders, shakes, and writhes powerfully. I've sprained fingers and wrists. Not mine. Mine are used to this.

Army Cowboy and Dark Cowboy both watched me until I calmed down. Then they looked at each other. Oh, how I wish I knew what they were thinking, although I have a damn good idea.

Army Cowboy pulled his fingers out and licked my pussy juice off them while grinning at me. Then he looked at his best friend. "Good stuff, man. You should try."

Dark Cowboy looked a little hesitant at first, but Army Cowboy had already hopped up on the bed to switch places. Dark Cowboy climbed off and stood between my legs.

His style was completely different. He took his sweet-ass time. I could tell he was a leg man by how he lifted each of my legs and studied them, like he was memorizing every square inch of skin. That's damn hot. I like when a guy does this because it makes me think that when he's masturbating to the memory later he'll be thinking about exactly what it was like when he pulled them apart that first time or felt them wrapped around his body.

During all this Army Cowboy was biting at my nipples and then kneeling above my head with his dick over my face. I had to strain my neck to reach up and lick the underside. It was extra hot that he was stroking it a little while teasing me with it. Mmmmm *I'll be getting that cock of yours soon enough, babe. You'll be begging me to take it.*

Once Dark Cowboy finished caressing and licking the inside of my thighs, he slowly went for my pussy. I encouraged him by wrapping my legs around the base of his neck and pulling him in toward me.

At this point his best friend started paying a lot more attention to what Dark Cowboy was doing between my legs. I could tell he had quite the voyeur tendency because he all but stopped teasing me so he could watch how I reacted to his friend. Me being the exhibitionist, it was a great match.

Dark Cowboy concentrated a lot more on using his tongue, but he was damn skilled (better than Army Cowboy) so I didn't mind that he wasn't nearly as hands-on. Besides, that left room for me.

I sucked on my index and middle fingers then slid my hand down toward my pussy. Dark Cowboy saw what I was doing but didn't stop. I could tell he was smiling by his eyes. Army Cowboy pretty much stopped moving (and maybe breathing) at this point. Dark Cowboy pulled back with his tongue just long enough for me to spread my pussy lips open and then dip inside. He licked all around and in between my fingers. DAMN, I'm sopping wet just thinking about it.

After a few seconds, I pulled my fingers out to let Dark Cowboy get back to what he was doing so well and presented my juicy fingers to Army Cowboy. He started stroking his dick again as he took my fingers in his mouth and licked them clean.

After the first time I cum, all the others are pretty easy assuming I'm properly inspired. But damn, I wish Dark Cowboy had eaten me out first because he had some fucking magic going on inside that mouth of his. It took no time at all for me to be on the verge of cumming again. This time I came *really* hard. My back arched so much that I had to hold myself up with my arms. My hips ground in circles against Dark Cowboy—and thank goodness for his resilience, he held on for dear life when it really counted. With one final shudder I fell into Army Cowboy's lap and felt my legs collapse on top of Dark Cowboy's shoulders.

A few seconds later I calmed down enough for my head to clear. I sat up and then leaned forward on all fours so I could kiss Dark Cowboy's lips and taste my pussy juice on his tongue, meanwhile giving Army Cowboy a nice long view of my ass in the doggy-style position. Hopefully, that would fuel a few ideas for what to do next.

While I was bent down on all fours it took Army Cowboy no time at all to grab me by the hips. He got up on his knees behind me. I knew what was coming, but it was still hot as hell to feel that huge prick of his brushing against my ass as I was bent over on the bed. His hands slid down from my hips to rub all over my ass cheeks, thighs, and arched lower back.

Instinctively, I started grinding against him. My pussy was dripping wet from the two orgasms, one from each of them. Only one? *Pshaw*. Let's fuck these bad boys and show them how Texas pussy likes to ride a cowboy.

Meanwhile, Dark Cowboy stood up and stretched his long, thick body. *Mmmm*. What a damn fine view. A big hard cock pressing into me from behind and another one throbbing in front of me. *Oh, sweet goddess of all holy and ungodly sex acts, what did I do to deserve this?*

I looked up at Dark Cowboy with my dirty whore eyes. He grinned. His dick jumped.

"I like the clit ring," said Dark Cowboy.

"Oh, really?" I asked oh-so-innocently.

Army Cowboy squeezed my hips hard. "Yeah. That's fucking awesome. I've never seen one before. Your tattoo is pretty sweet too." As he said that, he gave me a little slap on the ass, right where the tattoo is.

I offered my thanks by arching my back more and grinding harder against his cock. "Glad you like it."

"I haven't gotten a very good look at it," Dark Cowboy said with a little pout.

"Aww, poor baby. What*ever* can I do to make it up to you?" I bit my tongue and looked up at him, then at his dick which was at the perfect cocksucking height.

Dark Cowboy's face broke into a smile. He took a step closer toward me. With one hand at the base of his cock, he guided it into my mouth. Without thinking I moaned and ground my hips in tighter circles against Army Cowboy. A few seconds later I heard deep moans coming from above me and behind me. Damn. That moment right there. Just . . . *damn*. And we hadn't even gotten to the fucking yet.

With Army Cowboy grinding his big dick against me, I was about to scream if he didn't start hammering me, like, RIGHT NOW. A girl can only be so patient when there are two cocks within reach.

I let Dark Cowboy's dick fall out of my mouth and then I sat up. I looked at Army Cowboy on my left and Dark Cowboy on my right. "I want to fuck. *Now*. Who's it going to be?"

Army Cowboy and Dark Cowboy looked at me and then each other in amusement. Their raging hard-ons were pointed directly at each other. I giggled. To myself, duh. I'm not going to do a damn thing to jeopardize getting chinese fingercuffed by best friends. Slutty in the movies, but so fucking hot when it's happening to *ME*. SO LET'S GOOOO ALREADY.

Army Cowboy fake-coughed. "Well, I *was* already halfway there…"

Whatever. As long as somebody sticks it in me somewhere. I was already in the closet busy digging out condoms. I handed one to Army Cowboy, then eyed his cock. Crap, that's right he's a big boy. Good for me, not good for the standard condoms I have in my hand. I'd only ever seen two really thick dicks that required a Magnum (which they brought with them), so I didn't exactly keep small, medium, and large condoms ready in my underwear drawer (although I started to after this).

"Uh, will this, uh, be okay?" I asked Army Cowboy.

"Think so. May be a bit tight, but that will probably help me from blowing my load too early, right?" he laughed.

Then I looked over at Dark Cowboy. He's average, so we're good to go there. Wow . . . so this is just a tiny bit *awkward* . . . two best friends since childhood are shagging one girl at the same time and then one sees his buddy's dick is insanely huge in comparison to his. Well, if we do anal we know who is my first pick, *yowch*.

I pulled off a couple more condoms and left them on the bedside table. Then we all stood next to each other trying to figure out who goes where. *Mmmmm . . . I get middle! GO ME!!!*

I looked at Dark Cowboy. I pointed to the bed. "Lie down on your back." He did. I spread my hands out over his thighs to make sure I could reach his cock comfortably while his best friend pounded me from behind.

Bending over the bed, I put my face in Dark Cowboy's lap. My legs were spread wide so Army Cowboy could ram his cock into my pussy as deep as it could go.

Army Cowboy came up behind me. He placed his hands on my hips and rubbed his cock against the lips of my pussy. I ran my hands up and down Dark Cowboy's dick. My breath stopped.

He hadn't entered me yet. I looked around. He was really tall, so he had to bend down uncomfortably to get a good angle.

"Wait. I know what will help." I slipped out from between them and went to the closet. *Ah, there we go. Perfect.* I walked out of the closet four inches taller, thanks to the black leather heels I had put on.

"Niiiiice!" said Dark Cowboy, propped up on his elbows.

Army Cowboy whistled. His dick jumped.

Without a word I strutted back to my place between them and—like a pro—spread my legs and bent over.

"Mmmph. DAMN, girl!" said Army Cowboy. He gave me an appreciative smack on the ass.

I took Dark Cowboy's dick in between my lips, then stopped for a split second to lick my three middle fingers and rub the moisture against my other set of lips. I was already wet as hell, it's not like I needed the extra lubricant, I just know no guy can resist seeing a girl do that. That gesture exists in the realm of sex and nowhere else.

Army Cowboy's hands took their place on my hips. He rubbed the tip of his cock up and down and up and down my pussy—teasing me, the fucker. Since when don't guys plunge right in?!

Meanwhile I was licking Dark Cowboy's cock up and down, up and down, following the rhythm of what his best friend was doing to me. Dark Cowboy's hands were in my hair at first, then he placed them behind his head and lay back with a big grin.

Army Cowboy's hands grabbed a nice chunk of my ass cheeks right before he delivered a loud spank. "Ready, baby?"

OH, HELLS FUCKING YEAH!!!!!!

He entered me slowly. I could feel each inch of his beautiful cock as it filled up my hungry pussy. My nails dug into Dark Cowboy's skin. He moaned. I moaned. Then another deep throaty moan came from behind me. *Oh shit, it doesn't get any better than this.*

Oh, yes, it does. Army Cowboy began to thrust, slow, deep, hard. My entire body tensed to make the most of each stroke. As he increased in speed, my own sucking action increased speed on Dark Cowboy. I could tell he was already close. Mmm, this is why the young guys are nice. Always ready for more, no matter how many times you get them off.

I wasn't ready to be done. I stopped blowing Dark Cowboy. He looked up in protest. I winked at him. "You like fucking the same girl as your best friend?" His eyes went wide. Oh, right. Most guys aren't used to girls with a dirty mouth. He'll get over it.

"You like having me suck you off while he pounds me in the pussy?" I whispered to him. His eyes were still wide, incredulous. I stroked his dick with a single finger. "Are you thinking about how hot it's going to be when I get on top of you and ride you for all you're worth?" I flicked his nipple with my fingernail. His head fell back down to the mattress.

He started to moan. So did his best friend. Army Cowboy was fucking me HARD and I was taking him all in. Knowing that both of them were getting off on what I was saying—and doing—that *really* got me going. "You like knowing that while I'm blowing one of you I'm fucking the other? You're both going to be smelling my pussy on you tomorrow, the pussy that you both fucked. You like that?"

"Daaaamn," said Army Cowboy. He had slowed down so he could hear me better. I reached around to grab the base of his dick as it slid slowly in and out of me. "What do you think about me doing your friend as soon as I'm done with you? You're going to like watching that, aren't you?" He shuddered. He was close.

"Wait. I want to watch you come." Before he could say anything, I pulled away from him and flipped positions so I was sitting on the edge of the bed. I positioned myself so I was in Dark Cowboy's lap. Immediately, he reached around to play with my nipples. The guy knew to pinch *hard*. That's the only way I can feel it when I get this high on sex.

I leaned back against Dark Cowboy and raised my legs wide for his friend. Army Cowboy wasted no time placing them over his shoulders and getting back to pounding me.

This is really happening. I can't believe this is really happening. I'm fucking two hotties at the same time. I think I may die from too much pleasure. FUCK, *what a way to go.*

I dug my nails into Dark Cowboy's leg. "Harder." His fingers worked harder at my nipples. The pain felt so fucking good. I needed more. "Bite my neck." He did, but a bit too lightly for my taste. "I said BITE MY NECK. HARD." He paused, then did as he was told.

All this time I had been flexing my kegel muscle, but as he got closer to the end I started tensing the kegel so hard that my abs hurt (by the way "ladies"–if you can do that, few guys will ever forget you. They won't know what the fuck it was you did, but they will remember that you did it and *it was fucking awesome*). I was getting pretty close to cumming.

I looked up at Army Cowboy. Time to finish him. "You like having your friend watch you fuck me, don't you? Fucking me with that big cock of yours. Are you going to get hard watching your friend fuck me? I bet you will, you'll be just as hard as you are now with your dick inside me."

He was pounding me hard. I mean *hard*, the way a girl was meant to be fucked. He was damn close. I was close. I felt the waves begin. A moan slipped out. He groaned in response. *No! Don't cum before me!! Wait, wait!!* I bore down on the kegel and abs, trying to speed up my orgasm before he finished.

Dark Cowboy bit down hard on my neck and then whispered in my ear, "I can't wait to fuck you." That did it. I came, and I came hard. Dark Cowboy held me down for Army Cowboy while I writhed in ecstasy, nearly in tears from the indulgent ungodliness of it all.

It was only a few seconds later that Army Cowboy rammed into me with force I didn't know he had left. The groans grew louder. He froze above me and then let go. Nothing moved but his prick pumping inside me. I dug my nails into his pecs and unleashed the screaming.

After I finished grinding against him all over again, Army Cowboy pulled out and then slowly dropped down to the ground in exhaustion. He leaned against my leg that was draped over the edge of the bed. I felt the sweat on his forehead as he turned to kiss my calf.

"Wow," he breathed.

"Yeah. WOW." I didn't know sex could be like that. *Wow*. To this day, that's some of the best deep dicking I've ever had.

I saw a pair of hands move across my tits and stomach and then I remembered that there was another guy to tend to after this. Oh, FUCKING SON OF A *HELLS YEAH*. I looked up into Dark Cowboy's eyes. He was completely dazed. I bit my lip and gave him my knowing "I'm going to fuck you so hard" eyes. He leaned over and started sucking on my nipples while I wrapped my fingers around his thick bicep.

I have some very special plans for you, sweetie. You'll be getting your own Wow *soon enough.*

How To Break Up in Fifty Words Or Less

Valentine's Day is just around the corner, so hurry up and break up with your S.O.B. (Significant Other . . . SOB . . . not just a coincidence....) and save yourself all that money on silly romantic gestures that you could use on booze.

If you don't have the ovaries to break up with your SOB in person, here are a few clever "Dear John" letters you may copy for your personal use (if you credit this site and note the proper creative commons licensure, of course). FYI, if there is any possibility that your SOB may try to talk you into staying in the relationship, add some extra asshole factor by breaking up with him on a Post-it note, overdue electricity bill for your shared residence, or a panty liner wrapper.

1. Dear Jackass, I changed the locks and bought a twelve-pack of D batteries for Mr. Jack Rabbit. You can jack off, too.
2. Pookie Pie, I can't do this any more. It's not me, it's you.
3. I bought myself the dog you didn't want us to have. Rocky is the new man in my life. You are welcome to sleep in the backyard in the dog house until you find a place. P.S. If I have to live with a dog, it had damn sure better be one who cuddles at night.
4. You remember my new friend Nancy from the gym? We're lesbians together. You weren't man enough for me.
5. I've been faking it all this time.
6. I made your bed, did your laundry, and packed my bags. I'm leaving. P.S. Call your mother. She wants to know what you did to make me leave.
7. Dearest Fuckwit, I have nothing left to say to you except that I have killed your cat.
8. Shithead, I'm leaving you. I'll be back Saturday for my things. I trained your cat to shit on your pillow so that you will always remember exactly how much I despise your existence. (By the way, good luck with your job interview tomorrow!)
9. Dumbass. THAT IS NOT MY CLITORIS.

About Me: Raw, Ugly, Real

Aussie is out of town, having a Guys Weekend with his friends. No, not to Vegas, but that is pretty much the images that are going through my head. Tits, sequins, shots, pussy, phone numbers on napkins, and more shots.

So I text message him. Again, and again. He doesn't reply the whole first night. I begin to panic.

Obviously, he's at a strip club getting his third lap dance and deciding which stripper to bring back to the hotel. Obviously, his stupid friends are getting each other shit-faced and betting to see who can scam more phone numbers. Obviously, his sweet (usually confident) girlfriend back home is the last thing on his mind while he's being surrounded by friends who are egging him on, trying to get him to break away from the ol' ball-and-chain, just to see if he actually will.

Did I text message him too many times? Did I seem too desperate? He's just busy, right? He's not ignoring me on purpose, right?

At least I learned from last time he was out of town that calling him every two hours to make sure he's not in a strip club or in bed with someone else is *not* what cool girlfriends do. No, no, no, no, no.

Yes, clearly, I am very, very insecure. I was way more sure of myself when I was single because I didn't have a choice, really. It's social suicide for a chick to be insecure and not have a best friend or a boyfriend to watch her back. Since I had neither, I had to have my own back, and it actually seemed to go OK.

But, I have a boyfriend now! I'M NOT SUPPOSED TO BE DOING THIS *'WHEN IS HE GOING TO CALL'* SHIT! IT SUCKS! I want to be single again! I don't care what they say, it's easier to be unattached! Waiting for a guy to call, although a little pathetic, but come on everyone does it even though we know better, is way less Stalker-Girlfriend behavior when single.

The thing is, I know that I can trust Aussie. Fine magazines like *Cosmopolitan* and *Glamour* say that you should trust your gut, you shouldn't listen to the nagging voice in your head if all his actions suggest that that voice is full of crap. I know that Aussie is a great guy. He pays attention to me, he encourages me, he listens to me. He was the one who first brought up the "L" word, moving in together, getting a dog together, getting married, having kids, the whole Happily Ever After. Together. Even the little everyday stuff suggests he's nothing but completely trustworthy. And, as to be expected, the next day Aussie calls and tells me about his weekend so far and nothing sounds anything but normal and sweet in his voice, just like my gut was trying to convince me was the case. Everything is fine, nothing to worry about, go back to what you were doing.[1]

Which just proves that I am a big, fat, insecure mess. When did this happen to me? I used to be such a fucking *badass*! I could have been Angelina Jolie's bitchin' not-as-hot-but-still-totally-hot cousin. But something happened and all that badassness dissolved in a bottomless bottle of anti-depressants.

Seriously though. What happened to me? It's not Aussie's fault at all, I was already unraveling when I met him. Was it the depression? The chronic depression that has hit every single member of both my extended families—maybe. I've always been a tough broad, that alone shouldn't have taken me down this hard. Maybe I've always been insecure but was just too arrogant to see it until I was twenty and realized I was *not* the smartest, sportiest, toughest, funniest girl I previously thought I was. Frankly, I miss that arrogance. It was nice to believe in myself with such conviction.

I know I can't be the only one, single or coupled, male or female, who feels this way. I hope. Thinking that everyone goes through something similar to this is the last hope I have. Please, seriously. Tell me if you have felt this way too, because I need to know that I won't feel this way forever.

I feel like damaged goods. Severely damaged. That I'm not really that great, certainly not worth the trouble, and any day now Aussie is going to realize that and he's going to leave.

Which is similar to what happened to me with my college boyfriend. He was a great guy, until the beginning of my third year of college when I realized I was depressed. Apparently, I much later found out, he wanted to break up with me then, but he's a nice guy and didn't want to make things worse for me. How nice

---

[1] Later I did find out that he was cheating on me, but by that point in our relationship, I was so checked out that I didn't care anymore.

of him. Fucking bastard. So, he stuck around for another year, letting me cry on his shoulder when I had no idea what I was crying about, baking me cookies when I didn't want to eat, being the support that I desperately needed at that time in my life. Eventually, he couldn't take it anymore and I was dumbfounded. We'd hardly ever fought, we got along great, we had similar personalities and the same sick sense of humor, what was wrong? Why did he want to leave? He told me months later, "I couldn't handle you anymore. You were too much. You had so much going on inside of you and I wasn't strong enough anymore."

That has been fucking with my head for years now. As I type this, I'm crying. Not from sadness, but from anger and frustration. Partially at the college boyfriend, but more at myself for letting that get to me as deeply as it has, that feeling that I am just *wrong*. *I am so wrong that I am unlovable for anything more than a couple jokes and an orgasm.*

By the way, that's why I try so hard to be funny. If I can keep the friends and the guys laughing enough of the time, it will make up for the times when I'm an uncontrollable crying mess. That's the equation I've been living with. Now that I've written it down for the first time, it seems pretty clear how insecurity factors in to it.

But, this is the last time I'm going to cry over this. I am depressed, and given my family's history, I will probably be depressed for life, no matter how much therapy, pills, exercise, random fucking, self-help books, or full-contact sports I try. And that really, really sucks. But that's the hand I've been dealt and I'm sick of feeling sorry for myself all these years.

I probably should have told this story ages ago, when I first started my blog. But a large part of the reason I started it when I did was *because* I was so sad, I needed something fun and sexy and not-too-real to take my mind away from the medicine cabinet full of prescriptions that don't help and the people who don't understand that the laughing smile on the outside is meant to hide the raw weeping beast inside. So, I talked about sex, because that's what I know and it's easy to tell stories about it and it's fun to write cute little posts. At first, I wanted my blog only to be about that, but the depressed sardonic side had too much to say—it's just as much a part of who I am, so out it came. So for those readers who came to my blog solely in search of sex–well, fuck off. No one can be just sex all the time, not even an over-educated nympho.

What You Think *vs.* What You Say During Sex

What you're thinking: Ewwww get that out of my ear!
What you say: If you're that fast with your tongue move it south, buddy.

What you're thinking: My dog humps me better than this.
What you say: I'm a virgin. I love you. I'm going to call my mother and tell her that her delicate flower is no longer pure. Then you'll get to meet Daddy!

What you're thinking: I missed *Will & Grace* for this?
What you say: Get out.

What you're thinking: Ack! you smell like ass!
What you say: Let's start off with a shower . . . with LOTS of soap, you dirty dirty boy.

What you're thinking: Why are you kneading my tits like they're bread dough?
What you say: You lost your turn. –proceed to pinch your own tits–

What you're thinking: WHY AREN'T YOU GOING DOWN ON ME YET?
What you say: –put your hands on either side of his head, look sexy at him, pull his down head to proper location–

What you're thinking: Why the fuck are you licking my chin?
What you say: Why the fuck are you licking my chin?

What you're thinking: You're my bitch.
What you say: Tell me what you want to do to me and if you're lucky I'll let you . . .

What you're thinking: You are the worst fuck I've ever had.
What you say: Can you hurry? Leno's on in five.

What you're thinking: It's time for you to go home and you don't get it, do you?
What you say: zzzzzzzzzzzzzzz GEORGE, STOP THAT! MAMA'S GONNA WHIP YOU GOOD WHEN SHE GETS HOME zzzzzzzzzzzzzzzz.

What you're thinking: THAT IS NOT MY CLITORIS.
What you say: THAT IS NOT MY CLITORIS, YOU DUMB FUCK.

What you're thinking: You're sooo bad . . . you *must* be a virgin.
What you say: –start crying– I –gasp– think I'm –sob– a –cry– LESBIAN! –sob– I wasn't –hack– sure until nooooow! –waaaaaaaaaaaaail–

What you're thinking: THAT STILL IS NOT MY CLITORIS.
What you say: Get out. Get out before I shoot you on behalf of the rest of the female race.

What you're thinking: Owwwie! Wrong hole!
What you say: HEY, WATCH IT, ASSHOLE.

What you're thinking: You slept with someone else last night, you awful jerk.
What you say: Mmm . . . I never knew you liked handcuffs so much . . . and it's a good thing, because I'm leaving you here tied to the bed, you used maxi-pad.

What you're thinking: You sooo lied about how big you are.
What you say: Is it in yet?

What you're thinking: Dude, your sweat is dripping into my *eye*.
What you say: Time for me on top!

What you're thinking: I don't want to look at your ugly face anymore.
What you say: Time for me on top!

What you're thinking: Hmm, too fast.
What you say: Time for me on top!

What you're thinking: Hmm, too slow.
What you say: Time for me on top!

What you're thinking: I don't ever want to see your sorry ass again.
What you say: I think I'm falling in love with you.

What I Miss About Being Single

I miss having the confidence I did when I was single. I'm not talking about the daily validation from appreciative male eyes, but the fact that I had to count on myself. I didn't have a choice, really, about being fully self-reliant. Without a boyfriend or a best girl friend, I was just SOL. I had to be strong, even on the days where I crumbled into a huge mess. Somehow, I managed to pick up the pieces of my broken self.

But now, having a boyfriend, I've come to rely on him too much. I take for granted the fact that I can hold myself together just long enough to get home from work and see him and I just let all the pieces fly out of my hands in all directions. "Would you pick that up, sweetie? I can't seem to do it myself."

I miss never having to keep someone else in mind, whatever I do. Being able to go wherever, do whatever, whenever I want. Now someone expects me to be home at the same time every day to make dinner and follow the routine of watching TV together, then he sits on one couch with his computer while I lie down at another and read a book. Yes, of course I can come home late if I feel like running some errands or going to a friends' house or shopping, but then there's the pressure to cram in the bonding/intimacy/catch-up on each other's days in a shorter amount of time.

Being single really isn't that bad. So many people (and, yes, I've been there too, so don't get sassy and shake your shoulders at me) take their singledom for granted. I did too because I didn't know any better. But now that "forever, at least for the foreseeable future" is staring me in the face every day with morning breath—being single looks pretty damn good. I wish I could go back and do it again, being slightly wiser and in a better place in my life (*i.e.* completely done with school and having a real, grown-up job). Yes, I am sure I would feel differently if I had never been in a long-term relationship or if I had been single for longer or if it wasn't part of my disposition to have random sex when the need so frequently beckoned.

Even though I found a great relationship that could easily last my entire lifetime, I'm scared shitless. What if something better comes along? I'm not sure

I'm ready to settle down into a life of we! I didn't have enough fun being single while I had the chance! I want to be single and flirtatious and just be a me. Fuck *we*. I'm too selfish for that.

Sometimes I wonder if I was meant to be single for life. Or at least for a significant amount of time, more than the limited two-year window I actually had between three long-term boyfriends. "Oh, don't be silly," you say, "how can you be sure you're not a serial monogamist only months away from having a wedding registry at Crate & Barrel?" Because I was *good* at being single. No, I'm not talking about dating and fucking like a man. Although that too, but what I really mean is it felt so nice to be self-reliant, to have so many options with what direction to take my life, like being able to up and move to New York City within the period of a month, or considering getting yet another degree, or doing whatever I damn well please.

This isn't Aussie-specific. This is Significant Other specific. How do I know that I'm headed down the right path with a boyfriend, toward marriage and a 50/50 shot at Happily Ever After? How do I know I should be on my own?

What about the things that are Aussie-specific? Like when I told him my bottom line, that I would only get married and have children if my husband agreed to be the stay-at-home parent. Not only did Aussie agree, but he was delighted. "I always wanted to be a stay-at-home dad! This is perfect!" Well, shit, I thought to myself. I thought that would scare him off. There goes that plan.

And then I started hyperventilating, because I realized, he is for real. This is real. This is scaring the shit out of me.

Get That Thing Away From Me

Try as I might, babies scare the fuck out of me. Seriously. Being in the presence of a baby is the best contraception I have ever encountered.

I think I was one of the very few women born without a biological clock. For me it's not like it's a matter of when it will go off, perhaps five or ten years from now—it's more a matter of not having a biological clock *at all*.

Don't get me wrong, kids are cute and shit, I like them just fine–but in the same manner that I like my mother: from far away.

Last week at the end of the work day our office held a baby shower for one of the admin women, it was a BYOB invitation to all employees with infants. (For those who don't know, as I didn't until there was a *Sex and the City* episode explaining this, when BYOB is in reference to a baby shower it means Bring Your Own Baby, Not Bring Your Own Beer. Well, who the fuck wants to go to a party like *that*?)

The baby shower at work was optional, but it was the end of the day, I was too bored to finish out my last half hour of work, and there was cake. I was in. Until I sat down and a whole flood of coworkers with their adorable babies had me surrounded on all sides.

I lasted fifteen minutes of enduing excruciating conversation about wedding plans at my table, which apparently was the official LIKE, OH MY GOD I'M ENGAGED!! table and that was the only topic of discussion, even though I kept trying to bring the conversation around to cake/baby shit/how boyfriends are dumb, they wouldn't have it. In fact, looking back, I'm surprised they didn't kick me out of the table, especially since they didn't seem to appreciate my one endearing quality *i.e.* my sense of blatantly sarcastic humor. Bitches.

Then the goddamn babies swarm. Yes, they are fucking adorable, how many times are you going to make me say it before you'll get that damn thing out of my face already?! The mothers and fathers are taking the babies around to each table in the break room, bragging about the solidity of their bowel movements and how long they can hold their heads up on their own. Or something. I was doing my best to ignore them and loudly suggest to whomever was in charge that it was time to cut the goddamn cake.

One especially fat and happy infant was placed involuntarily in my arms (and what exactly about me screams I LOVE CHILDREN?! because I thought that trying to make the women at my table crack up at least once from one of my "dead baby" jokes was really enough) and, with a dozen pairs of eyes on me, I forced myself to coo at the baby and dangle something bright and swallowable in its face and tap him on the nose and tell him how freaking cute he was so that the offending father WOULD GET IT OUT OF MY FACE ALREADY.

I. am. scared. of. children.

Especially babies. They're too fresh-from-the-womb and make me think of my own super-fertile body (I'm from a Catholic family, *i.e.* we were made to propagate the world with more little Catholics and therefore our seed is made for conception under even the most unlikely of circumstances (which is why when I was single I was on birth control, used a condom religiously, AND used a diaphragm when I knew I was ovulating, just to MAKE SURE there was no Mini-Me brewing inside my baby hatch. As if the world weren't dangerous enough with one OEN running amok.)).

So, finally, I left, without eating cake. This is a big deal for me, by the way. Because I LOVE FOOD. I love it almost as much as I love sucking dick, which I love A LOT by the way. I was made to spend my days swallowing and eating, I swear to god. Love it. So, yeah, no cake. It's the end of the day by now, so I get in the car and start to drive home. As soon as I get on the highway I start crying. Softly at first (it actually took me a few minutes to figure out why I was crying), then finally I start sobbing. Meanwhile I'm fiddling with the radio trying to find a good stop-crying-you-drama-queen song like Madonna or Ludacris or shit even *Mariah*, just someone with a good beat who would help me out here, but no, and at the same time I'm digging through my purse to find my Xanax. So that hopefully I can stop crying in the fifteen minutes I have remaining before I'm home and Aussie asks me what's wrong and I have to either tell him, don't make me have babies, they scare me or come up with a good lie for why my mascara is totally fucked up.

I got home and inside easily enough (he was watching a baseball game and not paying attention to me, which was fine) and by then the Xanax had kicked in and I was nearly normal.

Since then I have started punching myself regularly in the ovaries in an attempt to stop them from releasing super-fertile spawn that will grow inside me and haunt me with horrible dreams about how I will fuck up the child before it has even left my womb. Because I can do that, you know. Any kid with my genes is just fucked.

My Tattoo

I'm thinking about getting another tattoo. The current one I have is tribal and doesn't mean anything. I wanted a tattoo, I walked into a tattoo parlor when I lived in the East Village in New York City and picked out the first thing I liked that I saw on the wall. It was about what the tattoo represented, not about the actual tattoo.

Now things are different. That tattoo was a couple years ago, when I was in a very different place and (if you can believe it) in an even more confused place mentally.

But, right now feels like such a crucial time where my life can go in any of very different directions. And that feels tattoo-worthy. What specifically?

The same thing that Angelina Jolie has just above her pubic triangle, *quod me nutrit me destruit* which is Latin for "what nourishes me destroys me."

How fucking true.

I like the idea of *quod me nutrit me destruit* as a tattoo, but I'm going to change it up a little to make it more *mine*. The current translation from the Latin is a bit negative and would just be enabling me to feel sorry for myself for having depression/ADD and being hyper-sexual, which is not the way to go at all. I'm trying to remind myself that being a nympho is a *good* thing, an AWESOME thing, that having depression makes me a stronger and more introspective person, that ADD makes me creative as hell and good at multi-tasking. But, as you can see, some days those things just make me want to self-medicate into a forgiving numbness.

So, I'm thinking of altering the Latin to say *quod me create me nutrit,* "what creates me nourishes me." I told this to Aussie and he gave me a blank look and then said "Huh? What is that supposed to mean?"

This might not be as understandable as the original, but, frankly, I don't care. Because it's mine. It makes complete sense to me and I like the idea of seeing it every day on a central part of my body where hardly anyone else will ever see it. I like the idea of seeing those words as a permanent part of me, because I *do* need a daily reminder that these aspects of myself that I struggle to understand, to ignore, to push out of my life—the depression, the ADD, the hyper-sexuality—are the very reasons I am who I am. Which is not a bad thing, even though these things often make me feel lost within the world and even more lost inside myself. For so long I thought that the parts of my identity that were so interesting—quirkiness, extreme creativity and imagination, super-sexuality. snarkastic sense of humor, artistic sensibility (*i.e.* moodiness/passion/intensity, for good and for bad) and utterly charming tendency to chatter on about the most random of things. Upon discovering a couple years ago that I had depression and only recently discovering I have ADD (which I have barely mentioned in my blog because I'm pissed at it as if it were a person whom I could beat the shit out of with a baseball bat and since I can't, I just give it the silent treatment and hope it learns its lesson), it forces me to wonder just how much of my personality is a simple equation of mental dysfunction.

And, when I put it that way, it's no wonder I'm depressed all the fucking time, look at the way I've been viewing myself. It's amazing I don't spend six hours a week at my therapist's office. But that really is how I've evaluated the factors creating my identity. Depression + ADD + horny = moody/quirky/horny chick. It was like I had been genetically pre-determined to be the exact combination of personality traits that I am and that I had no hand in choosing the person I came to be. This is the state of fuzzy psychological muck that I have been swimming through for so long. This is half of what I talk about in my blog, when originally all I wanted was for it to be a fun place to talk about sex, bitch about relationships, and tell funny stories—and temporarily escape all the muck in my head. That, however, was *VERY* short-lived.

But, I'm finally moving beyond that. At least I'm still trying. Yes, these so-called disorders have a hand in who I am today. But you know what? I'm a pretty badass chick. So, maybe that's OK. Besides, I know that with this same equation of factors I could have been a very different person. It's not by virtue of having depression/ADD/super-sexuality that I am this way, it's the way I handled these things and learned from them. So, I should really shut the fuck up and stop feeling sorry for myself.

Aaaaand this brings us back to the reasoning behind the tattoo. *What creates me nourishes me*. So much better than the original idea, so much more me. I can't change the genes that gave me depression and ADD. I can't de-sexualize myself (although removing the piercing on the hood of my clitoris probably *would* help, but let's be realistic now). These are the things that created me and made me into the person I am. It's time that I embrace them instead of apologizing for them again and again. May they nourish me into a stronger and better person.

The next day:

I went to the tattoo parlor and got my tattoo. I was so excited all day long, I could barely stand it. Which just meant I drank tons of coffee and emailed all my friends about it all day.

The final Latin that I chose is *quod me torquet me nutriat*, which translates as "what torments me, may it nourish me." Now, being the Latin geek that I am, there's more to it than just, well, *that*—the word *torquet* has many English translations: torment, torture, try, test, *et al.*; and *nutriat* is the subjunctive which has a different meaning that yada yada yada. Too intellectual for a tattoo, I know, which is why I'm not going to admit that I spent an hour and half last night researching translations and the subjunctive vs. indicative mood.

Because that would be sooooo nerdy. And I'm *not* just a nerd. I masturbate to memories of threesomes, not the latest anime feature. OK, I have that one fantasy about Captain Jean-Luc Picard and the captain's chair, but what nerd doesn't?

So, there we go. I finally got my second tattoo ("Finally?" Oh, please, I conceived of this what like last Thursday night? While drunk?!). I'm very happy with it. I got my first one several years ago when I had just moved to New York City for an amazing internship and was living on my own for the first time. It was time for another one, and this is just perfect.

There's a good chance that tomorrow while at work I'm going to be having flashbacks to when I was a little girl in the airport: running up to complete strangers, lifting my skirt to show my lacy panties, and screaming "I'M A BIG

GIRL NOW!!!!" Because how can you get a tattoo and not show it off to everyone? Never mind that it's on my crotch. I have a *lovely* crotch, thank you, and Mr. Cubicle Man from three bays over should be so lucky to see it.

Preparations

I stopped at the liquor store on my way home from work. I picked out three bottles of vodka (Skyy, Svedka Vanilla, and Tito's (the best in Texas)) and took them to the register.

Clerk: You having a vodka-tasting party?
Me: No. I'm breaking up with my boyfriend this weekend.
Clerk: Really?
Me: Yeah. The big bottle is for him, the small bottle is for me, and this bottle is for my friends, so they can keep up with me.
Clerk: —
Me: —
Clerk: You want a complimentary shot?
Me: Yeah.
—Clerk opens a cooler under the register, pulls out a small bottle of vodka, and pours me a shot—
Me: You're a good man.
Clerk: Good luck this weekend.
Me: Thanks, buddy. I appreciate it.

Part II

I read and walked for miles at night along the beach, writing bad blank verse and searching endlessly for someone wonderful who would step out of the darkness and change my life. It never crossed my mind that person could be me.

Anna Quindlen

Just Fucking Go For It

Some people throw themselves out there, take risks, and just fucking go for it. I'm talking about that average-looking chick at the bar who goes up to the hottest guy there and gets him. I'm talking about that young intern who stands eye-to-eye with the boss and doesn't let the fact that she's just a peon keep her from disagreeing with him. That girl who does what it takes to make the play even if she finds her body covered in bruises and blood at the end of the game. The daughter who tells her parents *I know it might be a mistake to move to a new city with no friends and no money but it's just something I have to do*. The woman who can tell her boyfriend of two years, "I'm sorry, but this isn't what I want."

Sometimes, you just have to go for it. Fuck the risk, fuck the *should*s, fuck the doubt. Fuck it all and go for it. It's the only way you can get what you really want.

That doesn't mean being spontaneous. On the contrary—I'm the sort who sits on a decision and mulls over it for ages and ages. No one sees that though, they see when I finally decide what I want to do and, I GO. Then everyone had better get the hell out of my way.

So, where am I now? Single and flirting with a new career.

I was with Aussie for two mostly great years, but I finally admitted to myself that wasn't what I wanted, at least not at this time in my life. Some of my family accused me of being a coward for that, for running away from commitment because it's scary. Nuh-uh. Nothing's that simple. Because, yeah, there are two ways you can look at that decision: being a coward, or having the balls to walk out on something good because ultimately it's not right. I don't need ten years and three kids to realize that.

Then there's the career that cost over a quarter-million dollars in eighteen years of education. I was always at the top of my class at the best of schools, and it's so hard to convince myself I'm not throwing it all away to try to be a writer. I have the talent, the background, and the ability, but there's no more drive behind my current career. I don't give a fuck any more. I want out.

Yet the idea scares the bejeezus out of me. Yeah, I admit it, there was some serious cowardice going on for a long time. There's a little bit of residual cowardice still. That's why it took me six months to get here.

Really, it's not the huge ordeal it feels like in my head, it's not like I'm quitting my job right now to be a writer and I'll be living off Top Ramen for ten years while waiting for my big break. I already have a solid foundation. Just keep doing what I've been doing and keep an eye out for someone to leave that door open so I can wedge my foot in and slam that motherfucking opportunity open.

So yeah. This is the other half of the explanation for my new tattoo. *Quod me torquet me nutriat,* what torments me nourishes me. The word *torquet* also translates as tests or tries, among other things. I love looking down every day and seeing this statement right there on my body where I have no choice but to face it.

Fuck yeah. Bring it.

Red Wine and Oreos

The first night I was alone in my new single-girl apartment I popped open a bottle of my favorite cheap red wine (Gabbiano chianti) and a fresh bag of Oreos.

The chianti was feeling extra smooth for being only six dollars. The Oreos have been a favorite comfort food of mine for as long as I can remember. Not for the creme filling, (Double Stuf? EW) but for the decadent texture change when submerged in milk and then popped whole into my mouth. (Hint: extra delicious when dunked in a latte! Beware the caffeine/sugar combination.) While living with Aussie I had practiced discipline with Oreos because occasionally I could see his eyes of judgment whenever I ate too many cookies. On these rare occasions he made me feel very self-conscious and it ruined the childish fun of being able to eat as many Oreos as I damn well pleased whenever Mom was out of town and Dad took care of us for the weekend.

That wonderful night in my new apartment, alone with my dozens of boxes, I opened the bottle of wine and brought the Oreos with me over to sit at the coffee table. *Sex and the City*, who would be my supportive and sassy older sister if anthropomorphized, played on my laptop (the DVD player wasn't hooked up yet and even if it were, there were a dozen boxes in front of the TV).

Normally I prefer my Oreos with milk, but there were exactly three things in my fridge that night: a box of Pizza Hut Meatlovers pizza, a bottle of Skyy, and a six-pack of Corona. I'd have to settle for eating my Oreos with red wine.

That night was my first time for the odd pairing. Let me tell you–it was *heaven*. I don't know if it was the cardboard box dust in the air or the high of newly-taken independence, but it was the single most wonderful taste combination I have ever encountered.

I stayed up until four in the morning, sitting on the couch with my wine and cookies contemplating the new life I had laid before me. A life of the cheap Italian wine I adored and eating as many cookies as I wanted—no explanation, no apology, no guilt.

On my way to bed, I rinsed out my wine glass in the kitchen and saw the cork from the bottle of chianti still on the counter. The first cork from the first bottle of wine in my new apartment. I smiled proudly to myself and tucked the cork away on the same bookshelf where I keep all my old journals and notepads, a bookshelf dedicated to the oh so many twists and turns in my life.

Cheers to the next twist in the road.

My Story in Boxes

I've been breaking down my moving boxes tonight to save in the closet for when/wherever my next move may be.

There are so many boxes, enough to fill up half the living room in stacks as tall as I am. I've moved so many times since the age of eighteen. Every time it has been a fun move, a welcome change, either into an apartment with cool roommates, or into my own beautiful apartment, or into a shared grown-up apartment with my ex-boyfriend, and now into something different than all the others.

While in college I knew I would be moving regularly, every year or two until I finished my degrees, which meant that I accumulated quite a collection of moving boxes. With each move I owned more things and had to find more boxes for them.

Over the years some of these boxes were used five or six times. The top of the box would have several different things written and then scratched out, the side would have notes on whether it went to my next apartment or to my parents for a garage sale. When I moved to New York many of the boxes said "NYC" while others containing slightly less important items, were labeled "TX" and were to be stored until (if) I returned and once again lived in an apartment of more than three hundred square feet, not much bigger than my current living room.

I had a helluva time acquiring all these boxes. Flirting with Spanish-speaking-only employees at grocery stores, swiping TV boxes from trash piles on the street, dumpster-diving at Barnes & Noble (yes, as in actually climbing into a dumpster to reach the really good boxes at the back, then being found by a store employee and trying to look like I was not a complete loser when I thanked him for dropping his pile of collapsed boxes on top of my salvaged stack on the hood of my car), paying off restaurant employees for the good plastic milk crates (I didn't know those still existed!), and raiding a stack of precious cardboard trash at a Lower East Side Dunkin' Donuts at 2 a.m. the night before my father was due to arrive to drive me back to Texas.

Over the years I became very attached to my boxes, which is why when I moved in with Aussie a year and a half ago I was mortified when he told me it was time to throw them out. He did not understand, I had been with some of these boxes longer than boyfriends, since the beginning of college! I pointed to one of my beloved boxes, covered in thick layers of packaging tape and large labels crossed then circled again and torn off.

But we have HISTORY! How can you make me get rid of them?!

"Yeah, I know, sweetie, but now you *and I* have a history and a future, and that future does not include you and your huge stack of moving boxes ever again."

So, I *did* throw out all my moving boxes. All of them. And I had a lot, mostly because of my extensive book collection. Aussie came with me to the recycling center, my SUV full of my darling boxes. He helped me pull out a couple at a time and throw them into the cardboard only dumpster over and over until they were all gone. In the car he gave me a reassuring squeeze before starting the drive back to our new apartment together. I resented him immensely and it pissed me off that he wouldn't acknowledge it.

Sitting here today a year and a half later in this situation, *i.e.* single again, I wonder if the reason I was so upset over parting with my box collection was because even back then I could feel the tiny tug of what if. That voice in my head trying to tell me, *Hey, Chica, you* are *going to need those boxes again! They lasted longer than your boyfriend of three years, what makes you think they won't last through your current boyfriend too?* Maybe I'm just projecting my current situation onto something that really wasn't about this at all. Maybe I wanted to hold on to the boxes simply because I'm a pack rat and I liked seeing my history of apartments, school, jobs, and relationships written and crossed out and circled again on box after box.

They're all gone now. I started this most recent move with a mere four boxes that I had taken from the mail room at work. Fresh boxes, their edges crisp and sides straight, the original tape over the seams–they didn't have the same magic that my old boxes had. I don't think it was entirely because of the less-than-desirable break-up situation, but because it felt like I was starting all over. Not just with the relationship thing, but with, well, everything. Starting fresh and looking at all the options before me, choosing what's right for me based on what I know I don't want. Not the ideal approach, but going for what I thought I wanted didn't work out too well, so who's to say this isn't a better method?

After I moved out of our apartment, I stayed with my best friend Sweetie Pie for the next week until I moved into my own place in her same complex. During that week I started to panic because I realized I had only a few days to find a good fifty boxes which I would then have to fill with all my books, clothes, and everything else. I had to accumulate the same number of boxes in seven days that it had taken me seven years to find. I managed, and this time it was not nearly so fun and anecdote-worthy as going dumpster-diving at Barnes & Noble. For some reason I felt like it was cheating. Or perhaps that I had been cheated.

My half of our apartment—my half of our life—all of it hastily packed up in one afternoon by my father, my brother, and a couple coworkers. It's really weird, wrong, seeing that—your life that you always thought was so *full* being packed up so quickly and effortlessly, as if it were really that easy to completely change the course of your life.

I wanted to go over to my father and smack him in the back of the head and demand that he slow down so he could mourn this huge change in my life properly. I didn't of course. I just drank vodka-laced Gatorade with a Xanax chaser and tried not to think about the piles of our things I was hastily separating: *his . . . his . . . mine . . . his . . . mine . . . his . . . mine . . . mine . . . mine.*

Just because I chose to leave the relationship doesn't mean that I don't feel a huge sense of loss that I wish desperately to push into a distant memory. But it's not that simple, is it? How many more moves and crossed-out labels on boxes before I stop feeling lost?

Three weeks ago, I looked at the four new boxes I held in my arms and wondered where I would be with them five and ten years from now. I hoped that I would be moving away from figuring out what I don't want and moving into something that I know I do want, where I wouldn't mind throwing out every last goddamn box because I know I got it right this time.

How to Get Your Coworkers Fired

1. Spend twenty bucks to hire a streetwalker to come to Coworker's cubicle during lunch and while she's pulling up her cheap-whore pantyhose, have her say, "You ordered the lunch special? So, you got a closet or somethin'?"

2. Put sleeping pills in Coworker's coffee. Wait till Coworker falls asleep, then place his hand down his pants. To bring prank to level of You're a Total Bitch, place Coworker in a vibrating chair and put other hand inside shirt to reach nipple. Run into Boss' office screaming, "HE'S DOING IT AGAIN, I TOLD YOU HE WAS A FUCKING PERVERT."

3. Have a slew of thirteen- and fourteen-year-old girls come into the office and ask for Coworker.

4. In important office publication that Coworker is in charge of, print as header "Spank me in my tightie-whities, please, oh goddess of the Kingdom of Come, I am your slave boy for all of eternity" (women love romance!!).

5. When Boss is within earshot of the break room, slam the cabinet doors and rattle the coffeemaker and swear under your breath, "Goddamnit, Coworker is always getting lubricant *everywhere!*"

6. Send yourself a basket of pussy- or penis-shaped cookies, then turn to Coworker and say, "Goddamnit, Coworker, I will NOT be in your amateur porn video with you! NO MEANS NO."

7. Spike Coworker's coffee with Everclear. Keep spiking until Coworker has either passed out in pool of vomit under the desk or is dancing on top of a file cabinet doing a strip tease.

8. In monthly office newsletter, include, "Congratulations to Coworker, for finally overcoming that triple-threat of STDs! Hope the swelling goes down soon, you rascal!"

9. Get a roll of quarters and spend day throwing quarters down Coworker's blouse. Keep throwing quarters until she stands up and screams, "I AM NOT A TWO-BIT WHORE!"

Having A Girlfriend Is Usually Considered a Cockblock

    I almost had my first post-break-up sex last night. Almost. Guys have a way of fucking up even the surest thing. *Idiot.*

    My friends dragged me out to multiple bars last night. I'm actually not really a bar sort of girl. I had planned on being in bed by 10:30 to make up for the past several late nights of boozing.

    At the last bar I was on the verge of falling asleep at the table while I watched my two friends Blondie and Sweetie Pie, alternated dashing off to say hello to all these random ugly guys they seemed to know. From what I can recall (at this time of the night my memory is hazy due to sleepiness, not drunkenness), they both ditched me at the same time and the group of guys at the next table over were laughing at my blatant lack of interest in being there.

    Then they started howling at me when Blondie led back the ugliest motherfucking guy I've ever seen (short of Danny DeVito), although there were eerie similarities)) and I shot her a look of death, which she ignored, so I stood up and started frantically making the cut-throat gesture to indicate my great displeasure at his presence. The three guys next to me were laughing so hard and the Penguin guy in front of me was so fugly that it was easy to decide who to talk to.

    I hit it off with two of the laughing men right away. One was hysterically funny, one was very funny, and the third guy was married and therefore never spoke to me or my two friends but was the dear lad who fetched beers for the six of us for the rest of the night.

    I alternated paying attention to Mike and John because it was one of those really loud bars where it's all but impossible to hear someone unless they're talking right into your ear. That worked out great because it's easier to make a guy feel special if he doesn't witness you flirting with his friends too.

    Blondie kept trying to get me to dance (which I declined for a while because it's been so long since I've danced (um, or fucked) properly) and I was not confident that my hips would remember how to move in the inappropriate fashion. After much of Blondie's sexy dance-action I relented. It's hard not to dance with your super-hot girlfriends who you'd kinda sorta really like to get on.

I dance and talk with Mike and John for hours. They're both funny, sweet, handsome, bigger than me (I'm tall and meaty and have a serious dominatrix alter ego which makes it all the more fun when I throw around a guy who's got fifty pounds and eight inches on me) but finally I settle on Mike when John seems a little intimidated by my level of cursing. If he's scared of that then *shit* I would have him rocking back and forth in the fetal position before we got to any good stuff.

Mike and I are dancing slow and sexy and saying all sorts of delicious things to each other that are making my nipples hard. I tell him I broke up with my boyfriend of two years recently and I'm looking for someone to help me "move on." I am also sure to tell him that I'm sober and nothing I'm saying is because of drunken stupidity. He appreciates that. And from what I feel down below, he appreciates many other aspects of my charm.

We leave the bar and walk out to the parking garage. As soon as I have Mike next to a brick wall I throw him up against it and start having my way with him. He's saying really dirty things in my ear that nearly make my pussy blush. I like this guy.

Suddenly he breaks away.

"Um, I feel I should tell you that I have a girlfriend."

Oh. Fucking. Hell. My nipples go soft.

"*What?!* You mean, like, a girlfriend that you, like, *love* and shit? WHAT THE HELL IS WRONG WITH YOU??"

"Oh, I knew I shouldn't have said anything. I'm an idiot. Why did I say that!"

"YES, YOU ARE AN IDIOT *AND* A HUGE ASSHOLE!! IF I WERE YOUR GIRLFRIEND I'D KICK YOUR FUCKING ASS!"

"Oh my god why did I tell you that why did I tell you that what IS WRONG WITH ME?!"

"Why does this keep happening?! The last time I was single I was always the girl that guys cheated on their girlfriends with! What the fuck about me screams CHEAT ON YOUR SIGNIFICANT OTHER WITH ME?!"

"Um, well you're really, really hot . . ."

"STOP SPEAKING. YOU ARE NOT ALLOWED TO SPEAK ANY MORE. How long have you been with your girlfriend? It's like just three months, right?"

"No. Um, three years . . ."

"OH MY GOD I CANNOT BELIEVE THIS IS HAPPENING!! I JUST WANTED TO BE IN BED BEFORE MIDNIGHT AND EVEN WHEN I WAS STILL OUT I THOUGHT, 'OH NOTHING WILL HAPPEN IT'S A GODDAMN *TUESDAY* AND NOTHING HAPPENS ON TUESDAYS' AND THEN OH MY FUCKING GOD HERE WE ARE AND YOU'RE TELLING ME, 'OH, SORRY SWEETIE I HAVE A FUCKING *GIRLFRIEND* BUT I WANT YOU ANYWAY' WHAT THE FUCK DO YOU EXPECT ME TO SAY TO THAT? I KNEW I SHOULDN'T HAVE LEFT THE APARTMENT, WHAT THE BLOODY HELL IS WRONG WITH YOU???"

"I know you're mad but I'm still going to try calling you tomorrow before I leave this weekend."

"LIKE HELL YOU ARE, BOY. DON'T YOU *DARE*."

"I'm going to call you tomorrow and hopefully you will have forgiven me and I really really want to fuck you. Please pick up the phone when I call you tomorrow, please?"

"OH MY GOD I TOLD YOU TO STOP SPEAKING!"

"Please! I'll break up with my girlfriend tomorrow! It's a long-distance relationship and we've been fighting a lot any way!!"

"DON'T YOU DARE BREAK UP WITH HER BECAUSE OF ME. THAT'S NOT THE POINT."

"I'm—"

"I SAID STOP SPEAKING. DID YOU THINK THAT JUST BECAUSE I'M PROMISCUOUS I WOULDN'T HAVE ANY MORALS AND I'D SLEEP WITH YOU ANYWAY??!!!"

"Well . . ."

"NUH-UH. NO. SPEAKING. WE ARE DONE HERE."

And I left him leaning there against the parking garage wall.

My pussy is totally dying. I am dying from the inside out. Oh my god. And if/when he calls, I probably will answer. Because we all know how it goes when there's a Celebrity Deathmatch-style fight between my brain and The Pussy.

Am I missing the Bride Gene?

I admit it. I've been a huge sap lately. Every TV show, commercial, song, and lame chick flick makes me tear up. Normally I'm not like this. Normally it takes nothing short of the depression beast to make me shed a tear. Most of my friends take two to three years before they see me cry.

Not so much now. The break up was what, six weeks ago? Long ago enough that I can't tell you for sure what day it was any more (progress!). And yet I still feel doubt. The funny thing is that my gut tells me from the very pit of my stomach that I made the right choice, yet my brain still insists on bitchslapping me every day as a reminder that I walked away from a really good guy. That's pretty fucking courageous (or dumb, depending on how much you have to lose I suppose) considering the small percentage of Nice Guys amongst all the douchebags.

Just now I was watching *Sex and the City* on TV. It was the episode when Carrie breaks off the engagement with Aidan. I couldn't help it—I started sobbing.

As much as I adore TV and my beloved TiVo (and yes, my complete pink velvet DVD collection of *SATC)*, I'm not one to tell stories of *Remember when..?* with TV episodes that I did not partake in like many people do, *i.e.* "Remember when Chandler told Monica that he loves her for the first time and she had a *raw turkey* on her head?" Um, yeah. Because that shit happens in real life all the time.

This particular episode has always hit me hard, ever since I originally saw it years ago (*i.e.* while single). The first time I watched this episode I started bawling during "The Big Fight" episode where Carrie is wearing her beautiful white evening gown and Aidan looks smashing in his tux in front of the big fountain. Such a perfect place for a guy to try to talk his fiancée into going to the airport and getting hitched in Vegas while he still has thirteen hours left on his rental tuxedo.

How _____ [I don't even know what word to insert here . . . maybe ironic? Fitting? Portentous (extra points for being an SAT word! Lame ass? Sad? Lifetime of therapy bound?]

I feel that I should admit that I am ever so slightly inebriated right now. Not drunk, because I can still type and think coherently. Just slightly tipsy, just enough that I'm at that state where I am utterly and unapologetically honest. However, I'm still depressed enough that I have eaten over half a block of smoked gouda cheese, my favorite non-chocolate comfort food.

In addition to the break-up scene mentioned above, let's not forget the scene in *SATC* where Carrie and Miranda go into the ugly-ass bridal boutique and try on "giant cupcake" gowns, and Carrie has an anxiety attack and breaks out in hives.

Yeah, that would be me, at least with Aussie.

While we're at, let's back up a couple episodes to the one when Carrie discovers her soon-to-be engagement ring in Aidan's bag. At which point she immediately throws up in the kitchen sink.

Again, that would be me.

So, what the fuck? Am I missing the Bride Gene?

Why don't I ever get giddy about the whole marriage and wedding bit? I tried so hard. The Ex and I discussed marriage frequently (keep in mind that he was the first one to bring it up way back in the day, after we'd been dating for like a month). But, if it's not there, it's not there. I tried so hard to make it be there, but if you have to force it then you're not being honest with yourself.

Not once in my entire life have I been the so-called normal girl when it comes to diamond rings and wedding gowns and *happily ever after*. Never. I never played wedding as a child or fantasized about what my wedding gown would look like or fantasized about The One. I never thought about centerpieces, invitations, or my engagement ring. It's just never been there for me. Makes me uncomfortable. (For those who are wondering, *no,* I am not a child of divorce. My parents were high school sweethearts and have been married for over thirty years. I think they still have sex. Maybe. There's no dysfunctional-relationship syndrome at work here.)

What does this caution about marriage mean? A lifetime of love 'em and leave 'em relationships? Loneliness? Or maybe, just maybe: happiness.

Maybe I'm not the marrying kind. Maybe I'll eventually find a great guy to be my life partner. And as long as the dreaded M-word doesn't come up, we'll be fine. Maybe I'll spend the rest of my life being coupled and being single in two- to three-year rotating increments. Maybe marriage is right for some and wrong for others, and maybe you don't know which one is for you until you're staring it in the face.

Meet The Triad: The Pussy, My Brain & Me

The three-way war between my brain, The Pussy, and me.

my brain

The uptight, goody-goody, "I told you so" one. No one likes him because he is the voice of reason and listening to the voice of reason is a good way not to get yourself laid. Very uptight. He's not right nearly as often as he thinks he is. Clearly needs to get laid.

The Pussy

The most powerful one. She is very scary. And sassy. And intimidating. Yeah, the Pussy is really just one helluva mean motherfucker. It is best not to piss Her off.

Keep in mind this is home-grown Texas platinum pussy. Which is not to be confused with West Virginia snappin' pussy. You do not want to piss off The Pussy in general, but you especially don't want to piss off Texas Platinum Pussy. She knows how to shoot a 12-gauge gun, beat the living shit out of someone with a baseball bat (thirteen years of sports will teach a girl how to handle any sort of equipment in the meanest of ways), and suffocate a man using only the kegel.

She starts getting short-tempered and antsy at two weeks without sex. She gets downright mean at four weeks. She's only made it to six weeks twice and the poor guys who were there at the end of that swore they saw the light of God. *From the pits of hell.*

Me

I am the pushover of the Triad. The one who tries to keep everybody happy, which of course usually leaves no one happy. The sole power I have among The Triad is that I am the only one with a mouth and a body, *i.e.* the vehicle for the greater conflict between my brain and The Pussy.

Complications: At times The Pussy gains superhuman powers and can actually begin to take over other parts of the body: the legs (spread 'em!), the hands (an extension of The Pussy to do all her evil bidding), the face (ever heard of giving good face? It's essentially using sex eyes, coy grins, raised eyebrows, etc. to one's advantage), and worst of all, She can gain control of my brain if it has been at least four weeks since She last fucked someone. I do my best to let Her feast about once a month so She's placated just enough to stay out of the way. Maintaining the delicate balance of The Pussy is a full-time job.

Meeting Apartment #41

The new single/dating life is looking very promising. On Friday evening when I was moving the first of many boxes into Sweetie Pie's apartment, the first neighbor I met was a smokin' hot black guy who grinned as he held the gate open for me.

Hot Guy: Are you moving in?

My brain: *Ding, ding, ding! Helllooooo, sexy accent!*
The Pussy: *Mmmm if his accent is that sexy, what is that tongue capable of?*

Me: Sort of. I'm moving in next week, but I'm staying here with a friend until my apartment is ready.
Hot Foreign Guy: That's great! Welcome. My name is—

The Pussy: *Mmm hmm, whatever, yada yada, WOW he has a nice body . . . I haven't been on a body like that in sooo long . . .*

Hot Foreign Guy: I live right over here in apartment number 41.

My brain: *Remember, 41, 41, 41, 41, 41, 41, 41, 41.*
The Pussy: *THIS IS VITAL INFORMATION 41 41 41 41 41 IF YOU FORGET THAT YOU STUPID BRAIN I'M FUCKING DISOWNING YOU 41 41 41 41 41.*

Me: Hi, nice to meet you!
Hot Foreign Guy: I'm from the Caribbean.

My brain: *Random. And* not *subtle. Loooooser.*
The Pussy: *Stop speaking. Don't ruin this for me.*
My brain: *Bitch.*
The Pussy: *Um, dry spell* much?

My brain: *It's been a week. Shut the hell up, you cry baby.*

Me: I was wondering what your accent was.
Hot Foreign Guy: Yeah, you know you should come visit sometime.

My brain: *Again. Subtle.*
The Pussy: *STOP IT, YOU IDIOT CLIT-BLOCK.*

Me: Yeah, maybe after I get settled in . . .

The Pussy: *HELLS YEAH BABY* —kegel muscle starts contracting uncontrollably—
My brain: *I don't believe you.*
The Pussy: O*h, go read a book, loser. We're single for the first time in two years. We's gonna get LAID, BABY.*

Me: OK, well I have a lot more boxes to move . . .
Hot Foreign Guy: You need any help?

The Pussy: *Oh, come now, that's too easy!*
My brain: *Oh god. Don't say it, don't say it, don't say it . . .*
The Pussy: *Oooooh, yes, I could use your help, I've only had two orgasms today but that was by myself and I could really use some help from A NICE PIECE OF MAN-MEAT LIKE YOURSELF, WOOOOOOOOOOOOOOOOOOOOOOOOOO.*
My brain: Please *don't say that, don't you dare say that, dontsaythat.*

Me: —swallows— No. I'm good. Thanks.
Hot Foreign Guy: You sure? Well OK, it was nice to meet you . . .

The Pussy: *Right back atcha, baby, SO very nice to meet you, you hot, hot hottie godDAMN I want to hit that so hard!*

My brain: *I am so not speaking to you anymore.*

Me: Nice to meet you too!

The Pussy: *Mmmmm HMMMM look at that nice ass walking away! COME BACK HERE SO MAMA CAN SPANK THAT SHIT.*

My brain: *Oh, dear god.*

The Pussy: *My panties are totally wet.*

My brain: *I so don't know you.*

When I did eventually make it over to Jean George's apartment, I found multiple black and white photographs of himself, all shirtless. I excused myself and never returned.

Douchebags At The Bar

It's really hard to find a winner, or even a runner-up, at a bar. Which is why I generally don't go to bars to try to find guys.

Last night only added to my conviction that it's pointless and double-fold nauseating to try to meet someone at a bar.

I met Sweetie Pie and Troublemaker at a bar down the street from our apartment complex. They were both there with the guys they're dating, which left me as the only single one. Actually, no, not true. Those guys had brought their friends, and I believe they were all single—but they were also all ugly and/or socially stunted[2]. I mean, *fuck*, if you're idiotic when it comes to speaking to people, just how idiotic are you going to be when it comes to things requiring *finesse*?

For the first hour or two I mainly talked with my friends and caught them up with who's on my dating roster (including my date tonight!). While doing so I kept an eye out for interested parties and began running mental analysis of who may be worthy.

Halfway through the night I was getting another bucket of beer from the bar when a guy eased in beside me and proceeded to *stare*.

Like, really staring. I did a quick check to make sure a boob wasn't sticking out or huge beer stain conveniently located on my "Save a horse ride a cowboy" T-shirt. Nothing. Check nose for boogers. (Only a small one.) Look behind me to see if there's a train wreck situation that's stare-worthy. Nothing.

I feel uncomfortable. I leave with my bucket of beers and find our crowd of people has moved over by the bar and DAMNIT! Troublemaker (earning her name yet again) has started talking to Staring Douchebag. I have no choice but to plop my bucket back down on the bar, turn my back to Staring Douchebag, and try to resume having fun with normal people.

---

[2] This was before I knew about social anxiety disorder.

Immediately I hear him asking Troublemaker about me. I feel his eyes of Stalker-ness on my back. And ass. Casually, I turn my head just enough "to look at the band" and *yep* he's staring intently at me. His eyes are raping my soul.

Doing my best to ignore him, I talk to Troublemaker's Guy and within minutes he has me laughing with his antics and forgetting that there is a *America's Next Top Stalker* behind me. Until I turn around for another beer.

"Heeeeey how's it going?" (His eyes now delighted to be able to do the full-body scan at close range)

Erp. I think I just swallowed a bug. Or maybe that was just me wishing I had so I would have an excuse for my face to turn blue and then promptly pass out on the beer-soaked patio. —sigh—

Troublemaker introduced us (and damnit, gave him my real name) and then left. BAD FRIEND. BAD FRIEND. I was stuck. I talked but revealed as little information as possible and tried to make it clear how incredibly not-delighted I was to be there. Which he took as a challenge. Oh, bloody hell, I got myself a little trooper, now didn't I?

Staring Douchebag proceeded to tell me about all the girls he's dating right now and how he's always having to keep track of who he sees when because none of them know about the others.

Is this shit really what you say to impress the ladies, you big manly 5'-3" douchebag stallion? When can I climb on for my turn. Please. Please.

The dumbfuck actually seemed confused that I wasn't eating his shit up. He switched tactics and started asking me for Troublemaker's story. "She's with that guy. That *big* guy. The one with his arm around her. That guy. Don't waste your time." So, he didn't. He went back to trying to impress me. S*hit*.

Finally, I couldn't take it any longer and my complete disregard for manners kicked in. "Um, excuse me. I have to go stand over there now."

And I went and stood over there.

A minute later Sweetie Pie came over and asked WTF was going on and we got our giggles at his expense. She promptly made me forget that I wanted those ten minutes of my life back.

For the rest of the night, Staring Douchebag continued to stare. Blatantly. Right into my eyes. I actually would have preferred that he stared at my tits or my crotch, because then I wouldn't have felt as violated as I did. It was *that* bad.

About every forty-five minutes Staring Douchebag maneuvered his way between my friends and came to ask me if I wanted a shot, a beer, and a ride home because I looked plastered. (I told him not to confuse disinterest with inebriation. He looked at me like he was surprised to hear big words coming from my mouth. I looked at him like he was a fucking douchebag.) He was a persistent little shit.

Finally, finally, about twenty minutes before closing I realized Staring Douchebag had left. I was a little surprised he didn't try to get in my pants one last time, but I was delighted to miss such an opportunity.

Enter Douchebags #2 and #3. It was a busy night. I was getting douched from all sides.

I had noticed Douchebag #2 earlier because he was staring at me too (although in a normal drunken-frat boy way, not a creepy buy-dirty-panties-off-eBay way). What had made me notice him was that every thirty minutes he and his friend moved ten feet closer. The first time he was on the other side of the bar sitting at a table. Then they were standing by the bar. Then they were sitting at the far end of the bar. Finally, they were sitting on my side of the bar, elbows on the counter and legs spread facing us. [Note to the chicks: this is classic "please approach me" body language from a guy if you're at a bar. Note to the guys: if you do this for more than three minutes, it becomes obvious you're too much of a fucking pussy to get up and make the first move, which means you're probably too much of a pussy to do much else, and you need to give up. As a chick who almost always makes the first move, let me tell you—this shit gets old fast.]

I had found Douchebag #2 to be dorky-but-cute, so I approached him over his friend who looked a little arrogant. At this point I had not yet classified either of these guys to be douchebags, but it quickly made itself apparent—

Between approaching them and actually saying hello, Douchebag #3 demanded to know if my friend Sweetie Pie was single. I was a bit taken aback. Like, *dude*, at least let us exchange names first . . . I told him that she wasn't, she was with that guy over there—the one kissing her neck—and Douchebag #3 scoffed with complete distaste, then began to break down all the points on which he *knew* that guy was gay. Yuh-huh.

Turning back to Douchebag #2, I asked him some of the standard questions and he seemed fairly normal. Until he asked me if after this I wanted to come with them to a titty bar down the street.

Oh. My. God.

I've got nothing against strip clubs. I know two girls who have been or currently are strippers and they are two of the coolest chicks I've ever known. I did, however, find it in very, very poor taste to ask a girl they'd just met to come with them to a strip joint.

I suggested we go to a great 24-hour diner I knew when the bar closed in a few minutes. They didn't get it. They were intent on "seeing boobies". Yes, that is verbatim.

At which time I started fishing out my keys. Douchebag #2 looked surprised and asked me where I was going.

"Home. Have a nice life." I patted him on the back and left.

Douchebags, man. I mean, seriously?

How To End a Bad First Date

1. When crossing the street, point at slutty girl standing on opposite corner, proclaim, "That bitch! SHE TOOK MY CORNER," and proceed to beat her STD-ridden ass into the gutter where she belongs. Your date will leave because no man wants a girl who can't keep bitches off her own corner.
2. Have friend call cell phone at pre-agreed upon time. Answer, "What?? There's an emergency with Pappy the hamster?! I'LL BE RIGHT THERE!" and run out door crying.
3. Clutch left arm, grab heart, gasp uncontrollably, fall out of chair, and shout "HEART . . . HEART ATTACK!" when concerned date comes to your aid, start giggling and proudly proclaim, "LOOKS LIKE MY LOVE FOR YOU IS TOO MUCH FOR MY HEART TO TAKE!!" and date will leave of his own accord over your bad and sick sense of humor.
4. "Accidentally" run into large guy. Start screaming at him that he should apologize for trampling on your twenty-dollar whore clear plastic shoes. Grab date and demand that he defend your honor. When he doesn't, start pounding date with your huge purse full of silverware swiped from restaurant. That'll teach him to respect a lady.
5. As soon as he asks, "How are you?", start crying with great heaving sobs and wail "He said he loooooooved meee!" If he's one of those Mr. Sensitive types who don't scare off easily, blow your nose on his sleeve.
6. Show up dressed in a wedding gown. Fling yourself at date, happily saying, "I could just tell from the moment we spoke that you were The One! Mama and Daddy are waiting in the car to meet you!"
7. If date has been making lustful eyes at you throughout the date, roll your eyes, throw him a wrinkled twenty-dollar bill, and tell him, "Here you go, buddy, the blowjob's on me tonight" and walk out.
8. As soon as you see date, look him up and down, groan, and tell him, "I'm sorry, but there's been some sort of mistake. Our friend must have gotten confused. I'm not a lesbian. I don't date women." When date replies that

he is not a woman, respond, "Sweetie, take the hint. I only date *manly* men."

9. Be very, very quiet all evening. When date asks what's wrong, take your steak knife and plunge it repeatedly into your palm while screaming "I DON'T CARE ABOUT YOUR FUCKING CAT! STOP TALKING ABOUT YOUR FUCKING CAT, YOU FREAK! I CAN'T TAKE IT ANYMORE!"

10. Shortly into date, lean over and ask him, "Look, I'm just on this date for the sex. I need to know upfront if you're cool with strap-on's, because otherwise there's this hot dyke over by the pool table I want to go home with."

Dont' mind me it's the wine talking

I really wanted to love him. Truly, madly, deeply. I really did.

I wanted to love him with all my being. Clichés, teary-eyed lovemaking, *schmoopies* and all. But it didn't work out that way. It would be so much easier if it had.

But wanting to love someone isn't reason enough to stay.

This isn't an especially enlightening truth, but that doesn't mean it isn't painful as hell..

P.S. You know youjve have too much to drink when it takes eleven tissues to wipe all the wine you spilled off the curtain oh well. At least the curtain smells nice now.

The Rules of Fuck Buddies

Sure everyone has their own set of rules for fuck buddies, some nicer and some harsher, but these are mine. Some may sound cold and objectifying, but these rules are intended to protect feelings, as ironic as that may seem. Listen to me, I speaketh the truth. I only have your next orgasm in mind.

Reality check: the rules of boyfriends and the rules of fuck buddies are completely different. In no equation does BF equal FB. Do not ever confuse them, that's when feelings start to get hurt. Yes, fuck buddies have feelings too, but you are only concerned about how his cock feels inside you. Got it?

1. No holding hands. Keep hands to the crotch-el region.
2. No spending the night.
3. Fifteen minutes of cuddling max. Affection is generally discouraged beyond, "Aww, you're such a great fuck!"
4. Do not enter upon a fuck buddy arrangement or situation while drunk. There's a difference between a one-night stand and a fuck buddy. Although entering either drunk is not wise. God forbid there's a beer-goggles situation. You don't want to go to bed with Will Smith and wake up with Steve Urkel, do you? Besides, don't you want to be sober enough to remember all the marvelous sex you had the night before?
5. No toothbrushes. Refer to #2. There should be no ties at all, even if they cost only $2.49 and secretly you let your other fuck buddy use the same one.
6. Don't discuss anything real. No family history, no favorite colors, no goals, no personal triumphs or tragedies. If you want to keep it real, you have to stay light: movies, bands, and favorite brands of booze.
7. He is not obligated to have sex with you while you're having your period. Most nice boyfriends will, but fuck buddies have the option to pass. If he doesn't mind, then cool.

8. No *sweetie, honey, schmoopie* allowed. The only pillow-talk is *fuck me harder, ride me, bitch,* or *suck this big cock.*
9. No dinners, no movies, no quality time of any sort. If you insist on going out at all, meet him at a bar for drinks no earlier than 10 p.m. The hour between nine and ten is the grey zone between when a real date starts and when it's just a hook-up. If you ever wonder why a guy asks you out for a date so late, it's because he doesn't want to have to go through the effort of buying you dinner and talking, he just wants to get to the good stuff.
10. Two guys in twenty-four hours is fine, just be discreet.
11. You still need to dress to impress. Just because you know sex is a sure thing doesn't mean you should answer the door in your pajamas unless they're really tight and sheer. Shower, shave, lotion up, smell good, and have some fun with that tight miniskirt you would never wear on a *real* date.
12. Break out the sex toys. Play up the freak factor and see how much you can get away with. Part of the fun of a fuck buddy is you don't care if he respects you or not, so you can let loose and reveal that sadist tendency of yours. Who says the nipple clamps are just for women?
13. Hide evidence. Throw out all condom wrappers (although you should no matter what, ew!), put the lube back in your goodie drawer, and for fuck's sake don't get any hickeys, bruises, bites, or scratches if you expect to date/fuck anyone else any time soon. If you have a collared-shirt job, keep all that shit below the neck line so you don't give your boss a heart attack. Or ideas. —shudder—
14. No liquid exchange. You're not a twelve-year-old girl in a convent, you know about condoms and birth control. Use both. If you're young and worry about telling your parents you want to go to the doctor, you can go to Planned Parenthood on your own and take care of things there. They understand discretion. Being scared of your mother is no excuse. Believe me, I understand scary mothers.

15. Pee with the door closed. Just because you're using each other for sex doesn't mean you can't keep some decency.

Sound harsh? Then maybe fuck buddies aren't for you. It's a rough game and not everyone is meant to play.

Abort Abort Abort: My Brain, The Pussy, and Me Reach Agreement

This guy hit on me at a pizza parlor the day I broke up with Aussie. He was so funny and witty that I couldn't resist when he asked for my phone number.

He opened the door to his hotel room wearing a sweat-stained polo shirt and droopy jeans. He looked half asleep.

Him (no he doesn't get a cute moniker because you will see his is NOT WORTHY): Hey gorgeous, come 'ere and give me a hug.

He opened his arms wide in anticipation of my full-frontal embrace, but really opening his arms just revealed that he had some severe love handles. So severe that they showed under a baggy polo shirt. Oh, dear. How is that even possible when you're in your early twenties?

my brain: *Run. Turn and run. Throw the bottle of vodka at him so that he can drink away the memory of the fact that his mere appearance made a girl turn on her heels and run for the elevator. For the love of all things wet and holy, run.*

The Pussy: *Erp.*
Me: Hiii.......
him: You look cuter and hotter than I remember, wow!
Me: —
my brain: No. Just no.
The Pussy: *Well come on, give him a chance. You were attracted to him for a reason, right? He's super funny.*
my brain: *Yeah. Because he is a GUY and he is SINGLE and he is WILLING. That is not enough of a reason to invite him Down Town for a Good Time.*
The Pussy: BUT WE NEED TO GET LAID. IT'S BEEN TWO AND A HALF WEEKS.

With that, all three of us came into his room.

him: You don't mind if I unbutton my pants, do you? I feel really bloated, ugghhh.
my brain: *OH NO HE DID NOT JUST SAY THAT.*

It went downhill from there. I kept thinking he would do something to redeem himself—rub my back and shoulders that are still sore from moving to a new apartment, throw me against the wall in a really passionate kiss, or at the very least make me laugh so hard that I piss myself—anything. I was very open to anything that would make him more fuck-worthy.

It got even worse. I started to think it really was bad when I was spending more time staring at my cuticles and wondering why I had bothered to touch up my chipped toenail polish than paying attention to what he was babbling about (but that was probably because he kept repeating himself).

It was then that I realized I would rather be at home with my dogs and my laptop than with him. I didn't doubt that he knew how to go down a girl (some guys just have that look about them, and he certainly did), but I just didn't care to have to go through all that other stuff to get to what may be the one redeeming moment of an otherwise *icky* encounter.

This is what I get for putting on makeup. The last four times now I've put on makeup for anything involving non-work-related male interaction, it hasn't been worth those five minutes of my day which would have been more enjoyed watching a rerun of *Friends*.

Me: You know what? I'm *really* tired. I think I should send myself home.
him: What? Really? Why?
my brain: *Lookie at that, he actually seems* surprised *that I don't want to stay.*
him: Are you sure you don't want to spend the night here in this swanky hotel? Please?

The Pussy: *No. Just no.*

Me: I'm afraid not, I think I should really just send myself home, I'm so —fake yawn— *tired.*

him: Hey, call me this weekend OK, beautiful?

my brain: *Yuh huh. Sure. You go ahead and wait for that call, buddy BECAUSE I DON'T FUCKING THINK SO.*
The Pussy: *YOU'RE NOT WORTHY.*

Me: OK byenow!

my brain: *Idiot.*
The Pussy: *I know, wasn't he?!*
my brain: *I meant you. YOU ALWAYS GET US INTO THIS SHIT.*
The Pussy: *Hmph. At least I* tried, *bitch.*
my brain: *Stop speaking.*
The Pussy: *Hmph.*

So here I am. Horny as hell and pissed that I'm so horny that I have Horny Goggles on which, therefore make all available male specimens look Fuckable in spite of their actual (lack of) qualities/capabilities. And, unlike Beer Goggles, you can't just sleep them off. The only thing that makes Horny Goggles go away is 1) lots of fantastic sex or 2) excessive amounts of masturbation. Let's keep our fingers crossed for option 1).

When I got home I took off my sexy, lacy thong and short, touchable miniskirt in exchange for a ragged, white tank top and some comfy boy short underwear (yes, actually, they *do* have Superwoman on them). There's laundry running in the washer. My tiny 13" TV is static-y because cable hasn't been installed yet so I can only hear every third word of *Everybody Loves Raymond.* And oh, lookie over there, the dog just piddled on the carpet.

What is the end to a nowhere near perfect evening? Masturbate a couple times, finish off the bottle of Pinot Grigio from last night and feel triumphant about the fact that even in my horniest of horny/desperate moments I was able to walk away from someone that would not have been worth my time or pussy juice.

And, you know what? It's all good. I would rather be in this situation of botched dates and lousy near-laids than in a relationship with someone I was staying with just because it was easy, comfortable, and expected of me.

I raise my wine glass to the preferred of two evils.

The Pink Toothbrush Situation

I posted this the day that it happened. In the morning, Aussie checked my blog and read this post about his new girlfriend. Being the chivalrous gent he is, he shut down my site because it was still in his name. I had to apologize profusely before he conceded putting my blog back up. This is the reason I started a second blog about all my post-break-up exploits, Single by Choice Damnit, for several months.

Even though the break up was nearly three months ago, I still had a lot of things at his (previously our) apartment. Why is this? I had one day to move out as much crap as I could, one week after the break-up and the day I moved into my own apartment. In spite of having many wonderful mover-monkeys, whom I thanked with pitchers of margaritas afterward), I have so much *shtuff* that I couldn't get it all in one day.

Which brings us to today. Aussie has been patient in waiting for me to get my act together and move out the rest of my things (mostly old books from grad school, clothes, and just *crap*). He told me he would be out of the apartment for the afternoon so I could come and get it. Great.

I entered the apartment and the first thing my eyes went to were a pair of women's shoes. Ugly ones.

Hmm. I turn the corner into the bedroom and see an overnight bag. A *girly* overnight bag. Oh. My. God. He has a girlfriend. He HAS A *GIRLFRIEND*?!

So, what do I do? I snoop. THAT'S RIGHT I unzipped the girly overnight bag and looked inside. Deodorant. Jeans. Brush. And a GINORMOUS BRA.

Eep.

I picked it up and unfolded it for the full effect. Whoa. My head would fit in one of the cups. I look down at my own boobs. Granted, they're squished into a sports bra, but they are still clearly NOT THE SIZE OF MY HEAD. I feel a little dejected. My poor boobies.

I go down the hall to the bathroom. "My" sink is empty, as I left it—not even a bar of soap.

Then I see the pink toothbrush. IN MY TOOTHBRUSH HOLDER. *IN MY TOOTHBRUSH HOLDER.* OH MY GOD. I know it's not mine because I was sure to pack my toothbrush when I left the night of the break-up. And I don't buy pink shit.

Trashcan. There is an empty toothbrush package in MY TRASHCAN. I PICKED OUT THAT TRASHCAN AT BED BATH AND BEYOND.

AND THERE ARE *TAMPON WRAPPERS* IN *MY* TRASHCAN. *GENERIC* TAMPONS IN MY TRASHCAN.

I nearly threw up. I mean, yes, I stayed up drinking with friends until 5 a.m. and so I was a tad hung over. A pounding headache, nausea, and emotional baggage are not what I need when I'm moving out of my ex-boyfriend's apartment, which was previously known as our apartment.

Back to the entry way for my purse. I open my pretty little pill box and, OH MY GOD THERE ARE NO XANAX IN MY PILL BOX. NOW IS NOT AN ACCEPTABLE TIME NOT TO HAVE XANAX. **THERE IS A PINK TOOTHBRUSH SITUATION**.

I turn to the freezer to pull out the I-like-to-drink-my-problems-away sized bottle of vodka that is always there. It's only 12:30 in the afternoon. Damn. Not close enough to beer-thirty. I put it back.

Standing in the middle of the kitchen (his kitchen, formerly known as *our* kitchen), I stood and stared blankly at the empty kitchen wall. Formerly known as our empty kitchen wall.

Huh. I don't know how to deal with unwelcome feelings without my trusty sidekicks, Booze and Xanax Chaser.

Then it clicks. I smile to myself. Shit therapy. An excellent way to expunge unwantables from your system! BRILLIANCE.

Yeah, I did.

I went back to the bathroom (previously *our* bathroom) and sat down and took a shit. A nice, long, stinky shit.

I'm just sorry I didn't clog the toilet.

My Future NYC Brownstone

Years ago when I first moved to New York City for a year-long internship, I imagined renting a small, yet glorious, apartment on the top floor of a beautiful brownstone. My room would overlook a quiet yet busy street where I would set up my computer, stare out the window, and write brilliant things every night.

Instead I got a shitty run-down studio overlooking a courtyard which held nothing but thrown out furniture and metal trash cans covered in muddy snow. My apartment was so small that the one exterior wall had only two windows. One housed the window unit, the other was covered with a huge iron fire escape gate to keep out intruders. As if the fire escape said intruder was climbing up wouldn't plummet to the ground under his weight.

Not exactly the glamorous Carrie Bradshaw, *Sex and the City* scene I was expecting. Especially not the rent-controlled apartment. Oh, *hell* no. I did not have the square footage, big operable window, apartment location, or even the nice laptop that made the ideal writing environment, at least not as I envisioned it. Instead I sat huddled in the corner at my ancient desktop computer, where I faced the tiny kitchenette with the sloping floor and cracked walls and tried not to think about the mouse I could hear scratching his way at the wall behind the fridge.

The other day while bored at work I searched through Flickr.com for photos of New York City brownstones. I found the perfect photo, a line of beautiful undulating brownstones covered in snow. A single window was open to the cold outside. That window, that window right there in that photo, is my happy place. That's where I imagine one day I'll have my laptop and writing desk, complete with my favorite mug that will mark the wood with years of coffee rings. That's the window where I'll write freelance magazine articles by day and novels by night.

This photo is now my computer background at work where it can be my daily reminder of what I'm working toward. Not this boring and unsatisfying (buthighprofileandveryrespectable!) job I have now, this job I worked so hard for for the last umpteen years. In all honestly, I'm not sure I would have had the skill to be a professional writer if I hadn't taken this current career path. Maybe all the years as a cubicle monkey will prove themselves to be worth the effort and the mindfuckery in one of those piss yourself ironic and entirely unintentional ways.

The writing, the New York City brownstone—is this a stupid, naive, and silly dream? Maybe. Probably. Fuck it. I need to have dreams, if for no other reason than to have something that keeps me going during the worst of cubicle monkey days. What about the off-chance it actually happens? What if it actually happens? If there's one thing I've learned as a Texan, it's that you never know when a big piece of *holy fucking shit!* will knock you flat on your ass.

According to every inspirational and entrepreneurial book I've read, one of the key steps to achieving your dream is to visualize what it is. Hold it out in front of you and feel out exactly what it looks like, the exact shape and size it is to become as you slowly form it with your hands. For me it's a desk at a window in New York City—a far stretch from the $13 Ikea table here in Texas with a window that looks out onto a parking lot.

When I'm typing at my computer at work, my mind is on anything but the monitor in front of me. Instead, I'm thinking about the stack of neon green Post-it notes tucked away under the keyboard, the notes where I have hastily scrawled out thoughts, post titles, excerpts, and outlines when the boss wasn't looking. Every night I slip this stack of notes into my purse and then at home piece them together into the evening's post. At the end of the week I tape each Post-it into a notebook and place it back on the shelf with all the others.

Sometimes I think what's the point? I'll never make it as a writer. Why the fuck am I hanging on to hundreds of stupid Post-it notes*?*

Because I wouldn't be doing this if I didn't *need* to do it. All these hundreds of stupid fucking Post-it notes are my story. Because every day I feel my spine tense up as I walk toward the office building, and the moment I pull open the heavy glass door, I remind myself that I won't be opening these doors forever. I'm writing my way out of here, one Post-it at a time.

Besides, won't it make for great interview material years from now when I'm an established writer and I can laugh about how I used to disappear to the restroom at work for twenty minutes at a time so I could write in the tiny notepad zipped in my knee-high boot? There aren't many girls in Texas crazy enough to suffocate their calves in tight leather boots in the middle of summer.

One day. One day I'll make my way back to New York City, and this time I'll stay there. It's meant to be. Not that I believe in fate or destiny or any of that nonsense. What do I believe in then?

Myself. I believe that if I want to live in my own brownstone in New York City, then I won't stop writing until I'm sitting at a desk looking out that window in the photograph.

Keeping the Mystery

I kinda sorta maybe just a little bit have a very good chance of sleeping with someone soon. More specifically, two someones. A couple. One of whom is a chick. I've never fucked a girl; and it just seems like something you should do to be a well-rounded individual, like knowing how to use jumper cables or speak another language or how to rename your wireless network.

The offer—It's not official, no one has come out and directly said it, but there's been nearly every possible insinuation and the invitations to meet them have started. I can't decide whether to meet the couple or not.

Background: I first heard about the guy through a friend. The friend factor is important because then you know he's not a fucking weirdo who will root through your trash and save your toenail clippings. Always a plus. I have not met him yet. We have emailed and talked on the phone a couple times. He made it clear his girlfriend is into freaky things like me. She does sound cool. And, from the time we've spent on the phone, the guy and I totally hit it off. They sound like good peoples. People I would enjoy getting to know and actually talking to between rounds of fantasgasmic sex.

So why not jump at the offer and jump on them? Especially since I'm fucking drowning over here, going on a record for the longest I've gone without sex since I was . . . nineteen? OUCH. I think I just felt my pussy kick me from the inside.

Why the hesitation? OK, partially the goody-goody inside me doesn't want to be a guest star in anyone's relationship, but he said they've done it before and it was no big deal. That puts me at ease, but you still never know.

That's not the real reason though.

Both the guy and the chick have been reading my blog since our mutual friend introduced them to it/me a while ago. He has admitted that they're both intimidated as hell about the idea of meeting me. That intimidates *me*. I'm sure that many people who read OEN have an image in their head of this total red-nailed/red-lipped *takes no prisoners* sexpot. With big knockers.

Nuh-uh. I'm, like, normal. Seriously. I can completely pass for a normal citizen among the greater society. I swear. I'm pretty sure.

I have a real/boring career, I have a real name that is not nearly as cool or vixen-y as Vix, I have smallish boobies (fantastic smallish boobies, but still. Not nympho/sexpot boobies).

But, very few people who come here know *me* and know *that*.

Now don't think I'm getting all high-and-mighty on myself, because I'm not. The opposite, in fact. I like the idea of being this really amazing cyber persona. Who is very much me, don't get me wrong here—there has been NO exaggeration in who or what I am or what I have done. But, there's still a little bit of fantasy inherent in any blog, no matter how much I may talk about depression or any of those many unsexy things. Simply by virtue of being anonymous, there's fantasy. Mystery. A mystique.

I don't want to ruin that. For them or for me. The fantasy is often so much more satisfying than the reality.

This isn't me worrying about how I would be in bed, because, –scoff– *that* I will never be modest about. Come on, now. I'm worried about whether they would like me, the flesh-and-blood-and-boogers me, and whether they'd wish they had never ruined the mystique.

I may be completely making too big a deal out of this, but I can't help it. I don't want them to be disappointed when they see me standing there in front of them with a pimple on my chin and scuffed fuck-me boots and then they find out I often make very decidedly *not-funny jokes*. The horror.

187 Wrongs Do Make a Right

So, so many things were wrong last night on my date with Handsome Nerd, best friend of Barbie's husband Ken.

I was ten minutes late to the restaurant.

We had to go to a different steakhouse because the first restaurant's wait was 45 minutes long.

He didn't wear nice "first date" clothes. Or do so much as tuck in his shirt, or wear a belt, and I believe he wore hiking boots or something of the R.E.I. variety.

It did not start well. It also took a while to get the conversation going, mainly because our HIMYNAMEISTAMMYANDIWILLBEYOURWAITRESSTONIGHTANDOHMYGODGUYSTHISPLACESERVESTHEBESTSTEAKREALLYREALLYIUSEDTOCOMEHEREALLTHETIMEBEFOREISTARTEDWORKINGHEREANDILOVEITSOMUCHANDIMSOHAPPYYOUDECIDEDTOJOINUSHERETONIGHT waitress was trying so very hard to be the perfect attentive waitress, talking so much and telling us cute stories and yes, she was very adorable, and I did give her a huge tip because she was an (otherwise) attentive waitress, but come on, woman, you're talking through my game, here.

It felt like every time Handsome Nerd and I got into a really great conversation she would come over (fine, she is a waitress and I *would* like more wine, thank you), and she wouldn't get that we were on a date, because she just kept talking. And talking. And talking. The first two times she did this we just kinda giggled toward each other, but eventually I started glaring at her, then not making eye contact, then glaring again but with greater severity because she's getting in the way of our really amazing conversation. I do not have many really amazing conversations with a guy, so *pardon me* for being territorial of our witty banter.

Once we ordered food and got over the initial oh my god I'm actually on a date what the fuck am I supposed to do nerves (and between interruptions from TAMMYTHEWAITRESS!!) our conversation went really well. Very few pauses.

Even during those we were usually staring at each other snickering, daring the other one to be the first to speak with a mouthful of steak, which of course only meant that we got into elaborate chew-fests and the first to finish had to speak. (It really was funny, I swear. Fine, you had to be there.)

Just as I remembered, he was funny as hell. And in exactly my type of funny. Which, Handsome Nerd divulged to me, Ken has told him was "a really sick sense of humor. Just like you." Awwwww, that's so fucking sweet.

The main trend of the dinner conversation (which lasted nearly two hours, probably because we kept getting into staring/chewing contests) was that he kept saying the exact wrong thing. I had been doing OK, but that was because I had spent the entire afternoon composing a mental list of things to talk about. At one point, I was snickering at Handsome Nerd because he knew it was his turn to talk or ask a question and he looked mortified because he couldn't come up with anything, meanwhile I'm helping him along by snickering (not at him, but toward him). I teased him for clearly not having prepared for the oral section of the evening, for if he had, he would not be so lost for conversation topic. He said he thought he could wing it. I snickered toward him some more and offered to let him borrow the notecard I had prepared to avoid such awkwardness.

Toward the end of the dinner, TAMMYTHEWAITRESS!! came by and said she had asked the manager to come by to offer us complimentary dessert because they always do that on birthdays and anniversaries. Both Handsome Nerd and I were too shocked to correct her (although I think most people would have picked up on the matching dumbfounded faces). After her departure we continued staring at each other before the snickers began again.

It was very much a snicker-filled evening. We jumped right over the nervous chuckling and, god forbid, the chortling. Over the polite chuckling when your date is trying to be funny but not quite making it through, but the poor guy is clearly trying very hard so you give a mercy-chuckle. Over the poorly-timed guffaw. This is in the case of someone trying to please the one making the joke and starts laughing before the joke/anecdote is fully delivered, or laughing much harder than is really warranted. Over the nervous giggling, which is independent of conversation topic. Nervous giggling can occur at any time, nothing having caused it, and nothing being able to end it. It is in this situation that someone like TAMMYTHEWAITTRESS!! is appreciated for her frequent interruptions.

Then there was Handsome Nerd's particular laughter. The silent laugh. Typically paired with shaking his head at himself for having said something he immediately regretted for its stupidity, inappropriateness, or lameness. He didn't even try to hide his embarrassment. Each time he did this, I became a little more smitten. It was cute as hell to watch him go from a suave and witty guy to a blushing dumbass in the span of half of a sentence. How could I be anything other than smitten? I'd found my match in dumbassery.

Handsome Nerd must have felt the chemistry as well, because he shared a particularly embarrassing secret with me (first he made me guess, and after I loudly squealed, "IT'S A THIRD NIPPLE ISN'T IT! SHOW ME! I'VE NEVER SEEN A THIRD NIPPLE!" enough times I think he realized his dirty secret wasn't so bad).

Except that it was. Nothing *bad*, but royally embarrassing, along the lines of still playing with his Teenage Mutant Ninja Turtle dolls or sleeping under Superman sheets. It was a doozy. I was kind enough not to laugh at him, just toward him, a kindness which he had already shown me many times throughout the evening. It was a delight-filled laugh, not one of mockery.

I told him I was honored to be bestowed such a secret. Before I even finished the sentence his face was back in his hands and he was shaking his head again, why, oh why, did he say that! He normally waited much longer before telling anyone that! What was wrong with him??

And I became just a little more smitten.

At the end of dinner, I asked Handsome Nerd what he wanted to do next: go see a movie, go back home and play video games by himself and wish he had chosen differently, or come to my apartment to watch TV.

He got a cute little naughty grin on his face, oh, yes, he did. That was all the invitation either of us needed.

Handsome Nerd followed me in his car on the highway aaaaaalllllll the way back to my apartment, where we watched *The Office* on TiVo. I had told him about the show earlier because I thought he would appreciate its sort of humor, and also so it wasn't quite so obvious when I asked him to go back to my place that I wanted to not get in—but be *near* his pants.

We watched two episodes before I felt that it was a comfortable time to make my move. Since it looked like he wasn't going to dare.

At the beginning of episode three I yawned, stretched my arms out, and so not casually placed one around his shoulders.

"I've always wanted to do that," I giggled. I can so pull off being lame.

The dog jumped in the way. *ARGHGHHH.*

Try again: yawn, stretch, shoulders. He looked . . . something . . . Not mortified, not shocked, not freaked out . . . I don't know but it was something IMPOSSIBLE TO READ.

I got nervous. My next I'm-trying-to-be-cool-by-being-lame move is too embarrassing in the light of day to admit to. Let's just say that that something-face of his got worse. Oh dear God.

I got flustered. RETREAT! RETREAT! RETREAT! "I'm sorry . . . I know that was—"

"No, it's cool. Come back here." And he shifted over to be closer for my arm across his shoulders. He tried putting his around mine too, but that was uncomfortable, so we started kissing instead. Much better.

Until I felt a second breath on my ear and looked over to see Lil' Lesbian inches away, peering at us from the top of the couch.

Naturally, I did what any polite horny hostess would do to make her guest more comfortable. Took him to the bedroom and closed the goddamn door.

It was so nice to make out. I hadn't made out with anyone in months. Even the couple guys I got a little sumthin' sumthin' from, we just did the obligatory amount of kissing before moving on to other things. This was different. I was not going to put out. Barbie told me I was not allowed to put out and so I was not going to because as much as I want *I know they are right*. MUST. NOT. PUT. OUT. Much.

Instead we kissed, and kissed, and kissed, and it was wonderful. I have not made out with a guy for hours like that since I was a teenager. It went from just kissing to pulling down my sweater and kissing my breasts, then pulling off the sweater and burying his face in my breasts, oh, it felt so nice, I could have stayed there all night.

I'm guessing Handsome Nerd hadn't gotten any in a while either because he was taking his sweet time relishing every square inch of exposed skin on my body. He quickly figured out that I love having my neck kissed, sucked, bitten, and spent what felt like hours just on my neck. Which now looks like a purple battleground in the mirror and I totally don't care. It has till Monday to clear up before I go to work. Eep. And see my father for dinner while he's in town. Fuck. Don't care, still worth it.

I told Handsome Nerd to take off his shirt and was delighted to see that he has a nice thick stature (meaning I don't feel obligated to be gentle because I weigh more than he does, I tend to go for only meatheads or lanky guys). Except, um, he kinda did not smelL . . so good? Needed a little update on the deodorant? Wooooph. Major party foul. But to be fair, at first, I didn't know if it was him or me (I sweat like a bastard) so there was some awkward maneuvering on my part to wiff myself to see if I was the culprit. I wasn't. Not that I let that get in the way. No sirreeeee I AM A TROOPER. And my troops wanted in that tent.

Lots and lots of making out, my hands were everywhere, enjoying being on a guy's body. That sad and desperate and all-too-true line from *Sex and the City*, "Please, just kiss me! At least, lie on top of me!" kept running through my head. Please, body, let's never go so long again without a nice male body lying on top of me (oh, who are we kidding, I want top. He can be underneath me and he'll damn well like it).

Handsome Nerd's hands were a bit more hesitant than mine. I'm not going to read too much into that, from my experience a guy can want you as bad as hell, but not dare try anything because he wants to be COMPLETELY

POSITIVELY SURE he will not get in trouble for putting his hand somewhere you don't want it to be. Which was fine with me. I'm a big fan of the take his hand and place in desired location method, which I implemented at the proper times. Eventually he got a little more bold and let his hands wander down the back of my jeans to discover a barely there thong, so after a while (must show positive reinforcement) I took off my jeans and was now mostly naked.

Let me tell all you guys out there—nothing makes a girl feel sexier than feeling you lose your breath as your eyes run up and down her body in nothing short of *wow*. The way he looked at me and caressed me and touched me made me feel like a goddess. I'm still swooning.

So, yeah, I let him get in my pants just a little. OK, that's a lie. I didn't let him get in my pants, I TOLD HIM to get in my pants. Which is so not the same as putting out.

Just one finger. OK, that's a lie. Two fingers. He found the clit ring. He enjoyed the clit ring and I enjoyed him finding the clit ring. His fingers had their dirty way with me and a couple minutes later I really felt like a goddess.

That was it. There was more making out, but I never went anywhere near his big throbbing Happy Place (but hopefully he could tell I really, really, really, really, really wanted to and was simply trying to be as good a girl as I can manage).

He never tried anything, and I'm glad he didn't because my willpower sucks. Throughout the whole gettin' it on portion of the evening, we kept joking around and teasing each other. It was fun to be able to do that while being sexy. Because, well, sex is often an ugly or weird thing that you have to have a sense of humor about. Especially when you put two semi-naked dumbasses like us together in a room. There were still many, many wrong things said, including Handsome Nerd bringing up college football at a very, very, very wrong time. Which made me all the more smitten, and which I will never cease teasing him for.

Handsome Nerd left my apartment around 1:30 a.m. to drive the long way back home. We were both all goofy as I walked him to the door. We hugged and he said he would be calling me soon and we looked at each other all goofy-eyed before I closed the door behind him.

The One-Night Stand Contract

Back in my heyday of singledom (i.e. when I got laid more than once every couple months), it would have been nice to have some sort of disclaimer/reality check contract to hand over to potential one-night stands so that there would be ABSOLUTELY NO CONFUSION ABOUT THE SITUATION. Attached to the One-Night Stand Contract would also be a copy of The Rules of Fuck Buddies since the rules are very similar. We want to make sure that there would be ABSOLUTELY NO CONFUSION ABOUT THE SITUATION, WHICH IS DISTINCTLY *NOT* A RELATIONSHIP.

Please initial in the margin next to every statement to indicate your compliance.

The One-Night Stand Contract
If you choose to go forth in the mutual act of using each other for sex on this night the ___ of _____, 20___, you must adhere to the following terms and conditions:

We are just fucking. We are not in a relationship. We are not dating. We are just fucking. If fucking leads to something resembling friendship or general good-will toward each other, that is acceptable; nothing beyond that will ever arise from this chance occurrence.

That means I do not expect you (and would prefer that you not) hold my hand especially in that couple-y way with the interlinking of fingers. Do not get jealous of anyone who may hit on me or give me their phone number in your presence.

If you think alcohol or anything else (including a very recent break-up) leaves you emotionally or psychologically hindered beyond rational thought, then please give me an IOU for another night or back out gracefully. Save the "it's not you, it's me" excuse for someone who hasn't heard it before.

If you currently have a (check all that apply) __girlfriend/boyfriend __wife/husband __psycho stalker ex __a parole officer or a little tracking box on your ankle __a "situation" (please explain on attached piece of paper; this includes having a boy/girlfriendesque-*thing*, an emotional separation but not a physical one, or "a complicated relationship" with your ex), then OWN UP TO IT NOW and not during sex when I ask why your phone keeps ringing every two minutes, or why you're crying and saying "My ex used to lick my balls just like that! I WANT CINDY!" That is not proper sexiquette, asshole.

Do not expect me to call you after this. It is called a one-night stand for a reason. Not the story of "how Mommy met Daddy." Nor do I expect you to call me after this. If I decide to call you because you were an outstanding fuck who followed all the rules, then we can discuss entering into a Fuck Buddy Agreement.

Assuming it remains a one-night stand, you may assume that any or all of the following reasons were why I never returned you call: __couldn't find the clitoris __wouldn't find the clitoris __broke any of the rules listed above __body smell __crotch smell __came across as a little bit gay (not metrosexual, I mean gay as jazz hands) __called too many times immediately after __sent flowers (sweet, but wrong contract) __said what we had was "something special" (MULTIPLE ORGASMS DO NOT COUNT AS "SOMETHING SPECIAL," A-HOLE) __didn't want to wear a condom (this situation makes for automatic rejection, if not immediate kicking of dumb ass) __accepted a call while in the middle of foreplay __talked too much __were annoying __didn't respect the Platinum Pussy __were a bad fuck in general.

The following reasons may also negate the possibility of turning a one-night stand into a fuck buddy: __I moved __I got a boyfriend __I got a girlfriend __cock pisses me off __I got bored. NEXT.

I, (please print)_____, being of sound enough mind and body swear on whatever it is I find holy [please check all that apply: __God __the heavens __Napoleon Dynamite __my four-year old child I neglected to tell you about __all my future orgasms __Cartman __Angelina Jolie __my foreskin] that I am telling the truth the whole Truth so help me please don't hurt me. I understand that all I am entering into is a one-night stand, which may or may not become a fuck buddy situation and will never ever put you in situation where I want you to meet my parents.

I understand that this is a binding contract not to be a dumbfuck.

Signature: _____ Date: _____

_____

Signature of person administering The One-Night Stand Contract:

_____

Fuck the Mystery

Yeah. I'm doing it.
I mean, I have to. For the blog. I'm doing it for the blog.

Bi-Curious or Bisexual?

Somewhere in the excitement of my upcoming threesome I forgot to ask myself the obvious question: am I bi-curious or bisexual?

Not that it really matters. Besides, if I had to label myself I'd have to go with one of the all-time best lines from *Sex and the City*: "I'm a try-sexual. I'll try anything once."

HELLS YEAH BABY. My girl Samantha knows what's going on.

Many, many people over the years have asked me if I'm bisexual. I guess over-sexed girls tend to be more likely to be bi? Or something? Or maybe there's just a big fat FREAK written across my forehead.

I've never said I was bisexual. Bi-curious, definitely. I have kissed many a girl in my day. Gotten some boob a handful of times (hee hee). I have to admit that I like looking at the pictures in *Maxim*. (And maybe sometimes masturbating to the pictures.)

But that doesn't make me *bisexual*, does it?

Well, if that doesn't, having sex with a girl will probably push me over the edge of curiosity into knowing for damn sure whether or not I like getting it on with naked chicks.

But, being full-fledged bi? I mean, I don't see myself half and half liking guys vs. girls (otherwise wouldn't that have come out sooner?). It's more like . . . 25% pussy and 75% cock. I crave cock. I just fancy girls. They're so *soft*. And *pretttttty*.

The thing is that I don't ever see myself being in a serious relationship with a girl. That's my qualifier for being bisexual vs. bi-curious. I'll make out with them and get my face down in the goods, but as far as waking up next to a chick and calling her *schmoopie*? Weird. At least for now.

The Triad Wants You to Take Off Your Pants

This morning I took my car to the mechanic again because it was making a weird noise. While I was waiting for the diagnosis (another part fell off? dead squirrel in the crankshaft?) I leaned against the wall and read a book. The little bell on the door rang. I looked up and saw one of the finest looking Southern guys I've seen on this side of the Mississippi. The Pussy fluttered.

We briefly made eye contact. Hot eye contact. He smiled shyly and walked to the counter. While pretending to read I sized him up: light-colored hair, nice build (slender yet toned, much like a volleyball player), nice smile, pale blue eyes, and –*happy sigh*– thick black glasses. I'm a total sucker for a guy in a good pair of glasses, which means a sucker for other things as well, if guys would only stop cockblocking themselves with their own stupidity.

The Pussy: I WOULD SO HIT THAT.
my brain: Oh, shut the hell up. Like you have a shot in Hell. You're at the fucking mechanic.

Guy: Hey.

Me: Hey.
my brain: Ah, the words of scholars. Stop making me look bad.
The Pussy: I want to hit that. I want to hit that right now. I want to hit that right fucking now so hard that he asks God to kill him because it doesn't get any better than this.
my brain: You would probably have a better chance if you came up with something more interesting than "Hey."
The Pussy: Like "Hey, you want to go get your freak on with me in the storage closet?"
my brain: Your stunning oratory skills are exactly why you don't get to be the one who talks.

The Pussy: *Au contraire.* I have FINE oral-tory skills.

my brain: So not the same thing.

The Pussy: Your oratory skills get you diddly-fucking-squat. My oral-tory skills get me in some delightfully compromising positions.

my brain: Shut up already and say something to him.

The Pussy: Like "Chuck Norris is in my home boy"? That would definitely get things started.

my brain: It's a good thing you look pretty. AHHH HE JUST LOOKED AT US! Say something!!

Me: —

Mouth opens, a gurgle comes out—

The Pussy: Tell him to take off his pants.

my brain: Have you looked at him? He's all icky. He's in a dirty uniform. His shirt has his name embroidered on it.

The Pussy: Then tell him to take off his shirt. It's only a hop, skip, and a hump away from getting him to take off his pants.

my brain: I do like his glasses.

The Pussy: He can take off his glasses too. Weee, Naked Tuesday!

Guy: —

Looks over. His mouth opens and immediately closes—

my brain: Maybe he is a good match.

The Pussy: Yes he is. He has a dick and doesn't mind getting dirty. I'm in, now LET'S GO.

Me: Soo . . .

my brain: This is the part where you're supposed to combine words in some sort of logical order to form sentences.

The Pussy: Or I can take off my pants. I'm good at taking off my pants. I do it all the time. Oooh, there goes the bra! Weee, it's Naked Tuesday every day!

Guy: —looks up in interest, waits for me to finish (or start) speaking—

Me: *You know it's going to be expensive when they have three mechanics looking under your hood at the same time.*

The Pussy: "under your hood" . . . heheeehehehehehehehehheeheehehe

my brain: At least we didn't say, "I like your haircut. Wanna fuck?"

The Pussy: I'll have you know, that worked once.

Me: —smile hopefully at guy—

Guy: *Oh, really? That sucks. Which car is yours?*

The Pussy: The one that has ample space in the back seat and condoms in the glove compartment.

my brain: Be normal. JUST BE NORMAL FOR ONCE.

The Pussy: Are you talking to me or him?

my brain: Yes.

Me: *That one over there.* —points—

The Pussy: The one that has a selection of snacks in the trunk for after we make nasty-nasty and need nourishment for another couple rounds of rocking the casbah.

Guy: *Huh.* —A minute passes. He stares out the window—

Me: —I resume pretending to read my book—

my brain: He isn't doing anything. He isn't talking! How did we fuck it up in so few sentences?

The Pussy: If I were allowed to talk we'd have his shirt off by now. Ooooh, I bet he has a tattoo. Maybe several. Mmmm. GET HIS SHIRT OFF.

my brain: What did we do? Wait, maybe he's married. Look for a ring but be inconspicuous.

—eyeball nearly pops out from over-extending peripheral vision—

my brain: Damnit, I can't get a good look.

Guy: *Is the manager here?*

Me: *I haven't seen him. But that guy is his brother, he may be able to help you.*
The Pussy: . . . help you double-team me! Now how do you expect to do that if YOU ARE STILL WEARING YOUR PANTS?
my brain: Keep talking! Get him to look at you and then The Pussy can send her kegel waves of cockquest out and maybe he'll get the hint.

Guy: *Oh. Is that him? He's coming inside.*

The Pussy: *That's what she said.*
my brain: Stop watching TV.

Mechanic: *Hi, can I help you?*
Guy: *—yada yada—*
After a couple minutes of them discussing car crap, I managed to work my way into the conversation. I've been to the mechanic so many times that we've gotten to the point that we can joke around easily. Eventually all three of us were laughing and talking, then the mechanic left to tend to another customer.
Me: *—yada yada—*
Guy: *—yada yada—*
my brain: Please hit on me! I'm sending you all the signals but you're either shy or scared or *clueless* and I won't want to make an ass of myself when you're being so hard to read.
The Pussy: Oh, he likes us all right. Didn't you see the eye he gave us when he first walked in?
my brain: He probably just had gas.
The Pussy: That wasn't gas you dipshit, that was sex eyes. Big difference, but you don't know that and *that* is why no one ever tells us "your brain is so hot."
Me: *—yada yada—*
Guy: *—yada yada—*

my brain: Just hit on me! I WANT TO FUCK YOU! How can you know I want to fuck you if you don't hit on me?!

The Pussy: Looks like I'm not the only one who's horny and pissed off.

my brain: So . . . why aren't we hitting on him?

The Pussy: Because we're pissed at the male species for being dumbasses, douchebags, and fuckwits.

my brain: Right. I'm supposed to be the one who says things like that.

The Pussy: It's okay. We haven't been laid in a while, I know you're getting stupid.

Guy: *Well it's time for me to get back to the truck.*

Me: *Yeah . . . I think my car is ready.*

The Pussy: Oh just give in and invite him to the party in my pants. It's been two and a half months. The party in my pants is feeling like an eight-orgasm guaranteed minimum. He may need to bring back-up.

my brain: Make sure the back-up has glasses too. *Raaawr.*

The Pussy: Don't do that. Don't *rawr*. Stick to thinking you know big words other than onomatopoeia.

Guy: *It was real nice meeting you . . .*

Me: *Yeah you too . . .*

my brain: HIT ON ME! HIT ON ME! HIT ON ME! HIT ON ME! HIT ON ME! HIT ON ME!

The Pussy: FUCK ME! FUCK ME! FUCK ME! FUCK ME! FUCK ME! FUCK ME! FUCK ME!

my brain and The Pussy: HITONMEFUCKMEHITONMEFUCKMEHITONME FUCKMEHITONMEFUCKME!

Guy: *Take care.* —he walks away into the polluted horizon—

Me: DAMN YOU.

my brain: You see that sexy man-strut of his? Dammmmn he has a nice ass.

The Pussy: Think about how good it would have looked if he had just TAKEN OFF HIS FUCKING PANTS.

my brain: Doesn't matter. I bet he has a girlfriend anyway.

The Pussy: Or kids.

Handsome & Pretty Twosome: A Proper Threesome Takes Nine Courses

The First Course: APPETIZING

I was already running late to meet Handsome and Pretty Twosome, the couple I had been phoning and emailing with for weeks in anticipation of our threesome. Not a goddamn thing to wear. This never happens to me. Usually, I have mentally prepared three outfits beforehand and it only takes me a couple minutes the night of to mix and match and pull together a killer outfit. Not so this time. Not that I expected there to be anything normal about this night.

I was running from my closet to the stack of clean clothes in the living room to the full-length mirror and back again for twenty minutes. What the fuck do you wear to meet the other two people in your threesome?

Finally, I chose something I hoped was sexy in a teasing way, not a putting-it-all-out-there way. My favorite booty jeans over knee-high, four-inch, black leather boots, a very low-cut, sleeveless black top that clung to my body and stopped just short of my belly button, leaving a couple inches of exposed skin. Texas is finally getting cool, so I tied a tight black sweater around my waist to cover up most of that exposed skin but still leave some peeks (hey I can pretend to be modest like a normal person, shaddyup). Make-up was just like what I do for work, simple and done hastily since I usually run late. Black beaded earrings and one of my many chokers.

I wanted to look as sultry as possible, yet still classy and smart. I have one helluva reputation to uphold, after all. These two have been reading my blog for a while now and I don't want them to come away thinking I was all talk and a prissy-pants walk. The horror!

On top of that, I was starved for sex. It would be three months on Tuesday. By far my longest record in years, and one which I do not plan on ever surpassing. I needed sex. After three months it's damn right I need two people to take care of me instead of one.

I arrived at the restaurant ten minutes late, but they were still another five behind me. Waiting at the bar where I could see the driveway and entrance, I people-watched.

Oh who is that? Chick with bad hair and guy with an LSU T-shirt underneath a blazer? Pleasedontbethem, pleasedontbethem, pleasedontbethem. Too old, OK we're cool. Who's this pulling up? Yummy black guy... two yummy black guys... Can I slip you my number in case this doesn't work out, eh buddy? Mmmm hmm you can walk right past me with a fine ass like that, damn. Who's this here? Nice clothes, good walk, DAH THE FACE! DON'T MAKE EYE CONTACT OH MY GOD. Sigh, OK that wasn't them either. I see another car... one head... two heads... two attractive heads with good hair... this is good, this is good... this looks like the photo he sent... YESSSSSS!!! NOT UGLY!! THEY ARE HANDSOME AND PRETTY TWOSOME!! I AM MENTALLY HIGH-FIVING MYSELF! GO ME!!!!!

I saw a similar sigh of relief on their faces. And then interest.

It's on.

The Second Course: SALAD

People have wretched first date moments over salad. There's lots of bumbling, stuttering, and general dumbassery. On most dates this is known as the "awkward" course. It's the beginning of the date, the beginning of the meal, you're still sizing each other up and trying to find your flow, assuming there is a flow to be found between you and your date.

Salad. Who are we fucking kidding. We're at a steakhouse. A real steakhouse. You come here for the meat. The salad is really just a technicality. I don't want the salad. Give me my fucking meat. Yesss, Mother, I know salad is good for me and I do genuinely enjoy a good salad, but tonight at this amazing steakhouse I don't want to allot unnecessary stomach space to anything other than red meat. And dessert. And booze.

The Third Course: MEAT

Then there are the couple, Handsome and Pretty Twosome. They are not the salad course at a steakhouse. They are the prime-fucking-rib. They are the signature dish you come here for. We're talking perfectly cooked and seasoned. If you're a vegetarian, this prime-rib would be the meat that made you switch teams.

That's how cool they are. The hours at the restaurant flew by because we were having so much fun talking, sharing stories, and making each other laugh. It wasn't awkward after the first couple minutes we sat down at the table (which meant our salad course was actually quite enjoyable). It felt like old friends catching up.

It felt so easy. There was minimal fear of fucking up somehow (my main first date concern). The mutual attraction was there. We'd already talked about the general guidelines over the phone. We knew we got along well, judging from the number of long phone calls and longer emails. I knew them equally well and had different shared interests with each of them. Handsome Twosome and Pretty Twosome individually were great, but together they were better.

There was no weirdness. We were able to talk to each other like human beings. Friends. Not at all what you might expect a threesome to be (or at least what I always assumed it would be for a girl-girl-guy three-way), where the guest star is a complete stranger, just some hot chick one of the twosome found through craigslist or a distant friend, who is only there one time for sex only.

Maybe there are plenty of threesomes that go down that way and it works out. But that was not at all what would go on between the three of us. This prime-fucking-rib came with the chef's personal guarantee and a four-star review.

The Fourth Course: DESSERT

I don't even know how long we were at the restaurant. I want to say it was three hours. Which meant we watched a lot of people come and go in that time. There were three birthdays with (free!) fancy cake and a lit candle.

Pretty Twosome and I were giggling about all the birthdays, saying we should say it was one of our birthdays so we could get the free cake too. Handsome Twosome, being the adorable smartass that he is, grinned and signaled the waiter over.

A few minutes later the waiter came back with a huge piece of fancy cake with a candle on top and placed it in front of me.

With horrible acting I fluttered my hands about in what I hoped was a convincing girlish manner and then lightly smacked Handsome Twosome on the arm and gushed loudly, "I told you not to make a big deal out of my birthday! Oh, you're just awful!" Meanwhile, I felt Pretty Twosome next to me trying to stifle her laughter before she outed all of us to the waiter.

I closed my eyes, made a wish (let's guess what that would be. Ahem, see Course Six. And Seven. And Eight.), and blew out the candle. Never mind my birthday was over five months ago. This make-up birthday was way better.

The woman at another birthday table next to us leaned over to ask me how old I was. I told her and said this was the best birthday ever (um, *yeah*). She gave me one of those great, heart-warming, old lady smiles and told me, "You should be happy to be spending your birthday with such great friends as yours."

I grinned. Hopefully, the naughty devil-girl inside didn't show herself to this poor unknowing woman.

Pretty Twosome split the fancy cake with me and Handsome Twosome ordered his own dessert. While eating, it occurred to me that dinner was almost over and that would mean, well, you know.

Perhaps Pretty and Handsome Twosome suddenly realized this as well, because there was a long break in conversation as we all ate our dessert, understanding that the real dessert was back at their house. This was the turning-back point, if any of us so chose.

Yeah. We didn't turn back.

The Fifth Course: DRINKS

I followed Handsome and Pretty Twosome back to the house where they live together. A house which happens to be five minutes from my office. Hmm, some great potential here . . . I'm telling you, the gods of fate are just throwing our naked bodies at each other.

Earlier Handsome Twosome had been telling me about his favorite TV show which he had triumphantly gotten Pretty Twosome addicted to as well. He pulled it up on TiVo while I went to the kitchen to talk with Pretty Twosome, who was preparing beautiful and elaborate cocktails for all of us.

So now, how to go about getting things going? Hmm. Cocktails were a good start. We'd all ordered plenty of drinks at the restaurant, but between the long duration there and all the red meat, they barely made a mark on me.

Some homemade cocktails were *definitely* in order. Except, well, either they weren't that strong or my tolerance has gone way the fuck up. Or both. An hour of TV, talking, and drinking and no . . . progress? In getting liquored up or getting some.

Not that I wanted to dive into things right away. That's weird. Unless you're with some fuck buddy asshole you want in and out and gone, it's best to take at least an hour to get situated before trying anything. It had now been a reasonable amount of time, how to get things going? Without vodka's magical powers of persuasion?

I was sitting between them on the couch, all our drinks lined up neatly on the coffee table in front of us. With each episode of *The L Word* we watched, we grew more restless. But, no one knew what to do to get things started. It was a three-way game of Chicken, each of us hoping someone else would be the one to break.

The Sixth Course: THE *REAL* DESSERT

At the restaurant earlier none of us had planned on ordering dessert because Pretty Twosome had a chocolate soufflé waiting for us back at the house. But the fancy birthday cake—it was hard to resist. No biggie. I always have room for more dessert.

After a couple rounds of cocktails, Handsome Twosome broke out the port to go with Pretty Twosome's chocolate soufflé. It was amazing. Wow. Not only is Pretty Twosome, well, beautiful, she's a genius in the kitchen. I wondered what other artistry she was capable of.

After we ate our homemade dessert (which was even better than the fancy birthday cake at the restaurant), we all sat back on the couch with our bellies out and satisfied looks on our faces. Which meant when Pretty Twosome went to the restroom, Handsome Twosome and I put our heads together to figure out how to get to the real dessert of the evening.

He told me Pretty Twosome was nervous as hell and that's why she kept leaving the room. I couldn't really tell she was nervous because she was still talking and making jokes like before, but I don't blame her for being scared. I was getting knots in my stomach too. Not that I admitted that. Eh, it was probably obvious to Handsome Twosome anyway, who didn't miss much.

He said she was especially worried about having to make the first move, which I was surprised at. I had assumed I would have to make the first move. I don't know why I thought that, but I did. Probably because I'm used to having to be that way around guys. At this rate, I'll marry the bastard who makes the first move before I do.

We whispered to each other about what would be the best way to get things going. Should I just jump her? Should I get all close and kissy on her? Maybe Handsome Twosome and I should start kissing and then he would pull her in and duck out himself? Or maybe he should start kissing her and wait for me to join in? Maybe we should be waiting for her to come out of the restroom into the bedroom and hope she knows what we're up to? We decided to go with that when we heard her coming into the living room. Crap. We needed to figure something out, before I fell asleep on the couch (it was a very comfortable couch).

Handsome Twosome and I looked at each other and immediately knew what to do. Unsuspecting Pretty Twosome sat down on the couch next to me. Handsome Twosome got up and went to the other side of the room to close all the windows and blinds. Before he even turned around I was on Pretty Twosome.

The kissing started slow. At first she looked shocked, but when I pulled back to look in her eyes they softened. I began kissing her harder as I changed position so I was no longer next to her but straddling her on the couch. Handsome Twosome came over (he later said he was bummed that he missed witnessing me make my move) and I felt him standing behind me. Then I felt his hands on me—on my waist, my hips, my ass, exploring the curves of my body.

He was murmuring things to us about each other that were making all of us even hotter. He said to his girlfriend, "Her skin is so soft, isn't it?" Then to me, "My girlfriend's so beautiful, isn't she?" Then as he continued saying these things it became hard to tell whom he was talking about or addressing, which just made it hotter.

Feeling two sets of hands floored me. I broke away from kissing Pretty Twosome on the mouth and pulled her long hair aside so I could reach her neck. Starting slow, I kissed and nibbled under her ear and then moved down to suck on her skin. The first thing I noticed was how amazing she smelled. So feminine. So different from all the guy smells I was used to. I buried my nose in her neck and her hair. Already my panties were soaking wet. Handsome Twosome's hands continued roaming over my hips and back as he began kissing me from behind.

It didn't take us long before we moved to the bedroom where things really turned to fire.

The Seventh Course: PITCHERS OF ICE WATER

Let me start off by saying that *boobies are so cool*. Seriously, now I get why guys are obsessed with breasts. Because BREASTS ARE AWESOME.

Pretty Twosome had quite a set, I found out once we moved to the bed to get things going properly. This was my first time with bare breasts, and I was loving it. Handsome Twosome hung back and assisted in disrobing so we could concentrate on what we were doing (What a sweetheart).

I'm not sure how it happened, but at some point during the making out I looked down and her shirt and bra were gone (Miraculous! I love having an assistant in the bedroom!) and I was able to ogle *ginormous* breasts. Not just ogle, but play with. Kiss and suck and nibble on and bite.

Duuuuuude.

I was such a horny teenage boy, I admit it. Breasts are just so cool. My first impulse (which I ignored) was to bury my face in them and give her a zerbert. I didn't, though. I'm not a complete idiot, I'm not going to do anything to get my boobie privileges revoked. No, no, no. I bow down to breasts.

It was cool seeing how Pretty Twosome's breasts were so different from mine. I mean, I've seen plenty of nekkid ladies in magazines and porno, but you don't realize how different each chick is until you're there with a breast in each hand. The size was different from mine, the areolas were completely different, the shape was different, oooh but let me tell you the reaction was the same.

I started by caressing her breasts with my hands and pinching the nipples to make them stand at attention. Once I felt bolder, I took one in my mouth and licked all over and around the areola and finally started gently biting the nipple with my teeth, which she seemed to like very much.

That's another difference between guys and chicks. A guy really only gives you verbal or groan-al (it's a word now, OK?) feedback during a blowjob, when it comes to most other things, they're silent. Sure after time with the same guy you begin to pick up on stuff, but what about the first time? You're flying blind.

This is why chicks are awesome. Or maybe it was just Pretty Twosome. She made it clear when she liked what I was doing. Which, of course, I liked, so I tried to please her more so she would speak and moan more.

Meanwhile, Handsome Twosome was quietly at work removing clothes. I looked down and, whoopsies, I lost my pants. And panties. COOL.

I kinda kept forgetting he was there, because during all this so far he was either hanging back and watching, removing our clothes, or doing things to his girlfriend. That wasn't much of a surprise, it was weird figuring out what was OK for me and him to do to each other without crossing that vague line of sexy into jealousy, not that Pretty Twosome seemed like the jealous type. There were never any comments or complaints the entire night, so that must have been OK with everyone. He always paid a little more attention to her than me, and she always paid a little more attention to me than him, is how I saw it. And I paid more attention to her than him because how often do I have a beautiful naked chick in front of me. WITH BOOBIES.

Eventually all of us were naked on the huge canopy bed together.

That right there is my new Happy Place. If only I had a midget and a unicorn and a bathtub of chocolate soufflé, I would have a better Happy Place than Happy Gilmore.

Things progressed as I expected, which was that Pretty Twosome and I were the main twosome, kissing and caressing each other. Handsome Twosome did a good job of keeping one hand on each of us (purely selfless of him, of course) and keeping those hands very busy. Every once in a while I saw them giving each other one of those adoring couple looks. It was very sweet. There are definitely not many couples in the world who are comfortable enough in their relationship and have a strong enough sex life to withstand a three-way.

Now I have to admit that things are kind of blurry as far as what happened when and who did what to whom. Not that it matters. It was all good. Hands and nakedness everywhere, weeee!

For the first orgasm of the evening (after Handsome Twosome told me they were not letting me leave their house without at least three or four), Pretty Twosome started things off with her fingers finding their way inside me. She has a little more experience with women than I do, so I was happy to let her lead the way. While she worked her magic she never stopped kissing me and rubbing me with her other hand. Handsome Twosome, very much the leg man, stayed down in that area for most of this, until the end when one hand wandered up the inside of my thigh and rode on top of his girlfriend's hand inside me. He slipped a finger inside so they both had me on the verge of cumming hard. At some point Pretty Twosome left the ending to him.

Excuse me, I just had to stop and masturbate again. Phew. Much better.] They moved around so that they were both lying in-between my legs. My left leg was up and around Handsome Twosome's shoulder and the other one was rubbing against his girlfriend. His fingers furiously worked my pussy but, well, I like it rough. VERY rough. It took two times telling him that before he believed me.

And I was off. With two sets of hands on and in me and two faces between my legs, how could I possibly not lose my fucking mind? My body doesn't stay still even when things are only getting started—I swear if there's a hint of sex in the air my pelvis automatically starts grinding in anticipation. So, when I'm actually cumming, my entire body goes insane. My legs are capable of a death grip on whoever is between my legs, so things got intense for all three of us. I might have nearly choked them.

Either way they seemed very pleased afterward. They did the cute couple eye exchange thing again (I could tell they were giving each other mental high fives) and we all took a breather.

And a water break. There were lots of water breaks during the five hours of sexcapades. Pretty Twosome and I had to send our assistant back to the kitchen for a refill of the water pitcher he'd originally brought in many times.

It was the beginning of a very long enjoyable night that would require many water breaks.

The Eighth Course: JUICE

After the first or second orgasm (or was it third? Hmm. So many between us that it's hard to keep count) Pretty Twosome got a devilish grin on her face. She got off the bed and went to pull a box out of her night stand.

"I bought you something . . . I know you like toys . . ."

"YOU BOUGHT TOYS??!!" —imagine me jumping up and down on the bed fully naked—

"My girlfriend was *so* excited when the package came the other day. You have no idea!" added Handsome Twosome.

With a proud look on her face she started pulling items out of the box: a small, rounded clit vibrator, another small vibrator with different attachments, a jack rabbit (may I add—THE jack rabbit), and finally, a double-ended dildo.

She looked a little embarrassed, I'm guessing because she didn't know how I would react.

"THIS IS SO FUCKING COOL!!! I CAN'T BELIEVE YOU BOUGHT US A DOUBLE-ENDED DILDO!!! SEE??? THIS IS WHY WE WORK SO WELL AS A THREESOME!"

Pretty Twosome beamed. Handsome Twosome rubbed his girlfriend affectionately on the shoulder. I hugged her. Our boobies touched. It was sweet.

"But we gotta back up, first. I came here to learn, damnit." With that, I pushed her down on the bed and seductively crawled on top of her body. I kissed her neck, her mouth (mmm . . . girl lips are so much better than boy lips). I took one of her breasts in my hand and began pinching the nipple the way I had found she liked so much just a little earlier. Then I worked my way down with my mouth so that I was sucking and gently biting at her nipple. The moans started.

Can I just say—hearing a girl moan is *so fucking hot*. Especially if she's beautiful and sexy and NAKED and UNDERNEATH YOU and you are the exact reason she's moaning so much. –shudder–

With her nipple still in between my teeth, my hand slid down her stomach to her thighs and back up to . . . wait, where is it . . . I can't see anything. I don't have my glasses on. And bless her heart she's clean-shaven but without the dark hair I CANNOT FIND HER PUSSY WITHOUT MY GLASSES ON.

I was so embarrassed. I'm not not sure if either of them noticed (oh, yeah, this whole time Handsome Twosome had one enthusiastic hand on each of us) that I like, *missed* her pussy. Twice. NO, it's not exactly an easy thing to miss but there were so many body parts everywhere, I was getting a little confused. And without my glasses, I didn't have a fucking shot in Hell.
THERE WERE SO MANY BODY PARTS EVERYWHERE I WAS GETTING A LITTLE CONFUSED. AND WITHOUT MY GLASSES I DIDN'T HAVE A FUCKING SHOT IN HELL.

Seriously. Such a horrible time to be near-sighted. Horrible. I have to get LASIK surgery. [And I did too, a couple months later.]

But, goddamnit, I'm not letting horrible eye sight keep me from pussy. With some finesse (I hope) I moved my entire body down a little lower so I could see the slit hiding between her legs, his hands, my legs, his mouth, her hands, all of which were gyrating or moving and making things quite impossible to work with. I mean really.

With one hand propping my body on my side, I moved the other hand all up and down her thighs until . . . Aha!! Found it. Wooo, that just slipped right in!!

Another aside—wow. Wet pussy. Just . . . WOW. Even better than boobies.

I had a finger inside her and I was surprised to find that hers felt exactly like mine. I'm not sure why I thought they would be different, I mean I know better, but I just thought it would be noticeably different. Hmm. Same shape, same ridges, and ooooh, lookie here, same sweet spot on me works on her. Mmmm hmmmmm yes it does.

After a few minutes of bringing her close with my finger, I lowered my entire body between her legs so I could be right up close and see everything. Very close, since I didn't have my glasses on and I'm blind as hell and I'll be damned if I don't see pussy properly.

I admit, I thought I would feel hesitant about getting up close and personal with a wet pussy as far as eating her out. I was worried I'd suddenly flip out and lose it and be like NUH UH can't do it, where's the dick please. But, no. There was none of that. After having my finger in a wet pussy it was just too hot not to dive in with my tongue.

Again. WOW. Pussy juice is so fucking cool. Why don't they tell you this in Sex Ed.?!

I had thought it would have a strong taste, and maybe it does sometimes, depending on the last time that she showered/time of month, etc., but this pussy tasted damn fine. Wetness everywhere, all over my tongue, my lips, her thighs, the bedspread underneath. A big beautiful mess of juice everywhere.

Maybe it was all the sweet girly drinks Pretty Twosome had prepared for us, maybe it was her natural taste, but the taste was amazing. I couldn't get enough.

Once I felt comfortable with my tongue technique (hey, it's not like I've done this before) I put my finger back in and started going for an orgasm. I was worried my amateur skills would show, or worse, that Pretty Twosome would sit up, roll her eyes, and tell me NEVERMIND, then take away my new toys because I didn't deserve to play with them.

Ooooh no, not so. Apparently, I was a natural. Just two minutes of tongue/finger action and she came, hard. By this time Handsome Twosome had swirled around to be up by his girlfriend's head so he could suck on her tits and have a good view of everything I was doing to her.

Once she came and I brought my body to hover over hers (so I could see her face better in my damn near-sightedness), I could tell she was in heaven. This was real. Her face was glowing and so was her boyfriend's. He looked at me in awe and said "Wow. She really came. I know when she's faking it. *That* was real. Wow. And it's hard to get her off . . . and you did on your first time . . . " They beamed at me. I kissed her forehead and stared into her flushed face. The flushed post-orgasmic glow that I had given her.

Now that is some serious WOW. No wonder guys love getting a girl off so much. That look she had, that look that I gave her, there's no other look like that.

After that I felt smug as hell. BECAUSE I KNOW HOW TO EAT PUSSY AND I KNOW HOW TO DO IT WELL. HELLS YEAH, BABY.

The Eight-and-a-half-th Course: A SECOND SERVING OF JUICE

The exact sequence of events that night is a little fuzzy—not surprising considering most of this took place between one and five in the morning, after a huge meal and a lot of alcohol. So, this account is not a play-by-play, it's a mixture of memories. And frankly, it's hard to keep track of who does what to whom. That was really just me bragging. OK, moving on.

Here are some recaps of what all went down (besides me) that night.

Pretty Twosome finger-fucked me and went down on me again. You know, I never really understood why guys are so particular about a girl having good hair, particularly long hair. But, now I get it. Pretty Twosome has loooong, natural red hair that she kept down the entire night (normally I prefer hair up and off the neck because I love long exposed necks, perfect for kissing and biting). When she started that slow sexy descent from my breasts to my pierced belly button to my pierced clit hood, watching that long mess of hair all over my bare skin damn near made me cum before she even got anywhere.

For awhile the mess of hair stayed covering my stomach and the Latin tattoo I have hidden below, but when she started licking me I had to see it. Just as I moved my hand to brush the hair out of the way, her boyfriend's hand reached over and pulled the hair away. Her eyes looking up at him were sexy as hell, almost proud (she did a damn fine job, she sure deserved to be proud, as proven by the fact that none of us could remember exactly how many orgasms I'd had by the end of the night. A fine night indeed). Each time a strand of hair fell into her eyes, Handsome Twosome tenderly pulled it back out of the way. Meanwhile his other hand alternated between finger-fucking her and rubbing me.

Which brings me to yet another super-hot thing about women. The pussy juice. Not just that, but—licking a combination of your own and another girl's pussy juice off your fingers. The licking of wet fingers quickly became a common occurrence that tasted exquisite.

It started earlier in the evening when Handsome Twosome had his fingers inside Pretty Twosome while she sucked on my tits. [OK, can we all just stop and take a moment to enjoy the irony that this beautiful sentence was just typed by a former teacher's pet/prep school nerd who was known to correct her Latin teacher's declension mistakes. Yeah, I bet all those boys wish they had asked me out now.]

As Handsome Twosome brought her closer and closer to orgasm (mmm so hot to watch . . . girls' orgasm faces are actually sexy. Guys . . . not so much. That's generally when I close my eyes.) I was getting quite excited myself. Handsome Twosome was lying on his side behind Pretty Twosome, both of whom were facing me. They seemed rather occupied, so I took matters into my own hands. Fingers, whatever.

At the moment Pretty Twosome had her eyes closed in her own bliss, but I caught and held Handsome Twosome's eyes as he realized what I was doing.

With two fingers inside my own pussy my body immediately began moving in its own familiar sex rhythm. After I had gotten myself good and wet, I pulled my fingers out and brought them to Handsome Twosome's lips. His eyes grew huge and then happily he took them into his mouth and sucked on the tips.

I only wanted him to have a little taste, so after a few seconds I pulled my fingers out and brought them to Pretty Twosome's lips, her eyes still closed. Instinctively, her mouth took them in and she sucked hungrily at the remains of my pussy juice.

It just doesn't get any better than this.

Well OK, yes it does, as I found out later but there were many wonderful things worth getting wet over.

Such as:

Handsome Twosome began fucking his girlfriend from behind. Immediately, their hips moved in the same back and forth motion. I didn't quite know how to fit into this. I could play with her breasts some more, but they'd gotten a lot of action already and I figured they were getting mighty sore. The ever-attentive Handsome Twosome noticed my displacement and maneuvered her onto her back. Then he breathlessly pulled me by the hands so that my pussy hovered just above Pretty Twosome's face. She reached up with her hands and lowered me down by the hips until I felt her tongue tickling my clit ring.

HELLS YEAH.

This has been my favorite way to get eaten out for ages. First, it's much less awkward for the eat-outer. Secondly the person can see what you're doing to yourself more easily, *i.e.* squeezing your nipples, rubbing yourself, or ever-so slightly rotating your hips in a circle (careful not to dislodge the tongue! YOU MUST RESPECT THE TONGUE). Then there's always grabbing onto the headboard and screaming when you cum. Very hot to watch that tension in the body. Oh and one of the best parts is that it's easy to make eye contact. So, so, very hot.

I am all about the eyes. Big fan of eye contact. Eyes have the potential to show prowess, hunger, enthusiasm, satisfaction, pleading, teasing, pleasure. Don't disregard the eyes, ever. Make the most of your eyes during sex (and during pursuit and courtship as well, but that's a post for another day). Which means when I have sex, I want the lights on. Sometimes I'm OK with dim lighting, or lots of candles in an otherwise unlit room, but really I prefer to see everything that's going on, every facial expression, every biting of the lip, every shudder.

Which is why hovering above Pretty Twosome's face as her boyfriend fucked her was extra enjoyable. Every pounding she received from Handsome Twosome reverberated its way up through me. I'm surprised the pussy juice didn't gush all over her face, I was so hot from all three of us going at it at the same time.

Then the elusive happened: Handsome and Pretty Twosome, in sweet coupled harmony, came at the same time. He shuddered, she shuddered, and with all of her shuddering frankly I was scared she was going to bite down on my pussy (remember the clit ring provides a handle of sorts), so I quickly raised myself above her face and turned around to get a better view of their double-orgasm.

Sadly, I did not quite make it to my own orgasm, so after yet another water break, Pretty Twosome turned her attention to me.

"I think it's time to bring out the new toys! Which one do you want to try first?" she asked eagerly.

I grinned. "Surprise me." She grinned back and then shuffled through the assortment of toys spread out on the floor amidst the abandoned clothes.

Closing my eyes, I leaned back and waited.

She turned something on. It was one of the vibrators, but that only narrowed it down to three. I tried to squeeze my eyes shut like a good girl, but I couldn't wait. It was the jack rabbit! The good one! I squealed and lay back down in eagerness.

For those who are not familiar with this wonderful piece of rabbit-shaped technology, the standard jack rabbit model has two pieces to it. The long shaft, similar to a regular vibrator except that it encases a bunch of small balls, which rub against that top ridged wall inside the pussy quite nicely. The other part, the famous part, is the rabbit ears coming out of a smaller arm attached to the main body. The rabbit ears split of course and, with an ear placed on either side of the clitoris, this is the key to the happy place. This gets me off easily every time.

Some vibrators, like this one, can be very filling. I have not used both parts of my jack rabbit at the same time in over a year because the thick, beaded part of mine broke (the poor thing, I've worn it down). I had not been laid in nearly three months, so the pussy was feeling a bit tight, but, with some coaxing, we were on our way. Filled and titillated. It only took a couple minutes with Pretty Twosome's knowing maneuvering before I came. Hard. (Maybe that was why she suggested the toys, because the previous time I came so hard I nearly broke her hand. Ha, no, I know that's not really it. I just wanted to brag some more.) Once again, she had me flushed, glowing, and aching.

Not a bad thing to be at five thirty in the morning.

The Ninth Course: RED WINE AND OREOS

I didn't mention this earlier, because it would have really fucked up the rhythm of all the sex taking place during Course Eight, but between each round of amazing fantasgasmic three-way sex, we talked a lot. And I mean good talking. The kind you don't normally have with people until you've known them a while. But, that's the thing–I *do* feel like I've known Handsome and Pretty Twosome for ages. I felt that way all throughout the long dinner, and then even more so when we went back to their house and hung out (somewhat awkwardly at that point, since we were trying to figure out how to get things going).

During dinner with Handsome and Pretty Twosome, I barely thought about sex. (OK, I did, that's a lie. I just mean I didn't think about sex much more than usual.) We were having such a fantastic time talking in person, joking around, and getting to know each other better that at the end of dinner, I could have gone home on my own and still called it a fantastic evening.

Although the sex made it three times more fantastic, but still.

This . . . this thing here . . . do I sound totally lame, naive, needy for saying that it's actually meaningful? Now DO NOT MISREAD ME, because there is plenty of room for that in a delicate situation such as this. What I mean is,

Handsome and Pretty Twosome already mean so much more to me than really amazing sex. We're friends. And, what more beautiful way is there to show you care for a friend than getting her off?

I've said it here before, and that's because I mean it. I can see the three of us being friends for years. Even after I get my own boyfriend, after they have cute-as-shit kids running around, after the three-way sex stops and it's clear it will never start up again. I think we'll still be friends. And I don't go around saying things like that.

This may be the first and only time I utter this term in reference to a relationship of any sort, but I see Handsome and Pretty Twosome as my lovers. Is that totally lame? Oh, I don't care. They're not my fuck buddies, they're more than friends-with-benefits, but it's not like I'm dating them—we're lovers.

For years I've read that word in contemporary fiction and I always thought it was fluffy crap, a nice way of saying "fuck buddy." Nuh uh, now I get it. It's how you express that special something that falls in that typically grey area. Wow, did I really just type "special something"? Oh my god, I'm smitten.

Sure, it sounds dangerous to many of you. This could easily be the pilot of a prime-time TV show about thee people who have sex and the guest star tries to weasel her way in and shove out one of the two in the original couple. Then when she gets sick of one, she goes to the other, meanwhile she's pregnant with someone else's baby but her new lover is ready to raise it as his own, but then, oh, no, he gets jealous and impregnates her with their own love-child they already have the 529 college savings plan set up for and yada yada cry my fucking eyes out yada yada.

Not my style. I hate the idea of screwing up someone else's relationship, however rocky or new or almost-divorced it may be. I've never been the kind to steal a man away from another girl, and I'm not starting now. However much affection I feel for Handsome and Pretty Twosome, they will forever be Handsome AND Pretty Twosome to me. They are great individually, but they're really best as a set.

Truthfully, for most people a slightly less dramatic version of the above prime-time TV paragraph could happen. That's why being the guest star in a couple's sex life is very tricky. In fact, both Handsome and Pretty Twosome told me that they would not have done this with any of their previous boy/girlfriends. That's because their relationship is so strong, they can withstand a threesome and ironically it brings them closer instead of driving a wedge between them.

One of the many things I enjoyed about being with Handsome and Pretty Twosome was watching them be all coupley together. They've been dating long enough to be past the annoying "Schmoopie!" "SCHMOOOPIE!" stage and well into the "yeah, we get each other" stage. It's nice. Refreshing. A well-timed reminder that there are fully functional, loving relationships out there among the douchebags, assholes, crazy bitches, and fuckwits.

They're also older than me, so it almost felt like they were mentors. I may have sex with them, but I still look up to them as a positive example for what a strong and healthy relationship should look like, and yes, my definition of strong and healthy DOES include feeling secure enough in my relationship that we can bring in a third person for sex and it doesn't fuck up anything. That's my new litmus test for when/if I ever meet someone worth marrying. Yeah . . . since nice, smart, and funny (and not a pussy) aren't hard enough to find already.

I've completely digressed from where I intended to be by four tangents. I blame the wine. And the fantastic sex that has left me at only 40% functioning mental capacity.

What I'm getting at is that this is not what I expected this threesome to be. When the thought was first thrown out there on the table, I thought it would be more of the Wham, Bam, Thank Ya, SLAM variety, which typically, is what I prefer in anything short of a serious relationship.

Instead it's this thing that has a set of rules all its own I've never seen the likes of. Instead of sneaking out or being thrown out in the middle of the night like I would normally do, they pleaded with me to spend the night, to keep talking and to let them cook me breakfast in bed in the morning! "Bacon!" she said. "Coffee!" he said. "Biscuits!" she said. It was touching. But, thanks to Lil Lesbian and Great

Big Pit, my two dogs who were surely flipping out at home alone, I had to leave at the end of our very long night. This was not without promising Handsome and Pretty Twosome that next time I would arrange for them to stay with a friend so that I could spend the night and we could all enjoy a lazy Sunday morning together.

As I was putting on my boots to leave, Pretty Twosome (now all sweet-looking in her plush white robe) reminded me to take home my presents.

I looked up at the coffee table and grinned.

When I had first arrived at their house, Pretty Twosome pointed me to the coffee table where there were two presents for me. One was a bottle of red wine, called Ménage à Trois, wrapped with an ornate bow around the neck.

"I saw it when I was shopping at Sams Club today and I just thought it was too perfect. I had to buy it for you!" she told me as I fingered the bow. "And did you see the other present?" She pointed to a second package which I had not seen. A package of Oreos, wrapped with a matching bow.

My heart grew three sizes.

"Awwww, sweetie!! You really do get me, don't you?!" And I gave her a huge hug.

Before I left that night (early morning, really), Handsome and Pretty Twosome signed their names on the label of the wine bottle, complete with a funny stick-figure drawing of Handsome Twosome falling off the bed (which actually happened).

"Are you going to drink the wine eventually?" Pretty Twosome asked as I hugged her one last time, bottle in hand.

"No. I could never drink this. I have something else in mind," I told her.

When I got home I took the bottle and I put it on that same bookshelf with my growing collection of journals and notepads, a wine cork from my first night alone in my new bachelorette pad, and the empty bottle of champagne celebrating my first big achievement as OEN.

Once again, as I have done so often these last couple months, I raise my wine glass to all the many unexpected twists and turns that make life worth living, no matter how boring the day job may be.

I Could SO Be a Model. If You Squint.

What? I'm dead serious. I could SO be a model, if I really wanted to.

You know that Katherine Heigl girl? Izzy Stevens, aka "Dr. Model" on *Grey's Anatomy*? Well I look *exactly* like her.

Ok, sure, I know I'm not all *model* skinny. I mean, I'd have to lose fifteen pounds. Twice. But other than that, I look just like her. The similarities are eerie. Or they would be, if I were blonde. And had better hair. And maybe if I were a little taller.

It would also help if I were pretty. Then I would be the *It* model. Forget Victoria's Secret Angels®, it's time for Vix's It's-No-Fucking-Secret Dominatrix®©¥ line of lingerie to run those glamazons off the fucking runway. Everyone knows leather and lace are the new blush and bashful.

So the skinny thing, and the pretty thing. Those are the only two tiny little things keeping me from a fantastic career in modeling, and then retiring at the old age of 32 to become a judge on *America's Next Top What's Her Name Again?*, cycle 27 and making mad whoopie with Nigel on top of the judging table.

Dude, it could sooo happen.

You still don't believe that I can be a model, do you? Well I'll have you know that when Barbie and I went to watch the girls auditioning for *America's Next Top Model,* there was a lovely young man with a clipboard who came over and asked us if *we* were models. Being the smart cookie I am, I did not trust this young fellow and therefore asked to see an application. He stammered and asked for our phone numbers so he could send us applications. But the clipboard!! HE HAD A CLIPBOARD. THAT MUST MEAN HE HAD SOME SORT OF MODEL-MAKING POWER.

That's ok, I can become a model on my own. I don't need Mr. Clipboard Man. I have natural talent! I have personality! Per-son-AL-I-TITTY. I am a great conversationalist. Go ahead, ask me about any prime-time TV show on ABC or NBC—I might know it.

Ohhh crap. The hips! Because, like, I *have* them. Okay well they can airbrush those out. And while they're tinkering with my photos, they can also clear up my skin. Sooo many pimples, where the hell do they come from?. Oh and that mole. It's gotta go. Not the discolored one on my shoulder, the other one–no, not that one, the *big one*. The one with the hairs growing out of it.

They may need to fix the eyes too. One is a different color than the other one. Dunno, birth defect yada yada the doctor said it wasn't *that* big a deal and eventually they'd be able to focus on the same thing without one veering to the left.

Also, my lips are kind of thin. Not very DSL-y at all. I can't afford collagen injections, at least not yet, not until I sign my huge modeling contract. So until then, I suppose I'll have to pinch my lips repeatedly to make them puff up. Or maybe I can have a dear friend punch me in the mouth every day to give me big, luscious lips. Oh yes, that's brilliant. I'll have to remember that tip for when I write my first book, *I Am So Much Prettier Than You: How to Look More Like Me Without Being a Reality TV Show Victim.*

I'd need to buy boobs, of course. The ones I have now are lovely, but they don't compare to the twin Heigls on the cover of *Maxim.* –looks down at breastises– Okay so that's one, well, two little things that aren't exactly model-ish either. Hmm.

Did I mention my toes? I forgot my toes. I would need toe replacement surgery. My little piglets are not the cutest things to get bright red nail polish slapped on them haphazardly (not to worry, I can pay someone to do all that for me once I get my big modeling contract). But glittery paint can only do so much. I need model toes. Make that model feet. My feet are kinda wide. And they sweat a lot. I can't have fat, sweaty feet. Not to worry, I can pay someone to find a way to make me stop sweating.

Okay, I hear all you bitches out there laughing at me. That's rather *rude*, don't you think? If the skeezey guy with the clipboard at the mall thought I was a model, *I could be a model*. Well, you know, except for that whole super skinny pretty thing. That's a bit of a pisser.

Fine, maybe you would be able to see my modeling potential if you just closed your eyes. Then I look *exactly* like Katherine Heigl.

TeXXXas Welcomes Porn Stars

This was originally written to go on the *Houston Press* blog HouStoned, but it didn't for reasons I never understood (it wasn't the writing itself).

It's not just any day when you find yourself holding a porn star's wang in the dark corner of a seedy swingers club for a photograph.

What? He asked nicely. Besides, I had to do it for the sake of the *Houston Press*. We are students of research here. How else am I to penetrate the --a-hem-- *mind* of a porn star?

For all the guys out there who want to know if they have what it takes to be a porn star: can you get a woody in two seconds flat just from rubbing a girl's fully-clothed hip? If yes then you may stand a chance against veterans like Dave Cummings, who is an actual veteran and a senior. He is just one of the many industry people I met during last week's four-day porn convention, the 1st ~~Anal~~ *Annual* Lone Star Pornutopia.

Here are just a handful of visiting stars whose websites I have bookmarked for, um, further research: Daisy Duxxx, Jade Simone St. Clair, Summer Haze, Lisa Sparxxx, Liv Wylder, Daphne Rosen, and Texas native Jessica Drake. I anticipate extensive research. And hand cramping.

Other gems you would not find out unless you were interviewing a porn star with one hand down his pants: 1) the trend of waxing pubic hair started with porn stars shaving their pubes to decrease their risk of sexually-transmitted diseases (that totally deflates the yuppie appeal, doesn't it?), 2) you typically find ugly/bald/old/fat guys in porn because that makes it easy for the guys to place themselves in the fantasy and whack off: *dude, that ugly a-hole is f****** that hot chick, that could be me!* Squirtsville.

Some of the other lucrative things I discovered under the guise of "journalism:" if you ask a girl what makes her successful as a porn star, she just might take your hand and begin drumming her tongue against the palm with such speed and expertise that you damn near renounce dick for life.

If this chick is someone as hot as Vivian West you may find yourself feigning drunkenness (never mind that the only drinks you have been slamming back are Coke and coffee), placing your hand on her thigh, and asking if she wants to make out. I'll be a sonovabitch, that actually worked. YUH HUH THAT'S RIGHT, BEE-ATCH. I made out with one of the biggest up-and-cumming stars of the year.

Our little kissing session was so hot and heavy that neither of us noticed a chick puke three feet away from our booth. Hey, it's cool! We were at the Penthouse Club. This place is so fancy that the attendant mopped up the mess, put out a CAUTION: WET FLOOR sign (hee hee, it says *wet*), and gingerly lowered the girl's head over a large trash can for her personal use. That's good service. He even produce a ponytail holder so she could keep her head back while she continued to yak her guts out.

This is so much cooler than my day job. Especially considering that all of the aforementioned happened within the first two and a half hours of the first night.

Oh, and Vivian West, like, *totally* touched my boob. Just thought I should rub that in a little.

The next couple nights were a blur of ginormous tits, camera flashes, and dodging the skeeze population following the porn stars wherever we went. Not that I didn't enjoy the many levels of skeeze-dom, my favorite being the *wanna-be pimp*: cheap ill-fitting suit, collared shirt with the top three buttons undone (to show off that sexy chest hair, BOO YAH), white fedora with a condom tucked in the band, a Bluetooth headset, and oh yes: white pimp shoes. The porn stars must have been getting in naked titty fights over who got to bag that fine piece of ass.

Ron Jeremy and Dennis Hof of the Bunny Ranch (a legal brothel) frequently came in and out to make an appearance. I gotta say: Ron Jeremy is an ugly m***** f*****. Whenever possible I avoided direct eye contact by standing next to him and letting him fondle my ass instead. Genius.

Then there is Dennis Hof... now that is one sexy bastard. He has that whole sex eyes thing *down*. Yeah I'm kind of getting a little excited remembering the other night in the crowded hotel bar when I was walking past him and *oopsies! Is that me pressing my scantily-clad body into you, sir? So sorry. Oh, you like that, well that is just fine with me, sir. Oh you want to stay here a little longer? Whatever you say, sir.*

Ok, give me a minute. I am in my Happy Place.

Not to totally brag, but Dennis Hof may have rubbed my hip, and I may have three-way made out with his girlfriend and Vivian West. All in the interest of journalism, of course.

A pajama party on the final night of a porn convention would be pointless without all of the following: strip Twister, an impromptu photo shoot of a topless porn star posing in a fire department uniform in a back storage closet with all the security guards watching approvingly, a boob job giveaway, a powerful vice president of a casino drunkenly fondling half the female party-goers, and oil wrestling between four X-T-C strippers and a club's general manager.

Yeah I bet you'll come next year, won't you? Shame on you, you sorry excuse for a pervert for not coming this year. You should come if for no other reason than to watch me try to get into girls' pants with the line "I'm straight, I swear, I just want to kiss *a little.*"

Now let us take a moment to appreciate all the many, many, beautiful things about naked ladies. Especially when they are contorted into all sorts of delightfully compromising positions. Oh crap who said that? *Bad feminist, bad feminist!*

To the many XXX stars who were kind enough to make their way to Houston for our first porn conventions: *Y'all cum back 'n see us now, ya hear?*

I need more photos.

Where Are You in the Blowjob Ring?

Before we start the blowjob tutorial, this guide will help you determine the appropriate level most suited to your taste. Repeat the following mantras. A special note to beginners: keep repeating until you can *actually* look the penis in the eye and not run away screaming.

Beginners:*

The penis is not icky.

The penis is my friend.

The penis likes me very very much.

I will look the penis in the eye.

I will not run away screaming.

I WILL LOOK THE PENIS IN THE EYE.

Intermediate:*

It is not a penis. It is a dick.

The dick is my homeboy.

A dick is not icky.

I'm down with dick. We're cool.

I like to make the dick jump with joy when it sees me.

I can get on that.

Advanced:**

It is not a dick. It is a cock.

The cock is kinda hot. Really hot.

I respect the cock.

I know how to make it happy.

And it sure does know how to make me happy.

Sex Goddess:**

I need cock.

I crave cock.

GIVE ME COCK NOW.

INEEDCOCKINMYMOUTHRIGHTNOW.

Every Guy's Fantasy Woman:***

"Hey sweetie, why don't I get you a cold beer while you put on the game, and during the next commercial break I'll give you a blowjob. Sound good?"

*only say these inside your head. Quietly. Inside your head.
**these are hot enough to say aloud.
***this usually leads to a drunken proposal. Not that I know. Twice.

Blowjobs Are Not Icky

How am I supposed to explain how to give good head if so many people are concerned about a much greater obstacle than jaw control? Apparently, there are many girls out there who think the penis is icky, ugly, gross, etc., and by association so are blowjobs. Which means we need to back up a little more before diving into the good stuff.

Now, I don't want anyone to think I'm saying YOU MUST GIVE BLOWJOBS BECAUSE IT IS YOUR DUTY AS A MODERN WOMAN. Nuh-uh. Some people just don't like them and have honestly tried themenough times to qualify as a fair effort. This post is meant to target those who are new to oral sex, scared of oral sex, scared of the penis, or generally squeamish around all things that jump unexpectedly.

Back to blowjobs. I can kinda see why someone would think they're gross. Although I am apparently the dirty dirty girl who loves to give blowjobs, so I will do my best to play devil's advocate here. Let's examine some of the common complaints and concerns:

There is so much hair.
Yes, an excellent point. More and more guys are trimming or even completely shaving that area, so there's a much lower frequency of pubic flossing than there was five years ago. I have found that it's fairly easy to talk a guy into trimming if you do it yourself already. Plus if he does it once he'll see how *huuuge* his dick looks without all the hair. (The most masterminded of optical illusions.)

It's so funny looking.
Eh, well, yeah. But they're all funny-lookin', so get over it. We girls are just as funny-lookin' down there. We have folds and ins and outs and stuff. Golly gee whiz, holy moly it's amazing any of us ever look at each other naked. Oh, right. Hormones or pheromones or some shit. Then there's the occasional weirdo like me who likes looking at hairy ugly funny-lookin' things that are waving at me. What?? They're fun to play with. Until they spit in your eye (rarely happens).

I don't like to see guys naked.
Um, there may be a much bigger problem at work here. One is that you're just not very sexual at all, and I fancy you don't much like seeing yourself naked either, orrrr you're into bush. Eiether is totally fine. You may exit the blowjob post now. Either way, both matters are way bigger than my little blog.

Blowjobs are degrading.
No, they're not. Sweetie, you're the one who's got *him* by the balls, I think it's obvious who's in charge here. Reminder: It's a unique position in which you can bite it off at any time.

But I'm a feminist.
CUT THAT SHIT OUT. I'm a feminist too. A fuck-me feminist. There are scary man-hating feminists and there are happy, normal, everyday feminists like your sister, your mother, your coworkers, the chick who makes your double tall extra foam latte, and nearly every other normal girl out there who thinks that men and women should have equal rights and equal say. Which includes equal time between each other's legs.

It tastes gross.
OK, I'll give you that, sometimes it does. Yech, especially if he's been drinking a lot of beer or anything sour. However, the taste of cum is easy to control. Have him eat anything sweet a couple of hours before getting it on: Fruit, fruit juice, maple syrup, etc. Although it's easiest if you just swallow him whole and the cum goes straight down your throat, thereby avoiding all taste bud zones.

I don't like swallowing.
That's OK, many don't. You don't have to swallow (although that's half the hotness factor right there, for both of you) and most guys don't expect it. They appreciate the hell out of it, but don't expect it. If you don't like swallowing

because of the taste, see my suggestion above. If you don't like it because it gets messy, that means you don't have enough of it in your mouth. When you do it all goes straight back. If you simply don't like swallowing, you can still get him to the Almost point and then finish him off manually, just make sure you give him sexy eyes while you're doing it. You don't want him seeing your disgust at the thought of his cum. That will make any guy lose his hard-on.

I don't get anything out of it.
First of all, it's not about you. It's about him. It's a really fucking cool feeling to be the reason for someone else's orgasm, especially if you were actively making him orgasm. It's all the better if you don't make the other person feel obligated to do something for you in return for your "selflessness". (This DOES NOT mean it's OK to make him go down on you but never give him a blowjob, or vice versa. That is mean, hypocritical, and generally bad sexiquette. Shame on you.)

He's uncircumcised! It's weird!
Again, get over yourself. A penis is a penis, whether or not it has a turtleneck. As long as the penis gets the job done, mm'kay? I've been with plenty of foreigners and seen plenty of uncircumcised dicks and it's really no big deal. Most guys will give you a quick run-down of how to hold it properly, so you don't stretch the skin the wrong way. In all honestly, I didn't notice half the time until afterwards when it was down to normal size and I was like, *hey, lookie there! Cool!*

How to Give a Blowjob

Only half of what makes a blowjob so great is the technique. What pushes a good blowjob over the edge into *sweetmercifulcrapWOW* is your attitude, *i.e.* making it obvious to the guy that you love sucking his cock. Let's go back and repeat that last part slowly: *Make it obvious to the guy that you love sucking his cock.*

Make it obvious to the guy that you love sucking his cock. I CANNOT STRESS THIS ENOUGH.

I have met/heard of very, very few girls who love sucking dick and were not good at it. Loving it and being good at it go hand in hand. Or dick in mouth. Either way, it's a happy coupling.

If you love dick, I mean really relish it, *crave* it—that shows in your eyes. And that is fucking hot as hell.

Before we go any farther: If you want to be able to give good head, first you need to get over yourself. I've been told that many girls don't want to give blowjobs because they feel insecure about it, that they won't do a good job. Well, you're kind of shooting yourself in the foot there. If you think you're bad, then you probably will be bad. Being self-conscious will fuck you up every time. And, let me tell you—the bedroom is the one place you should leave all self-consciousness behind. That's why sex is so fun, remember?

Just shoot the middle finger to your Insecurity Fairy and go for it. Don't hold back. Come on, you hold back all day at work, the bedroom is the place to let loose. Dive in to the situation with eagerness. You want to do a good job, you want to have fun, you want him to enjoy it. Holding back is *not* the way to get there.

This is the time you let your inner vixen come out. It's just you and your man. Don't you want him to know how much you want him? How much you want to ravish him, to suck him off, to lose yourself in him? That is *hot*. The main way that comes through is the eyes.

That's right. Nothing can make sex hotter than eyes that say, "I crave you and your body I want to fuck you hard, but first I'm going to suck you off and I can't wait another minute to taste your cum in my mouth." See? It's easier to see with your eyes than your mouth.

That comes through the eyes. Have you heard the term "giving good face"? Notice the ambiguity in the meaning? Yuh-huh, there's a reason for that.

Nothing is hotter than eye contact. Especially if the guy's own hard dick in your mouth is in the line of sight between your eyes and his.

Think about it—

Girl sucking off dick: Feels nice. Ooh la la.
Girl sucking off dick with enthusiasm: Yeaaaaaaah, baby.
Girl sucking off dick with enthusiasm and eyes that say all the dirty things she can't say verbally because her mouth is full: —insert orgasm face here—
Then team the fuck-me eyes with the three-point contact technique? No guy will *ever* forget you.

Many guys have said that (assuming there's no teeth) there is no bad blowjob because his dick in a girl's mouth is going to be good no matter what. Fine, that may be so. But my competitive side doesn't want to be just another blowjob. I want to be the best fucking blowjob he's ever had. I want to be remembered.

Here's how I do that:

First, down to the deepest part of my body I love sucking cock. I always have. The cock is a magical, wonderful thing and I adore it. I love to make it hard, I love to make it jump up and down, I love to make it shoot a big load, and I love the way it feels in my hands, my mouth, and especially my pussy. The cock is a wonderful thing that I can never get enough of.

Second (now we're getting out of the head and to the hands-on part), the build-up, *i.e.* the foreplay to a blowjob. As much as you want it, don't just dive in. Play it up. From the kissing take it slowly down the chest, stopping at the nipples (only if he likes that—about half of guys have sensitive nipples and the other half think you're fucking nuts if you touch them), down along the treasure trail (ummm, I love that little tuft of hair leading the way—like I would *ever* get lost en route, but whatever).

Another option: While making out, periodically break the kiss to suck on his fingers. Do two, not one. As you suck on the fingers pull them apart slightly with your tongue and lick between them—and I don't mean delicately. It will make him think about what he wants to do to you when it's his turn for some fun.

Yet another option is this: While making out or doing something above the belt, slowly but firmly move your hand up and down the side of his body, from the neck all the way down to his thigh and back again. Don't be fast. Go slow. With each pass increase the pressure and begin lingering in key places like the upper inside of his thigh, hip, and the base of the neck while you're kissing.

Of course, you could always do all these things and make him cream his pants before you unzip him. Then depending on his age/masturbation frequency (oh, come on guys, we are so onto you)/passion level, you can wait a while and start all over.

Eventually, on a pass, stop your hand on the upper thigh and leave it there, and begin exploring a little, perhaps even do a little ticklish teasing. Get very close, but don't touch it. Then go back to do another pass up and down the side of his body, with a lot of pressure now. Make it obvious you want to just *eat him up*.

The next time your hand makes its way down his thigh and moves inside, oh so slowly and firmly move your hand up the inside, squeezing his muscle just a little, maybe dig your nails into the skin just a little (if he can handle it and if your nails aren't those sharp scary-looking things). Meanwhile stop whatever else you're doing so you can pull back a little and let him see the naughty hungry look in your eyes. The eyes are what make this hot, so for fuck's sake *give him eyes*, the ones that say, *I can't wait to get my mouth around that big, hard cock of yours.*

Now would be a good time to mention the importance of not turning off the lights. Or, if you insist on turning them off, (I promise if you're doing these naughty things to him, he is not going to be looking at your cellulite, which even the loveliest of nymphos have), keep a couple candles and a lighter nearby, turn on a lamp in the corner, whatever. It is crucial that he can see your face and exactly what you're doing to him once you get started. Apparently, not many girls like it with the lights on? Is this true? When I tell a guy to leave them on, he's usually surprised. Come on now, I've got a hearty appetite and I like to see what I'm feasting on here.

Once you have finally teased him enough, move in for the good stuff. With your hand already on his thigh, slowly make your way over to his dick. Using just your fingertips, climb your way up and over the mound in his pants to the zipper/buttons/waistband and *get those damn pants off*. They are of no use here. Once his dick is exposed, alternate between caressing it with your fingers and stroking it with your hand. If you just like feeling how hard it is because a hard dick in your hand *is* really fucking hot. What*thefuckmenow*ever.

At this point, positioning is important. Between taking the cock out and starting the blowjob, you have to get comfortable or else you'll have a sore/dead back/neck/arm/side, something. Don't worry about stretching into some sexy Botticelli or Victoria's Secret pose—for fuck's sake get comfortable. And I do mean "for fuck's sake" because you don't want to have a sore back or dead arm from a blowjob and then go right in for sex when you're in too much pain to enjoy it, now do you?

Comfortable Position #1: Have him lie down on his back, legs spread. Kneel down in front of him. Note: *Do not lie down*. You need to fully support yourself with your legs. You'll be using both your hands in a minute, so don't bother lying on your stomach and propping yourself up with your arms. This one is my standard position simply because it's the easiest to transition into and the most comfortable. It may get to be a little uncomfortable for him, because if you're doing it right he'll want to be watching every single thing you do and his neck will get sore from looking up at you unless he has a couple of pillows.

Comfortable Position #2: Have him stand up so you kneel on the ground in front of him. This can be awkward on the back, depending on your relative heights. I'm tall so I often have to bend over a little too much to be at the right height. To avoid looking awkward, I push my ass back a little, arch my back, and stick my booty out. *Voilà*, sex kitten pose. The guy usually likes this because it's got that whole master/slave positioning (never mind he's at your mercy for his orgasm), and he has a fine view of every single thing you're doing. You can take advantage of this, while you're doing your thing by playing with yourself with one hand or grinding your hips a little in the air in anticipation of the heavy grinding you'll be doing to him later on.

OK, well a good blowjob is a good blowjob, but what I'm aiming for is being the girl he fantasizes about years later when he's thinking about the best head he's ever had. Just having that I-want-to-suck-you-off-like-no-one-has-ever-done-before attitude will get you far.

Don't believe me? I bet you half the guys who just read those last two sentences got a little hard. Attitude is everything.

Attitude is what gets the average-looking girl all the male attention in a room full of bombshells with DSL's (Dick Sucking Lips). When you have an enthusiastic attitude toward sex, goddamnit, it *shows*. You know what I'm talking about, those women out there who seem to ooze *sexsexsex* out of every pore. You know those women like sex and that they know what they're doing.

Bingo.

I cannot stress enough how important an enthusiastic attitude about sex is. It can make or break you.

For those of you who don't particularly like giving head but are great troupers and do it anyway: Keep doing it. Keep practicing. The more you do it, the better you get at it, the more he gets off on it, the more you enjoy it. It feeds into itself.

Time to get hands-on.

I like cock. I like to take it all in, in every possible way. I like devouring the mass of it with my eyes—and making sure he sees me savoring it—then devouring it with my hands, and I mean ravishing his cock with my hands. This is not a time to be a delicate flower. You're about to suck his dick. Gentle won't do.

Take his dick in both your hands and really feel the expanse of it. I don't care if this is the same guy you've been sleeping with for ten years. (Um, especially in this case, actually.) Approach it like you're enjoying it and appreciating it for the first time. Run your fingers, then palms and finally whole hand up and down the shaft. Do this a couple times, increasing pressure/coverage each time.

Play with the tip of the head a little bit. Circle a fingertip around the ridge, over the opening, and—scoop up that little bit of pre-cum before licking it off your finger while you've got the sex eyes coming out in full. You can alternate between going full-on with hand pressure and then stopping to do something teasing like this, or you can be firm with one hand and playful with the other at the same time. Variety keeps him on his toes.

After he's made it obvious he enjoys what you're doing [note to the male readers out there: You know how you like it when we moan? Well, we like it when *you* moan, so stop being so fucking quiet and help us out a little bit over here, eh? Don't make us drive blind.] make your way downward.

I'm embarrassed to admit I was nineteen before I found out that guys like it when we pay attention to the testicles. I was twenty-one when I found out that guys *really* like it when you have one in your mouth and suck on it. Hmm. Fascinating. [Where were all the sex blogs when *I* was figuring all this stuff out, huh?] I think it's safe to say that, in general, guys want us to pay more attention to the balls.

Start by fondling his balls with one hand while you're stroking his shaft with the other hand. If this is your first time doing this to your guy, go a bit slowly and watch his reaction to make sure you aren't weirding him out (actually, this is a good rule in general with a new guy, no matter what you're doing to him. But, if you're going to scare the *holyFUCKwoman* out of him, at least do it for something good, like sticking a dildo up his ass (more guys like that than will admit to it, by the way)).

Now with the balls you need to have a lighter hand than with his dick. The boys can be sensitive. Cup one in your hand and lightly massage it with your fingers. If he enjoys this, then cup the other one in your hand and continue. [Note: There is a huge variety in testicle size among guys and this has no correlation to the size of his dick. The balls can change size and hanging height significantly throughout the course of sex. Personally, I prefer smaller testicles because then it's easier to tend to both at the same time.]

[Another note to the male readers: We appreciate a little maintenance in the pubic department. That doesn't mean shaving, just keeping things neat and tidy with a trim. Nothing ruins the moment like when a girl has to stop sucking you off to pull a pubic hair out from between her teeth. For fuck's sake, if you're a hairy bastard, help us out a little here and spend some quality time with a pair of scissors. Now, not all women will agree with me, many like the hairy men. Just not necessarily below the belt. Ask her what she thinks. She may not care, or she may care a lot, but not know how to bring it up.]

In addition to kneading the balls, mix it up with lightly (and I do mean lightly) pulling them away from his body. Again, gauge his reaction here. If he shoots you a *what the fuck* look, pretend you were just exploring and move along to something else (like sucking him off. That will always make a guy forget whatever dumbass thing you just did. Jeez, why do you think I'm so good at it?). A lot of what I'm saying in this post varies between guys. One may love what another throws you out for. I'm trying to bring up everything so you have a good inventory to pull from.

As a precursor to sucking his dick, start licking the balls. At first lick one up and down with your tongue while you continue fondling the other in your hand. Gradually begin to take the entire thing into your mouth, if possible (there are some enormous testicles out there! If there's simply too much, save the effort for the dick instead). Once it's in your mouth, alternate between licking it directly with your tongue and juggling it around inside your mouth. It's OK if the whole thing doesn't fit in your mouth, just take in as much as you can.

From there maneuver the skin to be taut against the testicle so you can suck on it at maximum sensitivity. With your tongue push the testicle around inside your mouth while maintaining a slight suction. Hopefully at this point he's moaning and playing with your hair and wondering what he did to deserve his balls in your mouth.

Throughout this you need to be giving him sex eyes, those eyes that say, "I can't wait to feel your cock in my mouth."

The cock is not a complicated thing. Stroke here, lick there, suck here, and don't forget to close your eyes when he cums (that shit stings!). Although giving a blowjob isn't complicated, it ain't easy either, especially if you want to go down in his memory as the best head he ever had—and I mean when he hears your name or your favorite fuck-me song five years later he gets a distant, goofy look in his eyes and a little bit of a hard-on which he has to explain to his wife.

The key to good head is to mix it up. Keep him guessing what's coming next. Granted there are many types of blowjobs: The one-minute quickie (good for commercial breaks during the football game), the loving head (long and slow and a bit of *schmoopie* talk), dirty-whore head (fast, deep, hard and dirty), S&M head (biting, grabbing him by the balls, "you'll do what I say, you hear me, you prick?"; or he grabs your hair, forces your head down, "you'll suck my cock and you'll like it, bitch" (mmmm . . . sooo hot)), but what I'm aiming for here is the looong head (which in many cases only translates into five or ten minutes) that will have him whimpering, begging, and calling my name when I finally let him cum.

My method involves teasing the poor bastard right until he's about to blow his load–and then pulling back. Build up, pull back, build up, pull back, each time building up a little more than the time before. All the build-ups lead to a huge blow-out. He may hate you a little each time you do that, but he won't mind in the end.

Note: This post is not comprehensive. There are many more little tricks and techniques, but I'm writing this in one night and my left hand is already exhausted from masturbating.

Another note: You know there's no actual *blowing* in a blowjob, right? Don't they teach you anything at church camp?

After paying due attention to his balls (do not underestimate the orgasm-inducing power of the balls), it's time to work your way toward Three-Point Contact. Before I go into detail, I want you to keep the following mix it up styles in mind: *fast vs. slow, deep vs. shallow, long strokes vs. short strokes, and consistent vs. varied rhythm.*

FIRST POINT OF CONTACT: The hand. One hand, whichever one is the easiest to control and has the most endurance. Typically but not always, the hand that you write with. Clasp it around the base of the shaft and begin stroking up and down, slowly at first and then gradually increasing speed.

I'd like to take this time to point out that manicured fingernails look super hot when wrapped around a hard cock. I'm no girly-girl, but I know the power of vixen-red nails. Especially since I've now been on the receiving end of a glorious set of painted nails. WOW. They look even hotter going in and out of pussy (and I don't mean masturbating). But for fuck's sake, don't have those super long, pointy, *these-are-made-for-stabbing-you* acrylic fingernails. Those things are scary. I wouldn't want a set of those anywhere near my penis. —shudders—

Don't pump away on dick like it's a chore. It is not a chore, it is a privilege. You should be so lucky to have a dick standing up to say hello. Show him that you love having his dick in your hand. Get up close where you can see everything. If he's lying down, stroke his dick up and down while your face is directly behind it so he can see your hands, his cock, and your wicked smile all right there.

Every once in a while pull back to concentrate on a different area. The head and the frenulum (the tight little bit of skin on the underside of the head) are the most sensitive areas of the dick. Work this. Lightly circle the ridge of the head with your finger tip (your manicured fingertip). Tickle the frenulum ever so lightly (the sensitivity can work against you if you've gone hard faster than he was ready for). Bonus points if while you're stroking him you're giving yourself a little hand-action.

SECOND POINT OF CONTACT: The mouth. Just because the mouth is coming in, it does not mean your hand is done. Nuh-uh. We're building up, not making substitutions. No matter how good you are with your hand, the mouth is better. It simulates the pussy by virtue of being warm and wet. Besides that, it's fucking sexy as hell for a guy to see his dick in a girl's mouth, to see her taking it all in and wanting more. Remember the sex eyes? Make sex eyes. Although if you love what you're doing, the eyes will show it without you having to even think about it.

Pull back from his dick slowly, with your hand caressing the top as you pull away. Squeeze the tip of the head until you see a little drop of pre-cum. If this is your thing and you know it's safe, wipe the pre-cum up with your fingertip, look directly into his eyes, arch your back, grin like the cock-loving girl you are, and lick it off your finger.

Once his eyes have popped back into their sockets and he realizes you are for real, it's time to bring out your best stuff. Bite your lower lip and give him a naughty grin. Crouch down so you're hovering over or next to his dick. Starting at the base, lick the shaft ever-so-very-slowly with the tip of your tongue. End at the head with a little flourish of the tongue. Make eye contact. By this point he should be able to read your dirty, dirty mind through your eyes.

Go back down on the other side, with your tongue stretched out so he has the full luscious view. Come back up along the top, still slow, then bring your hand back in. Clasp the base of the shaft with your hand, put your head down in the position to begin sucking, but just before you do, look up at him.

Have you noticed I'm being totally obnoxious about the eyes? That's because giving sex eyes is the hottest and most under-utilized thing you can do, so *work it*, goddamnit. Flirt with your eyes, tease with your eyes, fuck with your eyes, *take him in* with your eyes.

Now dive in. You've been moving slow up to this point, so diving in with a visible hunger is a powerful contrast. Since his dick is mostly dry, take in a couple inches and run your tongue down the shaft to give it a little lubricant.

On the second run, take in as much of his cock as you can. The best way to do this depends on the proper positioning of your head/throat relative to his dick. For what I'm outlining in this post, the best body position is with him lying down and you kneeling so you can extend/crouch over him. You have to support yourself fully with your legs, because soon both your hands are going to be busy. If your head is directly over his dick (use your hand to hold it straight up into your mouth), it's your best shot to take in all of the average-sized cock. If you have a bad gag reflex—practice on a straight banana. If it makes you uncomfortable, go slow and try to relax. Being tense is not what you need to be right now.

To begin the licking and sucking, keep your shoulders steady and move your head with the neck only. As you get going, let your body follow the sex vibe. Kneel so that you lift up your hips to grind in the air. Arch your back and roll your ass around in small circles. Don't think about it too much . . . just let your body do what it feels inclined to do. There's a hard cock in your mouth. Enjoy it.

What to do with the tongue. At the beginning it's easiest to place it underneath the cock as you take it in. Don't let the tongue just *be* there, occupying space in your mouth. Press it up against the shaft. Once you get going, lick side-to-side with your tongue while sucking up and down. Lick all around. Meanwhile, you can bring in the hand as needed for another source of pressure/sensation or to act as a stopping point so you don't accidentally take in too much and summon the gag reflex.

Meanwhile with the mouth, keep it in a tight ring around his cock because they are yet another key contact in the blowjob. Just watch it, because lips can be the first thing to cramp up.

The mix of textures, pressure, speed, rhythm—there's so many options to try out. You don't ever have to give the same blowjob twice if you know how to mix it up.

THIRD POINT OF CONTACT: The other hand. This is why you need to be supporting yourself with knees/legs only. One hand is on the shaft, mouth is on the dick, and the other hand is what rounds this out as an all-round mind-blowing blowjob. While sucking and pumping, bring in your other hand, which hopefully up until this point has been keeping you nice and stimulated (masturbating, rubbing between legs, pinching nipples).

Start by playing with the balls again. In case you missed it: Guys like it when you play with their balls. Especially while you're doing all the other stuff. Lick them, strum against them with the tip of your tongue, juggle them lightly in your fingers, cup them in your palm, whatever. Don't be rough, they're sensitive, although the degree depends on the guy. Keep stroking his shaft with your hand and sucking on the head. You are now in scoring position.

BONUS POINT OF CONTACT: Exactly how good are you with your hands? Time to hit the magic sweet spot. (No, as much as I love poking something up a guy's ass, that's not what I'm referring to–not this time.)

After a minute or so, close your index finger and press it middle-knuckle first into the tissue just underneath the balls. I'm not sure what this is called (I don't think it's the same thing as the perineum, because that's farther away), but it hits the interior base of the shaft. If you apply pressure with your knuckle, according to some guys it feels amazing. If you're really talented, you can apply pressure with your knuckle or finger while continuing to fondle his balls. Massage the spot gently while you massage the balls as well. Not many people know about this magic spot, so it has a powerful effect on those who are fortunate enough to experience it.

THE ENDING. If you don't want to swallow, then you can finish him off with hand job only, or suck until the final thirty seconds and then switch to manual. Just watch your eyes!! Cum in contacts = *OW* motherfucker. Most guys are understanding about not wanting to take them in your mouth, whether for personal or health reasons. If you still want to finish with a flourish, you can pull my favorite porn star move of letting him ejaculate on your stomach or breasts. I think it's fun, but lots of people seem to think it's degrading. I don't care. I like it.

Don't ever take it in your mouth and then spit it out. That's just rude. If you don't want it there in the first place, fucking say so.

Note on taste: What the guy eats and drinks beforehand directly corresponds to the taste of his cum. Drinking a lot of beer (a lot, not just two) beforehand leaves a nasty taste. That is my only icky memory of a blowjob. In general, the healthier the food he eats the better (less bad, whatever) it tastes. Fruit and fruit juice has the best influence for a non-offensive taste. Let me just say again: Being able to somewhat deep-throat means you never have to worry about taste.

If you're comfortable swallowing, you can avoid the taste by taking him in as deep as you can right when he cums. That gets it past the taste buds. If you know the guy well enough to know his tells for when he's on the verge of cumming, that makes it a lot easier to time your technique. If this is a new guy, then you may need him to give you some indication or ten-second warning. Guys: This is why moaning, or, you know, SPEAKING like EVER during sex is beneficial. Why are guys always so fucking quiet? BLEH. Get over it.

When it's coming down to the finale, I like to finish hard. Up until the last couple seconds, going deep and fast helps the intensity. At the very end, take in as much of his dick as you can, ideally enough so that the head is pressed against the back of your mouth. The extra bit of pressure blows his mind—and wad. Continue licking the underside of the shaft with your tongue with as much pressure as the tongue has left in it. In the final second or two, move your head up and down just enough so that the tip of his dick rubs against the back/roof of your mouth.

As he cums, hold on. DON'T BREAK THE SEAL. That can make for a big sticky mess. Keep your mouth closed tightly around his cock until you're sure he's done, which can take as long as ten seconds. When you hear the post-orgasm sigh, slowly retreat. Keep the seal around his cock as you pull away. As you get toward the tip use your tongue to scoop up the cum in your mouth so it doesn't dribble out your mouth. Although, a single drop of cum can be damn hot if you lick it up with the tip of your tongue and then give your final naughty and self-satisfied grin. *Bon appetit*, ladies and gay gentlemen.

Ducking the Family Guilt Stick

I'm getting nervous about seeing my extended family at Thanksgiving. This will be the first time I will see all my many relatives since the big break-up four and a half months ago.

Considering that the last time I saw my family at our summer reunion, they were all teasing me and Aussie about when we going to get married. I'm worried. Very about-to-piss-myself worried.

My family is huge (I have twenty aunts and uncles, plus all of their progeny), Catholic (*i.e.* constantly fighting each other over who gets to smack who with the Guilt Stick), and opinionated.

Everyone has an opinion, and everyone feels entitled to share their opinion of your life because we're *family*.

Which means my body is already jumpy in anticipation of their blows. And I may be bringing whiskey in a flask to share with Dad while we hide from Mom's family in the corner. They scare me.

OK, now my mom? The MOM? She's the good one in the family. By far. She only gives *some* of her opinion, and only to a select few. I am obviously at the top of that list. But, in this case of *Vix* vs *The FAMILY*, where I am to be put on trial for *Why exactly did you break up with such a great guy? You know he was too good for you, right? So why didn't you marry him? He didn't like your nose ring, did he? We told you not to get the nose ring. What were you THINKING breaking up with him?!*, my mother will be my defense. The MOM is strong enough to take on the whole of The FAMILY. That's a tough broad right there.

She will be playing interference. I can already imagine it: Two aunts will casually sit down on either side of me to begin the grilling session. Mom from across the room will sense the change in tone (not that she ever gets it when *I* do that), turn with her paper plate still in hand, throw a piercing smile as she curtly tells my aunts, "I'm sure she doesn't want to discuss that now. But she has plenty of interesting things to say about work. Why don't you ask her about that?" and then turn back to her yams.

This is why in spite of being scared shitless of my mother, I have nothing but the highest respect for her.

Now this is in addition to all the behind-the-scenes things I have not seen. The many phone calls my mother has fielded from aunts, older cousins, and my grandmother, the matriarch, the holder of the Guilt Stick. My family is very covert. For all I know she has already answered questions from the aunts and cousins within the Circle of Trust and brushed off inquiries from all other relatives.

There may already be months' worth of brush-offs at play that I have no idea about, which may very well mean that Thanksgiving will only have one or two poorly disguised confrontations ("So have you talked to Aussie lately?") that I can dodge easily with only that great piercing smile I learned from The MOM.

At least when *she* smacks me with the Guilt Stick, I know she's doing it for my well-being. It's a smack filled with love.

What I'm Really Thankful For

We had been at Grandmother's for less than ten minutes when she said she had a surprise for me. She pulled out two beautiful quilts that she had made and told me to pick one to take home. I *ooh*ed and *ahh*ed while deciding which one I wanted. Silly me, I didn't think to ask why she was offering me one when I knew there was a long list of family members waiting for one of her prized quilts.

Suddenly, Grandmother's eyes got big. "Oh! Wait! There's another one I want to show you!"

With great excitement she motioned for me to follow her as she shuffled down the hall. She led me into the guest bedroom where she pulled out a half-finished quilt.

Grandmother spread it out over the bed. She looked at me with pride while I ran my hand over the curved pieces of fabric stitched together in interlocking circles.

"It's a wedding ring quilt. For whoever gets married next!"

Aw fuck.

I snatched my hand away from the quilt. Marriage cooties.

She peered at me over her bifocals. "Who do you think it will be?"

DAMNIT. I hadn't anticipated a sneak attack. Lured in with the promise of a quilt, damnit, she's good! I shifted uneasily, trying to figure out the best way to approach this. I knew she expected me to lay claim to the wedding ring quilt.

"Well, Grandma," I said with a big smile, "I don't think I'm in the running for that anymore!" and I finished with a hearty chuckle, like oh, silly, whimsical me, you never know what I'll do next!

Silence.

Eeep. I want Mom.

"I broke up with Aussie. A while ago. I thought Mom told you that?"

Hastily she pulled the quilt away from me and began to fold it up. "She did. I didn't think you *meant it*."

"What? Why wouldn't I mean it?"

"Young people. They break up and get back together." With that she turned her back to me and I ran out of the room to go find and hide behind my mommy.

A couple hours later my aunts announced that it was time to eat. We stood in line with our fancy silverware and Styrofoam plates and talked about the weather (So warm! So marvelous! So sunny!) to each other while waiting our turn at the food.

I usually wait to go until most people have gone through the food line before me to ensure that the dining room table will be full and I'll have to sit at the kiddie table. Ideally, the kiddie tables are also full, and I have to eat in the living room—safely out of sight and out of mind.

Perfect timing. All tables were full but none of the food had run out. I headed toward the living room to eat in peace, only to find my oldest cousin running interception. He pulled me back to the dining room where everyone was going around saying what they were thankful for this Thanksgiving.

Aunts and uncles said they were thankful for their kids having jobs. Older cousins said they were thankful for having jobs. Younger cousins said they were thankful it was almost Christmas.

As one of only two people standing (and partially hiding behind the door frame), I was last. What to say that would please my parents, Grandmother, not have anyone come to beat me with the Guilt Stick, and be remotely true? Oh, and it has to be a really good one because I'm last. Saying I'm thankful that it's a new episode of *Grey's Anatomy* tonight wouldn't do.

Since I didn't have a glass of wine like I'm used to (no booze allowed at Grandmother's), I raised my Styrofoam plate in a toast. What, we can toast really good stuffing, can't we?

"I'm thankful for Grandmother's excellent health, which means she'll be here cooking turkeys for many years to come–" (she may be the scary matriarch, but she's still my grandmother)

"–And I'm thankful for the many relatives we have, who couldn't be here today–" (haha, it's all in the wording!! I'm so clever!! I DIDN'T HAVE TO LIE.)

"–But, most of all I'm thankful for my great career, my current achievements, and all the many opportunities I see in my future."

. . . which I honestly don't think would be so promising if I weren't single and therefore had all the time in the world to devote to my dreams.

But, whatever. I don't need to explain myself, not to Grandmother or anyone else holding the Guilt Stick. I can just smile and keep it my sweet little secret.

This Is Why I Don't Like Bars

Because I SUCK AT THEM.

Seriously. The sexy confident OEN you see here does not translate well to the bar scene. At *all*.

OK, except for that ONE time I went home with two guys and had a super smokin' hot threesome. But how often does that happen?

Tonight, I went to a bar to see a buddy of mine perform. He was wicked good, high as a kite, and was half the reason I dragged my lame ass out of the comfort of my apartment.

The other half of the reason was that I wanted to get laid. It's been a couple weeks, The Pussy needs to be fed.

From the reviews of this place I read, the bar was rock n' roll yet hip and full of beautiful people. Which was no lie. Every which way I looked was another beautiful male specimen.

And next to most of these beautiful male specimens were drop-dead gorgeous girls. All of them were prettier than me. This is not me being modest, this is me being realistic. I ain't too shabby, but this was like a huge blonde bombshell exploded inside the bar. *Fucking A*, man. I might as well put a plastic bag over my head and call it a night.

This is why I don't like bars. When I go out with my girlfriends I am clearly the funny one. Being funny does not make itself obvious based on appearance alone, which is what you need to draw a guy out of crowd to come speak to you. I assume. I don't know, because it rarely happens to me.

That leaves me as the one to start conversations with guys. Especially on nights like tonight when I am alone. Ack! *ALONE!?* I didn't think it was that big a deal, but every girl I talked with asked, with more than a little pity in her voice, "Are you *alone*?"

Yes. I am alone. I would bring friends, but all my friends are prettier than me and that usually leaves me going home by myself. I figured it was worth a shot flying solo.

I don't do well in bars. There it's pretty much based on looks alone, and when I'm dressed like a normal person (like I was tonight, *i.e.* mostly covered) I don't get anywhere. I can dress trampy and get somewhere, but I have to be in the mood for that and that happens less often the older I get because most of the time I can't be bothered to give a rat's ass.

Besides, I depend on my witty banter and morbid sense of humor to win over guys. Sadly, how often do you get to that point at a bar?

When I first got to the bar I spent about half an hour scanning the place, observing people and making a mental checklist of people to talk to. At last I was ready.

I approached two guys sitting on their own in a corner. I will not go into detail about my line, what I said, or their reaction because it quickly sank so badly that it got to the point where I closed my eyes, waved my hand prettily, and said, "Please excuse me, this is not going well so I will just leave right now." They did not stop me.

Next, I talked to the most promising candidate of the night, a dashing young lad who was dressed well and smelled good. He was leaning over me to order a drink at the bar, so I used that as my line: "So, do you really want a drink that badly or are you just trying to get close to me? It's OK, I don't mind you invading my personal space." He laughed. I kept talking. I asked him if he was single, because if not I might as well save us the ten minutes. He laughed again and said I was funny. I took this as a sign to keep talking.

For some bizarre reason he left. He had another drink which he said he had to deliver to his friend. I smiled and told him to come back and find me later. Five minutes later he did, but to pay his tab, thank me for the laughs, and then leave.

Blimey.

I turned to my other side, where there was another nice-smelling guy leaning into my personal space to order a drink. I teased him that there was a charge for being so bold as to assume he was inside my circle of trust already. He laughed. We talked. He ordered me a drink when I wasn't even halfway through my current one. He introduced me to his female friends. We all talked and had a good time.

I spent most of the next hour with them, but this guy was just flirtatious enough to keep my attention, yet wouldn't do anything. I made the first move so it was his fucking turn (no more of this doing-all-the-chasing crap. No wonder guys winge about it, it's a fucking tiring pain in the ass).

There was one more guy I tried talking to, but it didn't go well so I backed out shortly after giving him my name. And it was my *real* name.

Before leaving I decided I would try to talk to one more guy. Just as I stood up to walk toward two guys I'd had my eye on all night, someone intercepted me. He was wearing a blazer. Who the fuck under the age of forty wears a blazer? To a *bar*?

But I gotta admit, the guy grew on me. He was funny and creative, which I had to give him props for. I took it up a notch and teased him. Hey, I like seeing if a guy can take a little ball busting. Apparently I took it too far because he muttered something about being shot down and left before I could correct him.

I didn't care that much because I was getting cranky and frustrated, so I went home. Home to the comfort of my laptop, where no one cares that I'm not the prettiest girl in the room or that I'm not even wearing make-up—because I'm funny and that's what counts here in my tiny little piece of the blogosphere.

Since, you know, I'm really a three-hundred-pound, middle-aged man named Larry. And ooooh, you should see my sweet-ass booty shake. I'll shake my Laffy Taffy for you any day, baby.

How Do Guys Measure Up?

OK, guys out there? Stop asking us what we think about your dicks.

Yes it's big enough, yes, it feels good, yes, it's bigger than my ex-boyfriend's (if saying that will make you to shut the hell up), *yes, I like it, NO I WON'T MEASURE IT FOR YOU.*

I get the impression guys have a skewed sense of average when it comes to the length of their dicks. The guys who think their dicks are small (maybe in comparison to a porn star's, although I know for a fact that not all porn stars have huge dicks) are usually average and the guys who think they're huge are often only average. Like, do you really think you're 8" long, buddy? . . . Uh, maybe if you measure from the bottom of your scrotum.

Average, average, average.

What exactly is average? I have read in multiple books and seen from plenty of personal experience that the average dick is 5 to 5 ½" (12 to 14 cm for all our foreign readers). I have seen very few that were less than 4" or more than 8" (10 to 20 cm). One guy triumphantly told me he was 8" but then naked time came and he was average, which wouldn't have been disappointing if he hadn't brought it up in the first place. I think he was measuring to the underside of Narnia.

Now it's my turn to ask a question to our male readers out there: How many of you have ever measured the length of your dick? Come on, 'fess up. Over half the guys I've been with have told me *to the quarter inch* how long they were. WTF? Dude, that's weird. Get your penis cooties off my ruler. Round to the nearest half inch if you don't want to arouse suspicion.

Let's dispel a few myths here.

Generally speaking, race *can* be an indicator of dick size. Some races tend to run smaller or larger than others. In *general*. But I have yet to meet a black guy who was hung like a horse—not that that stopped me from riding them cowgirl-style. Don't assume one way or another just because a guy is a certain race.

You can't tell how big a guy's dick is by the size of his hands, the size of his feet, or his height. There is no way to tell how big his dick is until you reach your hand down his pants and find out for yourself.

Size doesn't matter as much as you think it does. I'm not saying this to be nice (I'm not nice). I'm saying this because, for the most part, it's true. It IS the motion of the ocean that really matters. What's the point of having a big boat if you don't know how to steer the fucking thing?

I've been with smallish guys who knew the exact right positions to get me off. Doggy-style in particular, if you're wondering. If you're worried about him staring at the cellulite on your ass, get over yourself. Of all the many beautiful things on your body do you think he's going to be paying *any* attention to cellulite?

I've also been with guys who were hung and assumed *ipso facto* they were good in bed. Wrong, wrong, wrong, motherfucker. You might as well stick it in my ear for all the good you're doing with it.

Then there's girth. Girth does not get nearly enough credit out there. Having wide girth (can't reach all the way around when you grasp it) is, I must say, *a little piece of heaven*. Being narrow doesn't necessarily work against you. Some girls prefer narrow dicks, especially if she is of a petite frame and or if she's unusually tight.

Guys out there seem to be jealous of guys with big schlongs, but there's a few truths you may not know about.

How likely is a girl to have anal sex with the average guy? Low.

How likely is a girl to have anal sex with a guy who's well-endowed? Very, very low. You're better off getting her to stick a cucumber up her butt.

A big dick does not help your odds in the anal department.

Another little-known truth: Many girls (certainly not all) are intimidated as hell by a big dick. How the fuck is she supposed to perform fellatio on that big-ass thing? How is she supposed to let that thing near her, let alone inside her? Fuck, she may need to do a month of yoga before she's ready for that.

Not to scare off the guys out there with big dicks. There are many girls who delight in the challenge of a giant and tackle it with great enthusiasm. You may just have to exercise a bit of caution when it comes to initial penetration: Make sure she has loosened up with your fingers already, and lube is a help as well. Anal sex is always possible, but that takes extra caution. And one helluva good woman.

What about dicks that curve to the left or right? OK, granted it may look a little funny when out in the open air, but once you manage to maneuver it into the desired location it makes no difference.

What about dicks that curve up or down? This can work to your benefit, if you take advantage of the right positions for finding the sweet spot.

It is perfectly normal for dicks to curve in one direction, have a big head/ridge, have no ridge, whatever. It's like boobs. Every girl is different. Part of the fun of getting underneath her clothes is to see how she's different from all the others and what makes them so gosh darn fun to play with.

There are a few anomalies out there, I feel I must warn you. I once saw one that *I swear to the goddess herself* curved so severely it formed a perfect semicircle. Whoa. That was quite a maneuvering problem. That's the only dick in a sea of dicks that sticks out in my memory based solely on looks.

Now to address what all our male readers really want to know: How to make your dick look bigger, without a $49.99 penis pump.

In all seriousness, if you trim or shave your pubic hair, it makes your dick look bigger. That's the first thing guys always say when I finally talk them into taking scissors down the happy trail. Bonus: Now you don't have to worry about the other person stopping halfway through a blowjob because of a pubic floss problem.

To our "gentlemen" readers out there—stop asking us if your dick is big enough. Yes, it usually is. Now stop shooting yourself in the crotch by asking, because to do so is a sign of insecurity. Insecurity is not sexy. And it's annoying to assure someone *yes, babycakes, your dick is all I need.*

It's similar to a girl asking you, "does this make me look fat?" Save yourself the trouble and don't ask in the first fucking place.

As long as she's grinding and moaning, you're doing fine and that's what matters.

Are You *Sure* You Want to See My Place?

You can only avoid having the person you're dating come over to your place for so long before she starts accusing you of having another girlfriend, living with your parents, living with your wife, or living in a cardboard box behind the scary Taco Cabana, so at some point you have to suck it up and let her come over. Or, if you're smooth enough to pull it off, occasionally bring home a hook-up.

[Readers: please forgive me for addressing the male audience, but I assume more guys will benefit from this post than girls. I'm NOT JUDGING. My own apartment is a bit, well, *icky*. But, it's easy for a chick to get away with a messy apartment, all she has to do is take off her shirt and then a guy wouldn't notice if there were a feces-filled gorilla cage in the apartment.]

You should be doing most of these things in the first place, especially if you're well out of college and extra-especially if you're over the age of thirty. Your place should not look like the set of *Jackass* if you're middle-aged. If that's the case, you can stop wondering why you're still single.

Here are a few tips on how to make a good impression, whether you're bringing home a new girlfriend or a one-night stand.

CLEAN YOUR FUCKING BATHROOM

I mean get on your hands and knees and scrub every damn thing in the bathroom, especially the toilet. There needs to be NO ICKINESS in your bathroom. NOT A SPOT OF URINE. You think I'm kidding about this one? NUH-UH. HEED ALL THE ALL CAPS IN THIS PARAGRAPH. I once didn't sleep with a guy because his bathroom was so disgusting that I thought I'd grow warts on the bottom of my feet if I walked on the tile. Do you want that to happen to you? Not get laid because of YOUR BATHROOM?! Dude, don't be that guy, because then girls like me make fun of you.

DUST AND VACUUM

In that order, in case it's not obvious that gravity exists even for tiny dust particles. Get the pretty little vacuum lines in the carpet. Women like that. Vacuuming is the quickest way to make a big difference. By the way, you should vacuum more often than every time you think you might get laid.

YOUR POSTER OF JESSICA BIEL DOESN'T COUNT AS DECOR

Please tell me you have *something* on your walls (and I don't mean a Playboy bunny poster). It's kinda weird when a middle-aged guy has blank walls because it comes off as being too lazy to care. If you're too lazy to care about the place you live, how are you going to be about the women you date? All you need is a tasteful poster or two, a photo (black & white = artsy), or hell, even a big plant in the corner. Something to break up the big stretches of whiteness. This is where you're supposed to show off that charming personality of yours. No, a photo of yourself doesn't make up for a dull personality. Go to Target or Ikea for cheap art.

THE FRIDGE IS SUPPOSED TO HAVE FOOD IN IT

Make sure your fridge is stocked. It creeps women out when all you have in your fridge is beer and ketchup. Have some good cheese (gouda, goat, brie) to snack on, some chilled white wine (white, not red)(When in doubt, go for the fanciest-looking label), maybe some deli meat for a midnight sandwich (because you wore her out, soldier!), and something to drink other than beer. Major bonus points if you have things like butter, assorted salad dressing and condiments, eggs, vegetables, fruit . . . you know . . . things that *normal* people eat. The cherry-flavored lube on top: a pint of Ben & Jerry's ice cream in the freezer.

THE *QUEER EYE* GUYS WOULD SHOOT ME DEAD FOR THE ADVICE I'M ABOUT TO GIVE

If you're like me and you actually use your kitchen for cooking, it can get very messy very fast. Pots piled up in the sink, unidentifiable substances scorched onto pans, and dishes you don't remember owning let alone using. Yeah, you kinda have to clean those. Just throw them all in the dishwasher and set on "motherload" (that means "heavy" or "pots and pans"). For the really bad stuff you can't possibly clean in one day? Hide it in the oven. That's right, I said it. Just don't forget there's shit in there when you turn the oven on later, because that will probably happen when you have a girl over, and you really don't want an audience heckling such a magnificent display of smoking dumbassery. No one will believe that some random chick on a blog told you to do such a thing. Ha *ha*.

IF THERE IS A BAD SMELL YOU MUST IDENTIFY AND CONTAIN IT

Or at least mask it. It's better to find the source of the smell in case the girl outlasts the air freshener. If finding and removing the offensive smell takes more time than you have available, open the windows, light a scented candle in each room beforehand, and get a fan going. Do not spritz Old Spice all over your apartment.

DRINK LIKE A MAN

Having a nice selection of wine is sexy. Having a nice selection of hard liquor is, *well* . . . It makes me wonder if I would find a T-shirt that says "Alcoholics Anonymous is for quitters. I'm a drunk!" in your closet. You can also never go wrong with some craft beer. Hide your cheap beer in a closet.

CLEAN SHEETS HIDE A DIRTY MIND

No jerk-off stains on the bedspread, please.

IF SHE DOESN'T SEE IT, YOU DON'T HAVE TO EXPLAIN WHY YOU HAVE IT

Hide your porn. If she's a bit conservative, this includes *Maxim*, *FHM*, *Stuff*, and *Sports Illustrated: Swimsuit Issue*. (Even if she does know you use it, she doesn't need to know that you whack off to "Menage a Twat: Part IV".)

YOU'RE OLD ENOUGH FOR A BIG BOY BED!!

You are shooting yourself in the crotch if you sleep on a futon, a twin-size mattress, a bed you picked up off the street, or a box spring that sits directly on the floor. You can buy a real bed on craigslist or a new one at Ikea for cheap. Own up to a man bed.

IN CASE YOU DON'T FUCK UP ALL OF THE ABOVE

Have condoms nearby so you don't have to go hunting for them. Just a couple. Even if you have a huge box, don't let her see that because she'll think you're either a player or that you expect her to fuck for twelve consecutive hours. Or, god forbid, that you need two condoms to prevent premature ejaculation.

YOUR MARTIN SCORCESE COLLECTION WON'T IMPRESS HER

Owning chick flicks is a very wise move. I don't mean the entire Disney cartoon collection, but maybe a couple of the less lame ones like *Just Married* or *Spanglish*. *Hitch* is a guy's movie cleverly disguised as a romantic comedy. You can write-off *Pride & Prejudice* if you got a liberal arts degree. All it takes is a couple chick flicks scattered throughout *Fight Club*, *Die Hard*, and the complete *Dark Angel* DVD collector's set to show that you have a soft side. If you don't own any girl movies, go to Target or Best Buy and get *When Harry Met Sally*. It's worth the ten bucks if it helps you get laid—I mean, get closer to girls on an emotional level.

GOING FOR THE GOLD?

Bonus points! Have a spare toothbrush lying around. Just in case. Don't tell her you bought it specifically for her. Unless she asks, then say yes and be cute as a button about it. But, for fuck's sake, don't buy a pink one. Then it's obvious you put too much thought into it and your whole cover is blown.

Hey Dumbass, I'm Trying To Flirt With You

The other day I met my friend Barbie at a coffeeshop where she studied and I "worked" (meaning: I blatantly checked out all the nerdy-cute guys from behind the safety of a notebook). I may be a complete social retard in a bar, but the coffeeshop scene is where I'm in my element. Nerds, intellectuals, and closet freaks, all pumped with caffeine-scented pheromones. It was primetime, so every table was taken. My eyes scanned across the room several times before deciding on one guy in particular, conveniently seated at two o'clock. He had a good view of me, I of him. A very nice view. Mmm. Diggity.

Before I go any further I should explain that one of my New Year's resolutions was to stop trying so hard with guys. Ignore guys, if possible. (It's not. Obviously. The Pussy speaketh with frightening force.) This at least leaves me at a nice compromise of refusing to go out of my way for any guy in any way.

If a guy wants to talk to me, he can be the one to come over and introduce himself. If a guy likes me, he can pursue me. Sometimes I want to scream at these guys. Just come over and talk to me. I'll be nice, damnit. Of course, they never come talk to me, the fuckers. I'm sick of being the one who makes the first move and does all the chasing. I'm tired. It's not easy running in heels.

This means my new approach to coffeeshop flirtations like this is to sit back, give him the silent go-ahead with a strategic attack of body language and look-aways, and wait for him to come to me. I've been told this works, but I won't believe it until I see it. Preferably below me and groaning with pleasure.

First part of flirtation strategy: Look inviting. There's more to this than body language. Even though I was with my friend, we each had our own little table because of all our books. With no one sitting at my table, the chair was for the taking (a-HEM Mr. Cute Boy) and there was no friend-barrier to have to break through. It can be awkward as hell flirting with someone when there are two or more people there because then you feel a little apologetic for not having chosen them, like "Oh, I'm so sorry, sweetie, but maybe if you smiled a little more, or didn't smell like a frat party, maybe then I would have hit on you instead of your nice friend here."

Even though I often work better with headphones on, I intentionally didn't bring my mp3 player because that is one of the biggest fuck-off moves you can make, intentionally or not. It doesn't always mean that, but it takes a far smoother person than I to break someone from his focused music to try to chat him up with any sort of casualness.

The final way I tried to look inviting was in the body language: Begin by facing your torso toward him. Don't hunch over and pull into yourself, no arms crossed (the #1 fuck-off signal, which sucks because sometimes you're just cold), but leaning back, taking up some space, maybe arms stretched out along the back of your seat. I have long legs that I like to stretch out to the side, especially since when they're crossed they hit up against the underside of the table. Bonus: If they're to the side then they're easier to see, hint hint, Mr. Cute Boy.

Once all of this was set, I began flirting in the little subtle ways that a guy can easily miss if he doesn't know to look for them. If he does know to look, and he knows what they mean, you generally won't have to do it for very long before he finds a way to talk to you.

Um, except this guy in the coffeeshop seemed to be a bit clueless. He looked over more often than a non-interested person would, but he wasn't smiling back. Hmm.

Time to start throwing in the occasional look-away. I first heard this term on a little-known movie called *Whipped* [which is funny, but it can easily make you lose faith in all mankind. And womankind. But, if you can get over that, it's really good]. A look-away is distinctly different from a glance or a regular look. A look-away is when you look at the person you're interested in until he notices you looking at him, then you look away real fast, but—just for a moment, because then while he's still watching you, you look at him again (coyly this time) so he knows you were looking at him on purpose until he caught you. It's a stupid game of flirtation, but it's still flirtation. This is the most common form of flirtation, usually without either person even knowing it's happening.

With my cup of coffee as my prop, I held it to my lips and drank (or rather, *pretended* to drink. I had finished it ages ago), then kept it just below my mouth so I could peer over my glasses at him in a way I hoped was alluring. Mr. Cute Boy looked over at me, but still without *any* emotion.

Fine, I can turn it up a notch. In a short skirt (gotta love warm Texas winters), crossing and uncrossing yourlegs can be very effective, especially if done slowly and with a little slide of your hand up your thigh. This did get some attention, but from the middle-aged guy at ten o'clock and the skeezy guy from two tables over. RETREAT!

Hair's next. I've heard good things about hair-flipping. I try hair-flipping. I'm out of practice. It's been a while since I've had really long hair and was single at the same time. Hmm. He's still not getting it. That's okay, I've never been good at hair-flipping. Twirling? I try hair-twirling, wrapping a curl around my finger. No, I suck at hair.

Back to body stuff. I'm better at body. Ooh, arm stretch! This is an excellent move. Not always subtle, but it still works. I stretched my arms up, stuck the boobs out a little, arched the back, and pulled the arms down at an angle that showed off how toned they are. Mr. Cute Boy looked over, but it was just that. No curiosity, no heat.

Come on, buddy, you're like ten feet away from me! You should be able to feel my lust from there.

Fine. You want to play that way? Time to shed some clothes. I start to pull my sweater off. Barbie looks over at me in astonishment, "Are you actually *hot* in here?" She was wearing a long-sleeved shirt and a sweaT-shirt. "Yes, I'm burning up." No, I'm shameless.

There is an art to pulling off the sweater. Many women are hot as hell when they do this, whether they know it or not. Or, maybe, that's just me being a pervert and staring at boobies again. Taking off a tight sweater is another good way to get attention, albeit occasionally unwelcome from K-Fed wanna-bes.

The guy keeps looking over, but with neutral eyes. What the fuck? Come on babe, I've got a tiny little top with spaghetti straps on. Look at me. For longer than half a second. Look at me. Lookatmelookatmelookatmeeeeeee. Oh, your *friend* is looking at me, so why the fuck aren't YOU looking at me the way I want you to look at meeeeeeeee?

I had one move left. If this didn't do it, nothing would, and I'd call it a day. I uncross my legs and stretch them out in anticipation of The Strut. Loudly I ask Barbie, "HEY, I'M GOING TO GET SOME WATER, DO YOU WANT ANYTHING WHILE I'M UP?" Then I mentally prepare for The Strut. Gotta be in the right mindset. You have to work it, without looking like you're working it. Which I sometimes *miss*, hence the mental pep talk. *Be sexy, don't be a dumbass, be sexy, don't be a dumbass, AND FOR FUCK'S SAKE, DON'T TRIP ON YOUR OWN FEET.*

Slowly, I stood to full height. I'm on the tall side to begin with, then pair that with some killer heels and I'm an Amazon who's hard to miss. I smooth down my skirt, fix eyes straight ahead but not on anything in particular and begin The Strut. Slow, smooth rolling of the hips done by placing one foot directly in front of the other, shoulders back, and pretend you're the hottest thing in the room. I'm certainly not, but I pretend I am. That goes a surprisingly long way. Act like you're worth looking at.

I walk to the coffee area and reach for water. It's empty. The coffee people are too busy for me to bother them. I strut back but I'm kinda feeling like a jackass for returning empty-handed. I should have picked up some napkins or something. Shit.

On the way back I feel the eyes of the creepy middle-aged guy and K-Fed Jr., but nothing from Mr. Cute Boy. I sat down with a huff. Fine, motherfucker.

My old self was telling me to forget my new-found resolve and hit on him already. The worst he could do was laugh in my face and tell me I was a fucking moron for thinking I stood a chance with someone like him. The new, hopefully wiser, self was telling the older one to shut the fuck up and not waste any more of my time. This one won. Part of being a big girl is admitting defeat when it's time.

I resumed working for the next half hour until Barbie and I decided to leave. As we were getting ready, Mr. Cute Boy and his friend started to leave as well. Shit. *Don't waste your time, Vix! Your ego needed a beating anyway, it builds character! You don't need to try one last time on your way out!*

We ended up right behind them at the door. Mr. Cute Boy suddenly decides to look at me in the sexy way I had been trying to pull out of him all evening. He holds the door open for me. I turn for one last glance before I walk toward my car. There he is, giving me an appreciative eye and smiling like a goddamn jackass.

Does she look inviting?
- sitting/standing by herself
- not fully involved in whatever she's doing, *i.e.* looking up a lot
- open body language – arms open, doesn't look stand-offish
- smiling (or at least not scowling)

Does she look like she's trying to get your attention?
- the look-away (lots of eye contact, especially if she follows the look-away with a little coy smile)
- smiling a lot, especially in your general direction
- moving around a lot, like crossing and uncrossing legs, playing with hair, stretching
- if she's with a friend, is she: laughing a lot and looking in your direction when she does it?

Of course, you don't need to have all of the above criteria in order to have a clear signal that she would be friendly if you talked to her. Even if she's doing all these things, it may still not mean she's interested or even available. She may just be fidgety. Some people are natural flirts or simply want attention. I'm just saying that this list gives you your best chance of knowing whether a girl will welcome you or not if you make a move.

Now that I'm done with the pep talk, it's time for the begging. Guys, if you see girls doing these subtle flirtations, please grow a pair and GO FUCKING

TALK TO HER. You probably have a better chance than you think, and how will you know that if you don't try?

Fuck Prince Charming, Where's My Frog?

With each new guy I dated, I was always waiting for that magical first kiss, the one that (I'm told) sends tingles down your body and makes you lose yourself in that precious moment.

I have never experienced a first kiss like that, or any kiss. I am told it happens, and not just in the latest clearance chick flick. Or, maybe, I've never felt that happy feeling because I've never been in love. I thought I had been with my last boyfriend, but maybe not.

Orgasms and being in love follow the same line of questioning: "Have you ever been in love?" "I'm not sure. I think I have. Once . . ." "Then you haven't been. You'd know if you had."

Well, hell.

Maybe I've never had that magical toe-curling kiss because I've never been in love. Or, maybe it simply doesn't exist. Is it one of those urban relationship myths? A modern-day fairy tale with a Jennifer Aniston character living happily ever after? Because most of those go straight to DVD.

Not that any of that will keep me from going from frog to frog, hoping this one will be the one who makes me weak in the knees with his slurpy, fly-flavored kiss. I may be a cynic, but I'm not a hopeless cynic.

I gave up on the whole idea of Prince Charming years ago, well before I hit puberty. I was quite the precocious cynic. Although it may seem like it sucks that I have little hope in happily ever after, I think it leaves me far better off. How many women have you met who describe their Prince Charming as tall, dark, handsome, super smart, has a PhD, travels all over the world, reads *Gourmet* magazine, speaks five languages (three fluently), has a trust fund, but makes six figures a year "for fun", volunteers for Habitat for Humanity, and can cook a mean lasagna (from scratch, of course)?

Yeeeeeah. I tell ya what. While you're looking for Prince Fucking Charming, I'm going to be over here kissing frogs. It's not like I expect our blossoming love to magically transform my frog into the perfect guy. Life doesn't work like that. I've finally learned that no matter what you do, you can't kiss a boy into a man. He has to do that on his own while he's out in the wild eating bugs and wondering why he's alone. This applies to girls too.

I am also (finally) not naive enough to think that some wonderful prince will kiss me and turn me into the strong independent woman I knew was down in there somewhere. Girls come in ugly frog form too.

Say all the wonderful things you want about love, it's not magic. It takes more than love and a helluva lot more than a kiss to transform someone.

The next time I'm ready to look around the pond, all I want is a cute little boy frog who will look me in my big bug eyes and tell me "You're the greatest girl frog I've ever met." And then we'll smooch and I'll eat flies off his plate and we'll live froggily ever after.

Do Not Judge Me Based on My Impulse Purchases

Today on my way home from work I stopped at the grocery store. It wasn't a full shopping-for-the-week grocery run, it was a milk/Oreos/yogurt run. In and out in twenty minutes for twenty bucks.

It was while I was standing in the check-out line that I noticed the woman in front was raising an eyebrow at me. At me and my purchases. Whatever. She was the middle-aged, matronly type, the sort whom I regularly and effortless offend for far worse reasons than my eating habits. I'm used to ignoring this sort of attention.

However, when I turned around and saw the twentysomething guy behind me casting The Eyes of Judgment at my grocery cart, I began to feel self-conscious. Sure, all he had were orange juice, beer, and cereal, but he's a *guy*. The grocery standards are different for single guys . . . it's more like *Congratulations! You're eating something that doesn't come from a drive-thru window! Here's a gold star and a lime wedge for your Tecate!*

For chicks, we supposedly know better. I mean, I *do* know better. But, sometimes, I just don't give a fuck. Like tonight, for instance:

Frozen meat lover's pizza and chocolate chip cookie dough ice cream (extenuating circumstances! I bought these specifically for tomorrow night's two-hour premiere of my favorite brain-candy show, *America's Next Top Model*, during which my friend Barbie and I eat pizza, talk about how we are so much hotter than the wanna-be models (*hips are hot, bitches!*), and then pass the tub of ice cream back and forth). Although, I must admit, I normally have both these things in my freezer anyway. *Today* I just happen to have a reason.

A huge bag of shredded cheese. None of the other items in my cart have any association with this one-pound bag of cheese. The cheese stands alone. Tons of yogurt. Cereal. Healthy cereal! It was on the top shelf out of reach of children's hands! Only responsible bran-loving adults can reach the top shelf! I AM NOT A TOTAL PIG. Only a partial pig.

From the bakery: A cream puff pastry and a Texas-girl-sized cinnamon bun. Neither of these were on my grocery list, but as soon as I saw them I had to have them. I've always had a thing for cinnamony goodness, especially any cinnamony goodness that is so big I have to skip dinner just so I can finish it. Normally the one pastry would have been enough to settle my cravings, but then I saw (*dear God, has it always been here in my grocery store?!*), a cream puff pastry identical to the one sold at Le Madeleine. The cream puff pastry which I have driven twenty minutes out of my way to acquire—it lies here before me in the refrigerated display unit. I MUST HAVE IT.

Milk. To go with above pastries. Oh, and the cereal. Right. I was thinking of the cereal . . . not really. I hardly ever have milk, so on most mornings I eat dry cereal from a plastic cup between putting on eye shadow and finding my right shoe.

The final *fat* to go on top of the *ass*: A loaf of French bread. *White* bread. Which I like dipping in olive oil. Another impulse purchase. Oh, sweet purposeless carbs, how I adore you. It's a good thing, because I have to use your long, thin form as a sword to fend off the biting words of nay-sayers. Bite THIS, carb-haters. I know you want it.

As much as I would love to end this post by saying something inspirational like, I WILL NEVER APOLOGIZE FOR MY LOVE OF CARBS, THEY KEEP ME MEATY AND JOLLY, it would not be an entirely truthful declaration.

Perched at the front of the cart (not exactly an accident) was a lone bag of mixed stir-fry vegetables, which I plucked from the produce section at the last minute. I was a tiny bit self-conscious about the contents of my cart before heading to the check-out line, I admit it. I had absolutely no plans of making stir-fry this week, and there's a slim chance that I will even now that I have the vegetables for it. I thought the bright green and orange glow of health would fend off any wandering Eyes of Judgment, a task at which it obviously failed. Perhaps, if I had thrown in a bell pepper and some celery? An organically-grown cucumber? What does it take to mask the shame of pleasantly plump pastries and assorted dairy products?

Don't get me wrong, I understand the value of wholesome food habits. I can throw together a mean three-bean salad. But, I also understand the ugliest of late-night eating truths: Sometimes a nice, unsatisfying plate of healthy green crap leaves you finding yourself at three in the morning shoving your face with Girl Scout cookies by the glow of the refrigerator light (if you do it at night when no one sees you, it doesn't count. It's simple math).

If that happens, don't blame me. Blame the carb-haters. They're the ones who ran off Krispy Kreme, for which I WILL NEVER EVER FORGIVE THEM. I hope they burn under layers of molten icing.

Being Honest

Readers often tell me that they like my blog because it's so unabashedly honest. Over the course of the last year and a half, readers have said with varying degrees of awe and suspicion, *this chick can't be real. No one's that honest.*

Of course, no one's that honest, not face-to-face. Oh hell no. By "no one" of course I mean me. Hell, especially me. For someone who lays it all out on the computer screen, I reveal very little of myself face-to-face. It's those two opposing personas who make up me. Their separation grows by the day.

It's here in the blog that I make up for what I never say in my ordinary life. It's between the hours of 8 p.m. and 3 a.m. that I admit what I'm really feeling, and then it's only under the cloak of a dark room and a pen name.

In my ordinary life, I'm completely closed off. Sure, I talk about blowjobs and share naked stories with friends, but I won't go any deeper than that. That's the thing about talking about blowjobs. Most people don't talk about them with such ease, so when friends and new acquaintances witness me in such a way, they presume I'm really open. That's the word I hear all the time, open. I know that's bullshit, yet I keep pulling the same bullshit, fully aware of what I'm doing.

For almost all of my twenties, up to this point, I used to cry all the time. In solitude only. There were so many things I cried about, nearly all of which were depression-induced. Not so much lately. It's been a while. Which would probably explain why when I cried earlier tonight it came from deep in the gut, so much so that it had me bending over my knees with my head in hands sobbing as if something horribly tragic had happened. But, of course, there's nothing to really cry about. Everyone's alive and healthy, I've got money to cover all my bills, and I can't remember the last time I needed a Xanax. I should be Mary Fucking Sunshine.

I don't cry nearly as much as I used to. As much as I would like to think that this is because I'm happy, or at least satisfied for the first time in years, I wonder if I cry less because I hold back so much more. If you hold it in deep enough, it never reaches the surface, and people stop trying to get in to find it.

Not once in my life have I had a best friend, not even when I was a little girl. Best friends are easy to acquire at that age. "If you share your cookie with me, I'll be your best friend!" I couldn't even manage it then. I wouldn't share my damn cookie. Twentysomething years later, it's a hundred times harder to make a best friend. There have been a few attempts at best friends, but none stuck for more than a couple months.

Readers often tell me that they feel like they know me better than their own sister. That's so fucking wrong. I'm sure many of you *do* know me better than your siblings, and I'm sure the same is for my brother and most friends. That's like three degrees of fucked up, especially since I've been aware of this for months and made no effort to change.

Sure, there are dozens maybe hundreds of strangers out there in cyberspace who know me better than my own brother, and I *like* my brother. I told him once "So I kinda write a lot now. I'm kinda good at it." That was all I said. Of course, he knows me in ways that no one but a brother could. Like how much I weigh when I sit on his chest and hover a wad of spit over his faces (which I have done as recently as Thanksgiving, by the way. Siblings transcend maturity), or all the colors my hair has been over the years, or that when I'm in the shower and in a good mood I sing *yummy yummy yummy I got looove in my tummy and yada yada yadadadaaaaaa* (I do. For real. His room is next to the bathroom and he finds it incredibly amusing to wake up this way on holidays when we're home). He knows all these things about me but he doesn't know that I hate my career or that I'm way funnier in cyberspace than in person (sadly, it's true). Which makes me wonder, can anyone ever really know all those many different sides of you?

In this happy little brooding-yet-sexy corner of the blogosphere, I can be as open as can be. No consequences. If a reader calls me out on something that hits a little too close to home, I can brush it off as some asshole who thinks he knows me but how can he when he doesn't even know what color my eyes are? Never mind that regular readers probably *do* know what makes me tick better than most people who know what I look like.

It would be nice to get over my fucked-up mindset one of these days. I would like to be as honest in my real life as the average person, let alone my blog identity. I'm not sure where it originated, but I know exactly what fed the insecurity that has made me so closed-off.

This is one of the increasingly rare days on which I wish I had someone special. I want to be able to cry and feel a set of arms surround me with love. I want someone who knows me to care that I'm crying. I want to figure out how to find that one day. I'm not even talking about a boyfriend, necessarily. A best friend, my mother, a neighbor.

I am scared out of my fucking mind that if I don't get over myself soon and let someone—anyone—in, I will never let someone who knows my real name have the chance to know the real me.

Keep Your Happy Memories Away From My Soft Drink

The other day I stopped at a Burger King for dinner. I don't eat fast food very often because if I'm going to eat crap, I'd rather eat sugary or chocolately crap. Lucky Charms at dinner, for example. Colorful, simultaneously soggy and crunchy, and three bucks for an entire box that won't leave my car smelling like French fries for a week.

But, I was hungry and far from the two flavors of ice cream waiting for me at home. Burger King it was.

I ordered one of the meals. Chicken strips, onion rings, Dr. Pepper, $4.32.

The lovely woman in the headset handed me a paper bag and my drink. Before I placed the drink in the cup holder, instinctively I popped in the little raised buttons on the plastic lid. DIET *pop!* TEA *pop!* OTHER *pop!* You can't drink until you've done that. Really. You just can't. The soft drink loses its carbonated magic if you don't pop in the buttons. Which is why for as long as I can remember, I have popped in every button on each drink topped with a plastic lid that has come across my hands. It's just what you *do*.

As I drove off (steering with the knee, pulling out onion rings with one hand and sipping from my drink with the other (see? I am very good at eating. You can't learn that kind of knee-hand-mouth coordination, you know. That's what my grandaddy calls *gotdamn-given talen*t)), I looked at the Dr. Pepper in my hand and was suddenly filled with sadness.

How the fuck can a *fucking soft drink* suddenly make me feel like crying?

Popping in the buttons on my drink lid had reminded me of the very first time Aussie and I bought fast food together. It was our second or third day of constant togetherness and we were doped up on pheromone-driven puppy love. We each ordered meals. As soon as he passed me my drink, I punched in all the buttons. This lid had a lot. There were FIVE. *Pop! Pop! Pop! Pop! Pop!*

Aussie looked at me in bewilderment. I explained. He found my odd little habit endearing. But, of course, it was the early stages of love—I could have been doing cartwheels with a piece of bacon in my mouth while attempting to speak only in iambic pentameter and he still would have found me adorable. (Although

244

that image is kind of charming, isn't it? And something I would totally do if I could do a cartwheel without falling on my ass. Or if I could speak in iambic pentameter without reciting what little I can remember of some stupid sonnet I was forced to memorize against my will in middle school.)

The next time we bought drinks, Aussie popped in all of the buttons on his lid too. He beamed at me. For the rest of our relationship, he would pop in all the buttons on every lid on every drink we enjoyed together. He liked the popping noise. Eventually Aussie stopped making a cute show of it and grinning every time. He just did it. He finally understood the philosophy of *Pop!*

So, the other day, when I looked down at my drink with the DIET TEA OTHER dimples punched in, I had found myself wondering if Aussie is still popping in the same buttons on his drinks.

Had it become natural to him after years of soft drinks with me? Was he out there living his life, punching in the buttons, and remembering me every time he did? If he was, did it make him angry to catch himself performing an ex-behavior? Has he purposely stopped punching in the buttons specifically because he associates it with me, the evil ex? Does it fill him with sadness like it did me just now? Does it make him smile just a tiny bit, knowing that he will still find himself doing this twenty years from now and telling his wife about some quirky girl from Texas he dated once?

Or maybe he has forgotten entirely.

What's worse, it bothers me that I care one way or another. Why can't a drink lid just be a fucking drink lid? *Pop! Pop! Pop! Pop!*

My Careers Aren't Speaking To Each Other

If someone walked into my apartment for the first time, she would think two completely different people lived here.

The kitchen table is covered in neat stacks of white binders, thick textbooks, and four different colored highlighters. Post-its peek out the sides marking important pages. It is silent except for the sound of the coffeemaker. A lovely young woman sits in a metal chair (purposely uncomfortable to prevent falling asleep) and studies like the good ruthless ladder-climber she was raised to be. What a fine young professional! Clearly, she is responsible and orderly (the closet is *organized by color* for fuck's sake) and arranges all her toiletries on the counter by order of use in the morning. Her shoes are always polished and her hair smells nice. Let's call her Jennifer.

Then walk into the bedroom, where the other girl lives in a world all her own. Let's call her Vix.

In the corner is a plush, wing-back chair. It was once nice, *a valuable antique!* the mother gushed. *She doesn't know the dogs left matching teeth marks on it.* Three side tables are covered in spirals, books, a single piece of pink Bubbleyum bubble gum, a dozen pens with the wrong-colored caps, men's magazines dog-eared and marked up (it's called research), and always the previous night's coffee mug.

There is a red sticky tab stuck to the neck of the lamp. The table it sits on is covered in a thick layer of white Post-it notes, each of which is covered with scrawled handwriting running in all directions and occasionally onto the table. Peeling away the layers of Post-it notes, she writes out her latest thoughts—the precursor to peeling off the day's clothes before slipping into bed.

The bedroom is Vix's domain. Not just because of its sexual nature, but because the surfaces are soft, the lighting is soft—and a hard girl softens up in her haven of books and solitude. With a single lamp on, she spends hours every night writing. She puts off dinner over and over, *just one more paragraph,* until it's 10:30 p.m. and her stomach is growling over the music and two televisions.

She doesn't notice the huge pile of laundry even though she steps over it in the hallway to reach the bedroom. She's so deep inside her own head that she doesn't notice the phone ringing or the dogs whimpering to go out. She only acknowledges the messy apartment with a scoff. She has better things to do than clean. Like study *Maxim* while sitting back in her beloved armchair in mismatched socks and glittery Superwoman underwear.

One has a filing cabinet at work covered with bright green ferns and flowers. The other only recently noticed that her cactus died. Judging from the state of wrinkliness, the cactus has probably been dead for months.

From the looks of it, these two roommates couldn't be more different. It wasn't always like that. They remind me of two best friends who moved into the dorm and after a semester of living together arranged their course schedules so they never had to be in the same room at the same time. One smugly told me once, "I haven't seen the bitch in a week. It's fantastic."

It looks like it won't be much longer before Jennifer and Vix reach the point of leaving catty Post-it's for each other on the bathroom mirror. *You used the last tampon. BUY MORE.*

Sure, Jennifer is the bright-eyed one you want to introduce to your parents, "Look, Dad! My friends have a good influence on me! We talk about our dental plans over two beers max!" But Vix is the one you want to get to know during one of those great conversations that can only be had at two in the morning while sitting outside with cheap beers wondering how life got so fucked up.

I don't want to see two such different sides to myself. I don't want them existing in different rooms with the doors slammed closed. To a certain degree it's natural to have many different personas that come out as appropriate (the employee, the sister, the wife, the nerd, the daughter), but to this extent? They are both me. Both have always been there, just never before with such conviction. Now, so much is brewing, so much anger and resentment. They yell at each other *you're holding me back! this isn't what I wanted! You're screwing everything up! I HATE YOU.*

How can two such different people exist in the same apartment at the same time, let alone in the same *head*?

So, what now? I'm not worried so much about the careers—I'll be fine one way or another—but I'm scared as fuck about the growing distance between the two personas behind those career choices. Jennifer and Vix once lived together peacefully. Although different, they were complementary. At first the contrasts brought out the best in each other, then somewhere along the way the complements became opposites. It's only a matter of time before a mean-ass nasty chick fight erupts. Who will be the winner in the end?

Nympho Statement

This is an iteration in my Nympho Statement. They are different every time. Long. Just because you're born a nympho doesn't mean you naturally know how to wear it. But now? Now I wear it with ease. Which is why my latest Nympho Statement is one of the shortest posts I've ever published.

I am a nympho. I always have been and always will be. A lot of people don't get that.

This is about me and my sexuality, my sensuality, the fucking essence of who I am. This is not a slut thing or an identity issue or an intellectual matter. It's just *me*, pure and raw.

No apologies.

My Boyfriend TiVo Broke Up with Me

It happened a week ago, but I haven't been able to face it. My TiVo broke.

I'm heart-broken. We were together for so long! We got along so well! I LOVED MY TIVO SO MUCH! *How could my TiVo do this to me?!*

I LOVED YOU!!! I WAS NOTHING BUT GOOD TO YOU, AND *THIS* IS WHAT YOU DO TO ME?

—weeps over the discarded remote—

And with no warning! One day we were fine, he was playing all my shows for me and I was happy as could be, then the next day . . . I could tell something was wrong. He didn't light up when I clicked my remote. No! NO!!! How could this be?! What had I done wrong?

Frantically I pressed the cute little TiVo logo power button on the remote—the very button that had brought me so many hours of delight when I needed a pick-me-up after a long, boring day at work. *Maybe* Sex and the City! *He offered, or* America's Next Top Model *(a marathon!!), perhaps that would be better? No, my darling Vix, you need one of your favorites tonight, how about* The Office? *You like that episode where Dwight leaves Ryan stranded on a beet farm, don't you? Oh, that Dwight is so bizarre. How about that, would that make you feel better, my love? Here, let me put it on for you . . . or would you rather put on something brand new? You want to stop to make a sandwich? Go ahead, my darling. I'll be right here waiting for you.*

My boyfriend, TiVo, was so nice. So caring, so attentive!

Was. Prick.

After he first broke, I thought maybe he just needed some space. I unplugged him so he could cool off (we got very heated in our argument), and let him be.

The next day after work I dropped my work bag and went straight to my (ex?) boyfriend, TiVo. I plugged him back in and waited a few moments . . . the light came on!! There was hope for us!! I squealed in delight and wrapped my arms around his plastic casing. *My darling TiVo, let's never fight again.*

But the asshole wasn't done. Nuh-uh. *He was fucking with my head.* He clicked on, but the typical listing screen was frozen! *No! No, my love, don't turn your back on me, give me another chance!* I sunk to my knees in front of the television. Desperately, I pressed every button on the remote. Why won't he listen to me?!

In frustration I tore the cords from the back. I smacked him upside the head. *I AM NOT READY TO GIVE UP ON US. DO YOU HEAR ME??* —smack smack— *WE BELONG TOGETHER YOU IDIOT.* —SMACK SMACK SMACK—

In tears, I tried one last time. I plugged him in and hoped. *We can get through this.* Laying down on the carpet in front of him, I waited for what I hoped would be kind words.

The light came on. A few moments later I heard the familiar comforting *blip!* of TiVo. I hugged the remote to my breast. Could it be?! Was TiVo willing to give me a second chance?

I scrolled through the listings . . . wait . . . half of what was previously recorded was gone . . . IS HE REALLY THIS COLD-HEARTED?! MUST HE BE SO PASSIVE-AGGRESSIVE?! WHY NOT JUST DELETE THEM ALL AND BE DONE WITH IT? WHY MUST HE LEAD ME ON WITH FALSE HOPE??

Frantically, I pushed buttons to program a current show. He wouldn't record! But there was plenty of hard drive space, because HE JUST DELETED HALF OF MY FUCKING SHOWS. Why wouldn't he record?! I tried again. I pleaded with him. How could he sit there before me yet refuse to speak to me! What happened to my sweet TiVo?! He is but a ghost of the digital recording device he once was!

Since that dreadful night a week ago we have been existing in silence. I pleaded with him a few more times, *please baby, just record one thing! Show me you care! Don't break it off with me so suddenly, I beg you!* Alas, we have turned our backs on each other. He refuses to record, I refuse to admit that we will never be the same again.

I called my father for guidance. My father is a very smart man. He knows exactly where to smack each appliance to make it work again. We talked and talked about how I could fix it, but some things are simply too far beyond repair.

I know in my heart it's time to let him go. He had been around for so long, I was beginning to take him for granted. He would record so many things for me, which I would neglect for weeks or dismiss with ruthless rounds of deletions. Poor TiVo. All that effort, deleted without an ounce of emotion on my face.

I suppose it is remarkable he stuck around for as long as he did. It's been ages since I sat down and spent quality time with him. *Please, my love!* he begged, *I have so many things to share with you! Just sit down with your dinner for an hour! Half an hour! Twenty-three minutes if you fast-forward through the commercials*!

I sat down with him less and less. Often he'd play me beautiful things while I fussed around the apartment with chores and cleaning, but I didn't really pay attention to him. He could have been speaking in Spanish and I wouldn't have noticed. He'd be chattering away in the living room telling me great stories while I hid out in the bedroom working away on my laptop.

I'm sorry, baby, I told him so many times. *I just don't have time for you anymore . . . maybe this weekend? We'll watch a movie together, I promise! Just some patience, sweetie . . .* Maybe it is all my fault. I was so neglectful. We had our good times, and now it is time to go our separate ways.

I guess it's a good thing my boyfriend never found out that I've been seeing iTunes for weeks.

Sometimes Love Isn't Enough

The break-up with Aussie was eight and a half months ago. I haven't talked about the actual break-up that much. The aftermath, the random memories that pop up—these I have mentioned as they crept into my mind because talking about them is the only way to get them to go the fuck away.

Today, I had the movie *Prime* playing as background noise while I moved in and out of the bedroom with laundry and the vacuum cleaner. Suddenly, a familiar scene snapped me to attention as if someone had smacked me in the face.

I left the laundry on the floor and sat down at the edge of the bed. *Rewind.* Lil Lesbian lay down next to me with a reassuring paw on my leg (how do they know?). *Play.*

> Love is not always enough, not when you're talking about marriage and children and joint checking accounts . . . I'm not saying love isn't important, it is, but . . . I'm saying that—sometimes you love, and you learn, and you move on. And that's okay.

This scene threw me back to sitting on our blue couch in our living room in our apartment. Nine months ago, I was watching this movie for the first time. Aussie and I had rented it on a Friday night. He fell asleep halfway through so I sent him to bed. Some movies are better enjoyed solo anyway. Like chick flicks that you can sense don't end with the standard *happily ever after*.

It had only been a few days earlier that I had had a panic attack driving home from a baby shower at the office. So is it really a surprise that watching Meryl Streep say these things to her son brought on a forty-five minute fit of sobbing? It was bad. Really bad.

I turned down sex twice that weekend. Before that, I had turned down sex maybe five times *ever*. Didn't matter how bad my depression was or how busy I was, I rarely turned down sex. Aussie asked me about it. I waved him off and said

I was depressed and kept forgetting to take my meds (which was true, but not *the* truth).

When I watched this scene again today, it brought back so many memories that made my gut surge all over again. That weekend was the beginning of a two-week mental fog that ended with the break-up. It was such a miserable time, even though my friends were doing their best to keep me in good spirits with pool parties and countless pitchers of sangria. Not that it matters—all I remember was that I was just barely holding myself together enough not to cry at work. And that was with the help of my emergency Xanax pills hiding in the paperclip container on my desk.

I replayed the scene once more, taking it all in now that I remembered all the feelings that little twenty seconds of dialogue had triggered. I mostly remember the sobbing, the wails that came from deep in my gut. Aussie was asleep in the next room, so I covered my mouth with my hands and did my best to hold it in. I would have no idea what to say—other than the truth—if I woke him up with my crying. It only made me cry harder that I didn't know what to say.

I knew why I was crying. I just didn't have the strength to hold up that reason and examine it in the light. How was I supposed to hold myself together on my own when I could barely face the world with him at my side? Was I ready to learn from the relationship and move on without him? Would I really be okay?

But, I had to leave. Because sometimes love just isn't enough—and it takes more courage than I ever thought I had to admit that to myself.

He Had Me at Hello... And Lost Me Anyway

On Saturday, I went to the pool for the first time this spring. Ah, this is the fleeting and precious time that Texas has perfect weather, which means I will be enjoying it as much as I can before it becomes so hot and humid that I break a sweat walking from the car to my mailbox.

If you'll recall, last summer the pool scene was a source of great amusement (and blog material). So, when I went to the pool for the first time this weekend, I have to admit I was hoping for a little drama, a little something fun to kick off the swimming season. I was not disappointed.

Walking down to the pool from my apartment on the fourth floor, I noticed a hot guy getting settled at a lounge chair. I checked him out from head to head and thought to myself, *Oh this will do JUST FINE . . . mmmmm yessirreeeee get that fine piece of man-ass over here, babycakes.*

I spread out my towel on a lounge chair at the other end of the pool from the hot guy, thankful that my sunglasses could hide my eyes while I shamelessly stared at him. He had dark, dark brown skin (Indian heritage, perhaps?) and a fine muscular body. He had the potential to provide me with hours of poolside entertainment while staring over the top of my latest issue of *Cosmopolitan*.

Before I even had a chance to find a good magazine article, the hot guy had jumped into the pool and swam all the way across to where I sat. He came up out of the water and leaned over on the edge of the pool (exhibiting his fine biceps in a purely accidental way, I assume—not that I wasn't shamelessly posing with my long legs crossed, stomach sucked in, and breasts jutting out just a tiny bit to make the most of my itty, bitty, red bikini, but like, *whatever*).

He just *leaned* there. He didn't say anything, he didn't make eye contact, he didn't do *anything*. At first, I snickered because I thought he was nervous about talking to me, but he continued to NOT DO ANYTHING and so I began to think, *Oh my God, maybe I was being a cocky ass and he wasn't really coming over here to talk to me. Ohmygod, I'm so fucking conceited. Look at your magazine. Don't look up. Read your fucking magazine, you stupid ass and maybe he won't notice that you were staring at him like he was supposed to talk to you.*

"Uh, hi."

Yesssssss!!!!! I am not a conceited ass! He really was coming over here to talk to me! GO MEEEEE!!!

"Hey there." *I am sooo smooth. I am COOL, man.*

We stared at each other sheepishly.

"I'm David."

"I'm Vix."

He looked at me. I looked at my magazine. *I AM COY. I AM THE DICTIONARY DEFINITION OF COY. I AM ROCKING THIS COY SHIT.*

"Shit. I hadn't thought this far about what I was going to say once I got over here." He grinned with embarrassment. I was smitten. Awwww, *he's an idiot, and he 'fesses up to it! And he's SMOKIN' HOT.*

"Well, at least you admit to it. That's almost as good as having witty banter prepared." *Not really. I'm lying. I want in your pants.*

"Witty banter, that would have been good. Shit. Umm . . ."

"Well, you can cover for the fact that you don't have anything clever to say by asking me lots of questions." *I'm being such a bitch. I don't care. I'm used to being the one doing all the chasing. I'm just going to sit here and make him sweat a little.*

"Um . . . tell me about yourself!" And with that David pushed himself out of the pool in one smooth bicep-ridden motion. I forgot what witty banter had been forming in my head. He sat down on the chair next to mine.

He's sitting right next to me. I could reach out and touch his crotch right now if I wanted to . . . DAH!! Focus, woman.

I talked about how I love going to the pool. He dripped cold water onto my arm. In the middle of me speaking he stopped and said, "*Damn*, you have a nice body."

Um. Did he really just say what I think he said? I didn't know how to respond to that. You want a guy to think that, but it's weird to actually hear him say it.

"What's your name again?" he asked me. I stared at him.

256

"Are you really that bad with names?"

"Yes. What was it?"

"Vix."

"Vix. It's nice to meet you, Vix and *damn* you have beautiful thighs." He covered his mouth and looked away.

I busted out laughing. Okay, so he's not a creep. He's just a good ol' fashioned dumbass. I continued laughing.

"Um . . . I'm going to go back over there for a minute . . ." and he got up and walked away. I laughed harder. *I am so mean. And I so don't care. I'm double-mean.*

I picked up my magazine and pretended to read it, but of course I was watching him at the other side of the pool. He picked up his beer, took a long swig, and put it back down on the table. It tipped over and spilled everywhere. I busted out laughing all over again. He shook his head and leaned back in his chair, like *I totally meant to do that. I wanted to make you laugh, really.*

While David drank his beer, I looked at my magazine and started drafting out how things would go with my new lust-interest. Already I was outlining a blog post about how I met Dark Cocoa, my hot foreign neighbor who would surely become a fuck buddy and displace my hot Spaniard neighbor from when I lived in Manhattan as "the best next-door lay I ever had". I felt smug over my good fortune.

A few minutes later Dark Cocoa came back and sat down next to me. We talked about all sorts of things, all the while I was sizing him up in greater detail: well-spoken, good job, older (32), hot tattoos, hotter body, nice smile, looks like he won't be afraid to throw me around the bedroom a little bit—

But then . . . he went from being a cute ordinary idiot to a raving moron. He wouldn't leave me alone, even when I clearly opened my magazine and started reading, he knocked my taste in music a little too seriously to be mere teasing, he asked me three more times what my name was (it's a perfectly common name. Come on.), he didn't leave me alone after Barbie joined me at the pool and I kicked him off her chair (I had forewarned him a girl friend of mine would be joining me), he burped (Not sexy. Not funny. Not ever.), he wouldn't stop fucking talking (he spoke twice as much as I did, and usually I'm the one who talks more than my fair share), and finally—he shared his theory on homosexuals and how they're different from "normal people." At first, I debated with him, but quickly I gave up. He was a lost cause.

Finally, I pretend-napped. It took twenty minutes of pretend-napping to get him to go away. After he left, my friend shot me a look. I buried my head in my hands. She didn't have to say anything. I let out a huge sigh and cursed his idiocy. Does he realize *how close* he was to having me use him for sex? DAMNIT.

See? This is why I should move to a nicer apartment. I need higher quality guys to check out at the pool. Or at least someone who can keep my interest longer than an ad in *Cosmo* for a new facial cleanser. Woo-hoo, fight that acne! *Oh, I'm sorry sweetie, what did you say your name was again?*

Facing the Folks Again

Last weekend I went to visit my family for Easter. I was nervous as fuck because I planned on telling The MOM that I want to be a writer.

I fear the wrath of The MOM. You probably think I'm exaggerating The MOM, don't you? Nuh-uh. I speaketh the truth.

About six months ago I visited my parents in an attempt to tell them I don't like my current career and am thinking about becoming a writer. The weekend trip did not go well. She had me crying before I even started. I went back home with my tail between my legs and my head in my hands.

A couple weeks later in a wonderful weekend of bonding over spareribs and beer, I got the ovaries to tell my father that I write and it's beginning to show a lot of promise. I very vaguely may have perhaps mentioned when he was on his third beer that I would like to have a career as a writer. I'm not sure how much that registered.

Since then, whenever we talk, Dad asks me how the writing is going, to which I respond with something vague. My father does not need to know I write about blowjobs or make sales commission on sex toys. Nonetheless, it means a lot to me that he asks. He has seen my face light up when I talk about my writing. He gets that, and that means a lot to me.

He has told The MOM about my writing, which she asks about with less concern than when she asks if I received my AAA card. Which is why I'm hiding behind my father and telling him to go forth with my message, hail The MOM. This is how a lot of information is passed along between my mother and—through Dad. It's not like we hate each other or get in screaming matches, it's just that weird love/hate mother/daughter thing that I would really like to grow out of.

I drove up to my parents' house on Good Friday. After eating a hearty meal worthy of its heartburn, we settled down to watch a couple episodes of *The Office* over bowls of Blue Bell ice cream, just like we always do when I visit. We laughed in unison at Dwight's funny antics and shared our own stories of crazy coworkers. It was nice. It was a perfect little family moment, minus the smell of my father's bare feet.

This is the time, I told myself. Do it! *Your brother isn't here! It's just you and Mom and Dad! It's perfect! Tell them, tell them, tellthemtellthem.*

I couldn't do it. Several times I straightened up and looked at Mom, sighed, and then sank back down into the comfort of my armchair.

The next day we celebrated Easter. On the drive to my grandmother's house, my parents were telling me what to say to my eighteen-year-old cousin who is trying to decide which college to go to.

"This decision is very important, make sure he understands that."

"Tell him it can determine the course of the rest of his life!"

"You're so lucky you got into the program you did, I was surprised you did because it's so competitive."

Thanks, Mom.

"Thank God you did, look at how well you're doing at your job now! And you just got a raise!"

It's only 10:30 a.m and I've already been blind-sided with the family Guilt Stick. Fuck. This does not bode well for my little speech.

After our official Easter meal, all my aunts and uncles stayed chatting at the table. For the first time I can remember, none of my two dozen cousins were there. BECAUSE THEY KNOW BETTER. This means I had no one else to talk to or hide with. The elders in my family (elders is defined as the generation that knows what's best for you) are very career- and education-oriented. Aunts and uncles constantly compare their children's grades, spouses, salaries, or any other semi-quantifiable criterion to each other's. None of my cousins feel this competition personally. We are simply pawns in the scoring of I Raised My Child Better Than You. Which, I must say, is a fantastically boring game when you've heard it over and over for years.

As usual, the conversation turned to which of my cousins were in college/grad school and had a promising career. Everyone gushed over one particular cousin (my main competition, in the eyes of our mothers) who is graduating from an Ivy League university this summer and she is just *so* smart and *so* talented and *so* driven and it's such a blessing to have her in our family.

SHE WAS A TOTAL POTHEAD IN HIGH SCHOOL, BY THE WAY.
If I told my aunts and uncles that, they would probably gush, S*ee? She's so smart! She still made salutatorian while STONED.*

—sigh—

Eventually The MOM started talking about my high school cousin who's choosing which school to go to, one of which was where I attended undergrad. I straightened up. Finally, we get to brag about *me*. The MOM talked about the competition there and once again said something about how I was never as smart as my cousins or my brother—*what was your SAT score, honey?* (which she knows perfectly well was among the lowest in my class, because she won't let me forget it)—but I'm just so *well-rounded* that I got in anyway.

Say what? What the fuck was that? Did I just get a back-handed compliment? I tried to jump in to ask her to explain, but she kept cutting me off to talk about my high school cousin. Dad noticed my jaw tighten and offered a sympathetic look. *You know how your mother is. She didn't mean it like that.*

Then why the fuck did she say it, I thought. Again, AGAIN. I've heard her say that bullshit so many times, like I'm the dumbest person in the room. I got up and left before anyone saw the tears in my eyes and they urged me to come back and talk about my issues. I don't have issues, I HAVE RELATIVES.

Fortunately, I had one of my dogs with me, so I mumbled the excuse, "I have to take her out to piss." HA HA, I SAID "PISS" IN MY GRANDMOTHER'S HOUSE! HOW YOU LIKE ME NOW, JESUS CANDLE?

As I walked around the backyard with my dog, I wondered if I would ever grow a spine around my mother. I know she's not a bitch, I know she means well, I know she's proud of me, sometimes, so why does it still get to me so much when she says crap like that? My mother is a good woman, so why the hell do I always leave town wanting to choke her? I love her, I respect her, I would love to have half the strength she does, and yet I wonder—why don't I ever feel good enough for her?

Now I can't tell her I want to be a writer, not this weekend. Not after that shit about how lucky I am to have *slipped in between the cracks* to a good school.

Not after my aunts and uncles bragged about their kids with fancy science degrees and PhD's in things I've never heard of. My mother probably thinks writers do nothing but drink booze, write poetry in a field of a flowers, and commit suicide. They certainly don't have PhD's in Aeroneurophysiobionauticalology, and their parents definitely did not spend a fortune on an education for them to be known as the blowjob queen of the blogosphere.

After we left my grandmother's house (and I swallowed my first Xanax in months), we went to a party at my uncle's house. This is the side of the family that drinks, laughs heartily, and doesn't give a rat's ass what you do with your life as long as you're a decent human being. I'm glad we ended the night here. Brisket, booze, and no one giving their unsolicited opinion of what you should do with your life. These are my people.

Driving back that night, we stopped at a grocery store at Mom's request. That left me and Dad alone in the car. Due to this and my tongue loose with tequila, I had the talk with my father. It also helped that I was in the back seat and didn't have to look at him head-on.

"You know this whole writing thing I always talk about, Dad? Well, I'm kinda good at it. Kinda really good at it. I want to try to be a professional writer. I've been told that I'm good enough that I should write a novel, and it might have a chance of going somewhere. I'm good, Dad."

"Wow, a novel? Really?? That's great! What about?" His face lit up with a smile.

"Just . . . the last couple years of my life. Depression, school, dating, not dating, trying to figure out what the hell I'm doing with my life, the stuff everyone goes through in their early twenties . . ." *Like sex. Lots and lots of sex. With the occasional Xanax chaser or side of GIRL.*

"Wow, that's great!" He looked genuinely excited. So I kept talking.

"And . . . I have a blog. Like from that article in *Wired* you were reading? It's getting big. I have about a thousand hits every day."

"WOW." His jaw dropped. "What is the address so I can check it out?"

SHIT! RETREAT, RETREAT!!

"It's, uh, too personal, Dad. That'd be weird. But I'm working on other stuff too." Also too personal, but whatever.

"Oh, OK . . ."

"Don't worry, I'm not quitting my day job or anything, but I just want you to know that's what I'm working toward in the next five years."

"Well, kid. As long as you can support yourself." He smiled at me. I beamed.

"This next year is really promising, Dad."

At that moment Mom returned to the car. I hid my face in a book.

The next day was Easter. Whenever my brother or I visit, our parents take us to a nice Sunday brunch to fill our bellies before making the long drive back to our respective cities.

Over coffee and Texas-sized omelets, we chatted about the usual stuff. My parents asked me about my job and the annual review. From there I managed to segue into telling them about my friend's business idea that he wants me to be involved in when they start in a couple years. I hadn't mentioned this to either of them before.

"So, that's one thing that may happen in the next couple years . . . and there's the writing thing . . ." I looked at Mom. She put her fork down. Eep.

"I have an idea for a novel I want to write, Mom. I'm good. And I have a lot of other little writing projects in the works over the next couple months. Who knows where all that could lead in a few years . . ."

The MOM stared me down. I was now talking to my half-eaten omelet.

"Mom, I really like writing. And I'm good at it. In a couple years—after I finish the training program at work of course, because I know that's important—I may like to do that. For work. And I can still do consulting work on the side, so I'd still be in my current industry too . . ." My pleading eyes had no effect on my omelet.

The MOM looked at me, face blank.

Dad started running interference. "That's a really smart way to go about it, sweetie. Making your own opportunities and being prepared for whatever comes your way. I always knew you'd be better off working for yourself."

"Mom? I'm really good at writing . . . I could do both . . ." *Could I? Shit, I don't even know.*

I glanced over at her. She turned her head in the opposite direction to hide her pursed lips. Her silence said exactly all the things I was afraid of hearing.

I looked back down at my plate and resumed eating. I didn't know what else to do.

When we came back from brunch, I started packing up to make the long drive back home. As usual Mom was sending me back with boxes of stuff—a lamp, a DVD, some clothes, a blender, some books, leftovers. Because of all the stuff Mom was bringing in to my room, Dad offered to drive my car around to the back, so I wouldn't have to walk as far to load everything.

I was busy sorting through all the random things Mom had left in my room (including an issue of Oprah's *O* magazine with a Post-it note marking "Warning: Moving in Together Could Be Hazardous to Your Relationship." *Yes, Mom*) so I didn't pay much attention to how long my father was gone. A few minutes later he came for boxes to start loading into my car.

It wasn't until I was in the car making my way out of the neighborhood that I noticed my gas gauge. Normally I can make it door-to-door on exactly one tank of gas, leaving me driving up to my parents' house with a bright "E" glowing from the dashboard.

There was no "E." In fact, it looked like I had a quarter tank of gas. Impossible. I *know* I saw an "E" when I pulled up in front of their house on Friday.

Dad. I bet Dad put gas in my tank because he knew there was a good chance I would forget to stop for gas before I got on the highway, and there wouldn't be another station until outside the city limits. Awww, *Dad.*

I filled up at a gas station and then headed for the highway. As I accelerated up the entrance ramp tears filled the corners of my eyes. Good ol' Dad. He's always watching out for me, no matter where my journey may lead.

Part III

Life is like topography, Hobbes. There are summits of happiness and success, flat stretches of boring routine, and valleys of frustration and failure.

Calvin & Hobbes, Bill Watterson

Depression Is a Big Fat Motherfucker of a Blessing

With each new mental *what the fuck* of depression, ADHD, bipolar suggestions, whatever the hell other neurological demons are being unearthed, I feel that much more . . . distanced? Not normal? I dunno, *SCREWED?*

It makes me wonder—how much farther along could I be in my life if it weren't for depression and ADHD? What if I had been happy—or at least NOT depressed—for the last six years instead of sinking through all the levels of brooding? What if I had not been miserable with my own inner demons while working in New York City? Could I still be living there now instead of in Texas, wondering how and when I'll be able to go back? Would I have been more open to relationships? Would I have been strong on my own instead of expecting a boyfriend to make me happy? How much better could my life be if it weren't for depression?

Here's where I choke on the irony: Maybe my life is *better* because of depression.

Recently, I realized that all the good things that have entered my life are because of depression. Hours and hours of crying make for a lot of introspection. One day you get sick of crying and you ask yourself, W*hy the fuck am I crying so much? What's wrong? What do I have to change so I don't wake up and want to go right back to bed?* And then you get off your ass and do something about it. Of course, it takes a while for the depression cloud to lift, but it does. Eventually. And then you wonder why you waited so fucking long to listen to that little voice inside your head.

I'm thinking that depression can be a blessing if embraced as an opportunity for change. I don't mean for this to sound all Tyra-trying-to-be-Oprah, my intention is just to say, well, *why THE FUCK didn't anyone tell me that six years ago?* I got "Aw, poor you! Here are a bunch of books on depression that will make you feel worse than you already do because they are utterly uninspiring and make the guilt feast on what little remains of your soul! Kisses!!"

Seriously. Why didn't anyone tell me that depression doesn't have to suck? I mean, duh, by definition it sucks, but it doesn't have to suck *forever*. It can be a motivator to change. I think I've become a much stronger and wiser person for going through depression than if I had coasted through my life on normal, I really do. I'm positive my life would be very different now if I hadn't gone through so many cycles of depression. After so much time spent silent, complacent—I finally feel like I'm moving forward.

Depression is the reason I started writing. Depression is the reason I left a sucky job. Depression is the reason I left my last relationship. Depression is the reason I'm busting my ass so I don't spend the rest of my life as a corporate whore.

Depression is the reason I'm happy now. It didn't let me cruise through life. Over and over again it held up a mirror to me and said, *Can you face the person you see before you.*

For the first time in years, the face in the mirror is looking at me straight in the eye, and the cheeky bitch is winking.

Perverts Perverts Everywhere

As you may have guessed, I have become quite an expert on the world of perverts (does that make me a "pervpert"? *eeee tee hee hee heee*).

As a self-proclaimed nympho listed very high on Google searches for assorted sexual terms and phrases (including "goat sex midget porn". I think midget porn is funny, OK? *It comes up in everyday conversation*).

Throw in the goat and a bag of Cheetos and that is one slammin' Friday night alone on your couch with your hand down your pants (NOT in response to the goat midget porn (see the Just Stoppin' By Pervert below), but because that is your hand's default resting position. Hey, do not judge me. You are the weirdos Googling "goat sex midget porn.").

Many perverts cross my path. Many perverts are so dedicated to the cause that they throw themselves into my path with promises of driving across the country[3] to meet me "for dinner", flying me to their native country[4] (one of which I still can't find in an atlas), and sending me photos of their naked hairy ass[5] (see The Hardcore Pervert listed below).

Before we proceed: I've said it once. I've said it twice. I'm saying it again. DO NOT PROPOSITION ME. I WILL SAY NO. And then I will make fun of you for the general amusement of others. It's how I heal the pain. And, babycakes, I got *a lotta* pain.

All emails posted below are REAL. I have done NO EDITING except remove names and shorten one very long email. Everything listed in this entire post has actually happened, much to my amusement, displeasure, and occasional overwhelming disgust. I added my own commentary, but really the poetry oozes from the perverts themselves.

---

[3] This happens regularly. Which I find especially amusing because I don't think many people realize that driving across Texas can take fourteen hours.
[4] This has also really happened. Oddly, most of them seem to be offers from Britain.
[5] Sigh. This has also really happened.

If any of the people I make fun of actually read my blog more than the one time it took to see fuck written everywhere and find my email address and you are offended that I'm taking such delight in ridiculing you: Um, have you *read* what you wrote me? Yuh-huh. Now, excuse me, I have to get back to my pointing and laughing.

THE DUMBASS PERVERT

The most common type of pervert in the blogosphere, at least from what I've seen. The guy (they are almost always guys . . . of all the weirdos I've encountered, only two were chicks) can be identified by the following characteristics: inability to spell, poor grammar, and assume a girl will be happy to jump his bones simply because he asked.

Email #1

> *Subject*: Wassup so ur single huh hmmm I stay in dallas tx maybe we should get together sometime cuttie
> –[name]

That's it? Dude, can't you at least wait until the body of the email to hit on me? Gotta do it in the subject line? Really? WOW. I'm guessing you're the kind of guy who ejaculates before you manage to get your pants off? Oh, my apologies, I shouldn't assume that you wear pants. You probably walk around in your boxers all day (if anything at all) because that provides easy access and one less garment to get your man love juice on. Hell, sweetie, sounds like you don't even need me, except perhaps to provide laundry tips for those stubborn stains.

My response to Email #1

> *Subject*: RE
> No.
> Dude, I don't do random propositions. If that were my intention, I'd be on adultfriendfinder.com.

P.S. . . . and it's "cutie". Learn to fucking spell.

Comment by Anonymous:
> I still don't get why aint getting laid woman,which part of Tx r u cos am in Tx and there r a lot of ever ready walking dicks around here including me .
>
> Dang why don't I just meet chics like u.Well u can buzz me up on [upmine@idiot.com] and maybe we can do a lil' smth smth.

OK, readers, I know you're disappointed in me for not jumping all over this hot piece of man-ass. It was very hard to keep my hand out of my pants, because his lyrical words wooed my previously cold and unfeeling heart into the throbbing fiery ember it is today. I had to handcuff myself to the bed to keep from throwing myself out the window in desperation that I can't find quality guys like this in my daily life and cover them with grateful kisses.

Again: take the time to spell out the entire word. If you can't take the time to spell out "your" or "because" (at least do "b/c" if anything), what makes me think you'll take the time to do anything else properly? Besides, it's annoying as fuck.

THE PERVERT NEXT DOOR

Then there are all the emails which start off normal and then somewhere slip in an address to a MySpace page "in case you want to know what I look like". Um . . . thanks? But not really? This happens a lot from the more normal perverts out there. They are often the guys who ask if I can mail them a pair of my panties (sure, babycakes, you want a blood-stained pair with SpongeBob SquarePants or some stretched out ones I've had since eighth grade? Neither? Aw shucks, watch me cry on the inside and punch you on the outside.).

These are the perverts who have only 50 gigs of pr0n in addition to a bajillion DVDs and a much-loved old school collection of VHSs, including a copy of the original *Debbie Does Dallas*—which is nothing short of pure 70's-style awesomeness, complete with bush so full you think she's still got underwear on.

THE "JUST STOPPING BY" PERVERT

This is made up of Google searches. All of these sadly are real. I'm hoping that most were done in jest and not out of genuine curiosity. But, it's really best not to dwell on this kind of pervert for too long, because then I might start to cry in fear of the state of mankind. Not humankind. Mankind.

> over forty women sucking teenage son
>
> midget doing goat
>
> making your balls into "the goat" [OK, not perverted but very funny.
> Goats make me giggle every time, especially if testicles are involved]
>
> tampon string camel toe
>
> midget delight
>
> fuck mom tits
>
> eurotrash tattoo
>
> my dad spanks me but when he does he practically humps
>
> are you a pervert quiz [Ah, too bad I hadn't written this post yet. But safe
> to say: If you have to ask, you probably are]
>
> fuck thirteen boy
>
> dental floss bikini
>
> granny licking balls and dick

EWWW! Ew, ew, ewwwie ew ew, EWWWWWWW. THAT IS YOUR GRANDMOTHER. Grandma can probably give some fine head when she takes her teeth out, but, like WHOA. Gummy granny smiles ain't pretty, boy.

THE MYSPACE PERVERT

Confession: I was on MySpace for about a month. I posted a profile as the Over-Educated Nympho in the hopes of driving traffic to my blog. I have never been a fan of MySpace because it seems like one huge hook-up network, which was why the first two sentences of my profile summary were *DO NOT PROPOSITION ME. I WILL SAY NO.* In spite of this, I received dozens of propositions in that one month. WTF? Can't be bothered to read a person's summary? I had like, *nothing* on my profile. It was pretty much the little blurb I have on my blog right now and a link to theovereducatednympho.com. I guess all anyone needs to see is *Name: Over-Educated Nympho, Age: 26, Orientation: Bisexual, Status: Single.* Never mind that I said for networking only. Perhaps people thought I was being a challenge? It's not a fucking challenge. It's me sick of creepy emails filling my inbox with reasons to sew up my pootang.

THE WTF PERVERT
Email #2

Subject: Re [What was the Re: in response to? This was the first time I was aware of his existence.]

–*Yada yada yada yada yada yada yada*– [Loooooooooong email. One of the longest ones I've ever received from a complete stranger, It was full of many unusual things, but I only included the ones that made my skin crawl off my body and then bathe itself in a bucket of bleach and anti-creepazoid]—

My two fetishes: women pissing, preferably standing, and non-gay men with foreskins. [Um, that's great? Good for you? I'm glad you know what you want out of life?] My being an uncircumcised American Baby Boomer has powerfully shaped my entire sexual persona. I note that you happily take intact men in stride. [Ehm . . . leave ME out of YOUR fetishes.] I suspect that the sexual value of the foreskin has yet to be understood. [Okay, agreed.] Rest assured that the foreskin is vryMind you, I suspect that a condom obliterates any added value from the foreskin. [Uh, WHY THE FUCK IS HE SAYING THESE THINGS. I HAVE NO IDEA WHAT IS GOING ON. THIS MUST BE SOME SORT OF RIP IN THE SPACE-TIME-PERVERT CONTINUUM. JEAN-LUC (you sexy, sexy man), SAVE ME!!! (and then sit down in your captain's chair so I can show you who's really in charge) Mmm . . . oh wait. No, I was in the middle of Pervsville. ICKINESS!!]

The webcam has made it possible for tens of thousands of women to post explicit snapshots of themselves on the web. [WHAT THE FUCK. This is so random. I very much do not like where this is going.] The women photograph themselves, or have a trusted friend do it. No need to develop film. [I KNOW, BUT I STILL DON'T UNDERSTAND WHY THE FUCK YOU'RE SAYING THIS ACTUALLY I THINK I DO KNOW, BUT I'M TRYING TO STAY IN MY HAPPY PLACE, WHICH IS FAR, FAR AWAY FROM A WEBCAM] The pictures can be uploaded using a Gmail or Hotmail account. [I DO NOT NEED INSTRUCTIONS FOR HOW TO DO SOMETHING WHICH MAKES ME MISS THE PARAGRAPH ON GOLDEN SHOWERS] The websites fully respect the woman's anonymity. [YES, BUT YOU DON'T. YOU ARE CREEPING ME OUT] Many women who do this are not coy about revealing their faces. [IS THIS SUPPOSED TO MAKE ME FEEL ALL WARM AND FUZZY?! I ALREADY OWN A BATHROBE. IT'S PURPLE AND SMELLS NICE AND I SUSPECT YOU DON'T, IF YOU LIKE GOLDEN SHOWERS] I also note that full pubic hair is very much out of fashion. [WHAT THE FUUUUUUUUUUUUUUCK THIS IS THE WEIRDEST EMAIL I HAVE EVER RECEIVED IN MY LIFE, OH MY GOD, JEAN-LUC PICARD *WHERE ARE YOU!*] This gives rise to the possibility that pubic hair is what women have been most ashamed of: presumably they see it as very unfeminine. [I DON'T THINK IT'S THE UNFEMININE THING, I THINK IT'S THE PUBIC FLOSS THING BUT WHATEVER BUDDY, I DON'T CARE, I NEED TO GO FIND MY SKIN, WHICH CRAWLED OFF TWO PARAGRAPHS AGO.].

Margaret Thatcher naked on a cold day is sooo much hotter than this.

THE "I'M A WOMAN, I SWEAR" PERVERT
Email #3

Subject: Serendipity for real [Oh my God, like *for real* for real? i like totally heart you, will you be my new BFF??]

Howdy,

I recently split from a 6-year relationship and found myself reading your blog site No, I'm not asking to meet you, we are 2 peas in a pod [No we're not. I don't say crap like, "serendipity for real"]

I'm 11 years older than you originally from ny and have 2 residences in houston [One for you posing as your ex-girlfriend, one for when you live like the creepy guy you really are?]

I live a very extreme lifestyle and enjoyed your innermost thoughts on self love and self esteem [Ooooh, is this a poem? Is there a leprechaun in your poem?! I LOVE LEPRACHAUNS!!]

Baby girl . . . [Ack] You are not alone [Wait, is this an ad for Jesus? Hey, man, we're cool. JESUS IS MY HOMEBOY. It says so right here on my forearm tattoo.]

Have you ever considered skydiving? [What the fuck. Is that a euphemism for swinging? Bush-diving? Vodka body shots?]

I quite enjoyed the blog on the twosomes [You mean "threesomes," sweetie? You really need help counting that high?]

Have you ever been with a partner who could go for 4 to 6 hours without a break? [Aw, fuck. Here we go.]

Or had multiple gushing orgasms for 4 to 6 hours without a break? [Why does this sound like a bad personal ad. Did you get booted off adultfriendfinder because you are the human equivalent of a pop-up advertisement?

Yep, I wouldn't have believed it either except he taught me how to have orgasms that legends are made of... All hail the kegel! [LIES, LIES, LIES! NO WOMAN SPEAKS SO HIGHLY OF AN EX! And in so many clichés! Ugh, okay, you've sunk below a bad personal ad and now you're the wretched generic diet pill company that fills my spam folder]

He has no idea I am writing this [Doesn't he, now?]

He is a beautiful person inside and out [Mmmm hmmmm. I'm sure that will hold up in court]

It didn't work out BC of me and my drive to do it all [What? You have issues with British Columbia? It is *lovely* this time of year. Almost as lovely as your skydiving/gushing/maudlin sunshine-colored vajajay.]

If you want to find out how to contact him, let me know [No no no THIS IS A TRICK. MY MOMMY WARNED ME ABOUT PEOPLE LIKE YOU]... He doesn't have a computer but certainly knows how to keep an over educated nympho satisfied for long periods of time [I just rolled my eyes so hard that I'm sure you were able to sense it on some sort of serendipitous level, and so could he even though he is (conveniently) so backwards he doesn't have a computer and yet YOU are emailing me from a fancy Blackberry device, according to your address]

And I would feel blessed knowing the two of you would truly enjoy each other [WHO THE FUCK SAYS SHIT LIKE THIS?]

Search your heart and you will know [THIS *IS* A JESUS AD, I KNEW IT! Hey man, WWOEND? I'm sure it would send me straight to Hell and I'd be screaming HELLS YEAH all the way down, you cheeky cheeky thing.]

–[woman's name]

["her" phone number]

I kinda wanted to meet him just so I'd have an excuse to pee on someone for once in my adult life.

THE HARDCORE PERVERT

This type of pervert is few and far between (or at least better hidden), which is good because I still haven't recovered from the photos that attached with this email (which I am not posting for the good of eyeballs everywhere).

Subject: hi

hi,

love your blog. no idea what you look like but your writing is hot.

i'd totally let you fuck my ass and mouth with your strapon.

take care.

[pervert in another country]

see attachments

There was not one, but two photos, which I refuse to post, look at ever again, or acknowledge after publishing this (and thus providing opportunity for all the world to mock). Again: Humor is how I deal with my inner pain. And outer ickiness.

Revenge of the Cubicle Monkey

While sitting at my desk late last night I realized what great potential I had to get into mischief. It was midnight and I was left in a huge, empty office full of things to fuck with. My very creative and vindictive mind had no choice but to wander and cackle maniacally as I ate random people's food from their desks.

Oh, what a damn fine time to be a cubicle monkey. Dozens of little schemes came to mind throughout the evening, followed by more this afternoon when I was fuming over my boss surfing eBay (while I get glared at for spending more than forty-five seconds on Weather.com). I will have fun at the office tonight deciding which to do to a few targeted coworkers:

1. Fully cover target's monitor with any or all of the following: Post-it notes (placing them with extreme precision seems to induce the most fury), Avery labels of assorted sizes, business cards, baby shower wrapping paper (most effective if the male coworker has a dickdo situation), aluminum foil (best if has food remnants), and, my personal favorite, panty liners. Very stickable. Available with wings!
2. Leave a big box of Q-tips on desk of Annoying Coworker who seems to prefer digging out waxy build-up with his fingers instead. Like, all the fucking time. —shudders in ickines—
3. Take all items on the target's desk and flip them. If the computer is on the left side, move it to the right. If the poster of a bejeweled and bedazzled Elton John is on the right, switch it to the left, etc. This must be done all the way to photos and paperclips. It is best if this is done to someone who is not a morning person and therefore a little shifty to begin with. Bonus points if you relocate all items on his desk to an entirely different row of cubicles.
4. Stapler in Jell-O. Classic.
5. Fuck with the office candy bowl.
6. Jam all fax machines with a TPS Report.

7. Find the most anal-retentive coworker's desk. These can be easily identified with the neat stacks, everything placed parallel to the edge of the desk *just so*, and things are often color-coded to nauseating extent. The key here is subtlety and selection. Choose one small, yet crucial, piece of desk decor/equipment to leave askew. If there are three pens at the left side of the keyboard (always ordered by frequency, black, blue, red, maybe a highlighter), leave one *ever so slightly* slanted out of alignment. Or reverse the caps between two pens. Change the orange highlighter to a yellow one. The anal-retentive people are the most fun to fuck with because it's all in the details. And they scream the loudest. The limbs flail about and such. Love it.
8. Fix it so that someone's Bobblehead Dwight never stops bobbing.
9. Fuck with the office candy bowl some more.
10. Using every single paperclip in the entire office, make a paperclip chain. Suspend it from the ceiling in an artistic manner (festive lights, especially the ones shaped like chili peppers, make it extra classy), and then charge coworkers five bucks to view it. Then charge them a nickel every time they demand a paperclip.

This is why cubicle monkeys should never be left free to roam the office unattended. Let that be a warning to bosses everywhere. In case the flinging of monkey poo weren't clear in expressing our great dissatisfaction with being held in captivity eight plus hours a day.

Does Your Cooch Smell Like Rose Petals Too?

We all know one of those people. Someone *perfect*. She is smart, gorgeous, sexy (yet modest), funny, and sweet. Most people can't hate someone like this because she's so nice. But I can. That's the great thing about not being perfect—no one is surprised when you say things that prove, yet again what a far cry you are from a decent human being, let alone respectable or perfect.

That person swimming in fabulousness is so fucking perfect it makes me gag on her designer perfume. She got married at twenty-two (and will probably live happily ever after, damn her), got the perfect job right out of graduation, by age twenty-six has saved up enough money for a down payment on a beautiful house in an area with an excellent school system for the wonderful 2.3 children they will have (also perfect, right down to a short labor and getting potty trained as soon as they can stand), and by twenty-eight has an amazingly successful career without having sacrificed her family or her sense of self. And, to top it off, when she's fifty years old I'm sure she will look fantastic (no Botox or Spanx necessary) and still have orgasmic sex two to three times a week.

The *bitch*.

And then there are the rest of us. As I approach my twenty-seventh birthday, I still feel kinda goofy-grinned about this whole "Hey, I'm-kinda-like-a-grown-up!" thing. I'm smug that I have more than forty-three bucks in my savings account. Then I look around at all these people my age who totally have their shit together. What is wrong with them? Don't they know they're supposed to be fuck-knobs throughout their twenties? What the hell is this bullshit, being all *respectable*? STOP MAKING ME LOOK BAD. MY MOTHER DOES NOT NEED ANY ADDITIONAL HELP, THANK YOU.

I don't like these people with their bright smiles and sunny dispositions. They're perfect. They give me no writing material. I have no use for them. They often make me feel like a miserable excuse for a human being because the coolest thing I have to brag about is that Ron Jeremy grabbed my ass. Can't tell THAT to anyone at the office Christmas party. Not sober, at least.

Seriously, how are the rest of us supposed to compete with the perfect people who make everything look so easy? I'm proud that I haven't bounced a check in six months. I started taking vitamins again (and managed to resist the Flintstones Chewables that are nothing short of pure fruity awesomeness). I only occasionally show up more than fifteen minutes late for work. And this all fills me with a tiny bit of pride. *Look, Ma! I'm not in jail! I don't smoke up my rent money and then turn tricks on the corner! GO ME!*

How do these beautiful, perfect people make everything look so fucking easy? Sure, they struggle here and there with a bad break-up (often remedied with a a new girlfriend who's even hotter) or not making their first million until they're thirty-*one* (haHA take that, "Thirty Things to Do Before the Age of Thirty"!!), but, for the most part, they make it look like beautiful spouses and wonderful jobs fall in their laps. For this, I hate them.

Perfect people are infuriating. I want to break into a perfect-man's house at three in the morning in a futile attempt to find him in his study drinking a glass of cheap scotch and masturbating to porn. But, no, I'm sure if I peered in his window from a tree branch. I would find him sleeping in his youngest daughter's bed to comfort her after she woke up crying from a bad dream. What a perfect freaking fuckhole.

Sure, I've met plenty of people who seemed perfect and gradually knew them well enough to see that this was bollocks. I'm thinking specifically of a coworker of mine: She is mid-thirties, beautiful, sharp, owns a home, is climbing her way up the corporate ladder with great tenacity and confidence, and has an equally successful boyfriend. She has been pressuring him to propose for quite some time. Three years, according to the gossip I've heard floating around the office. Being the assertive and determined ladder-climber she is, she applies the same principles to dating. Unfortunately, this translates into nagging, at least in her particular situation.

Ages ago, I ran into this woman when I still lived at the old apartment I shared with my now ex-boyfriend, who was on my arm when I saw her. We chatted and, since then, whenever we spoke in the office she asked me about my "handsome boyfriend" and if we were getting engaged soon. Imagine her surprise when I responded once with "Um, we broke up . . ." Her hand flew to her mouth in shock. "Oh no, what happened?!" "Well . . . he wanted to get married eventually. I didn't. So I left."

Her eyes nearly popped out of their little Kate Spade sockets and threw themselves at my face in a whirlwind of bloody-eyed bitchslappery. "Excuse me?" She said not without some judgment. And by some of course I mean a shitload. Her thoughts were so loud that they were all but leaking out her ears: You left a nice, handsome guy? Who wanted to marry you? YOU?! IF I HAD THAT HANDSOME FOREIGN BOYFRIEND OF YOURS I WOULD NEVER THROW HIM AWAY.

Eh, well. Tough titties. You're still prettier than me. And older and wiser-ish and make more money and other than the boyfriend who is NOT a husband thing your life seems pretty fucking awesome. As I said earlier, I've met plenty of people who seemed perfect and gradually knew them well enough to see that this was bollocks—and in spite of this, they are still five times more together than I could hope to be.

I'm not perfect. I have cellulite on my ass. My feet smell. I have been known to eat three bowls of Lucky Charms for dinner. I hate doing dishes, vacuuming, or pretty much cleaning in any form. I'm ten minutes late for everything, especially work. My pussy smells like pussy, not rose petals. I say stupid things all the time, often offending people accidentally instead of on purpose, which is not nearly as fun. Considering the good breeding I supposedly come from, you'd think I would act it a little bit more, or at least not mistake our biggest client for the air-conditioning repair guy.

For a while, I hoped the perfect thing would kick in eventually: after I graduated from college maybe, then after I finished grad school, or maybe after I got the great Nice Guy boyfriend. I always wanted to be one of those fantastic young women who has created a wonderful life for herself and is the envy of all her peers for managing to pull off the near-impossible and at an extraordinarily young age. Oh, right, that will kick in ANY DAY NOW, I can feel it to the core of my size-six pants.

Sure, there are plenty of people who seem to have their shit together and, really, it's just that they manage to hide their inner turmoil better than the rest of us, but there are a few people who seem to have been chosen for greatness or something. Is it too late to sign up for that? Who do I have to bake cookies for? What, registration closed already? Well, fuck.

Recently, I've started to understand—really understand—that it's OK not to be one of those perfect people who make the normal struggles of life look so easy. Fuck them. That's not real. That's not life, because life is never easy. It's varying degrees of suckiness and hopefulness. I think that being perfect is boring. But imperfection? That's what life is made of.

One Of Those Godforsaken Days

Today is one of those days when I am so sick of staring at my computer at work that I feel like crying. Nothing bad has happened today, it's just another ordinary day. Which is exactly the fucking *problem*.

I'm a cubicle monkey. I have three bosses, and today I found out I have a fourth (who will tell me what to do but won't answer my questions (that only he can answer)). I check the clock every two minutes, although sometimes I check it so often that the time hasn't changed, proving that time can stand still. I have a closer relationship with my monitor at work than I do with two of my four bosses.

The thing is, I work at a *good* office. It was five times worse when I worked at Douchebag Incorporated, and my Xanax intake has decreased dramatically since changing jobs.

I wish I could excuse the bad mood with lack of sleep (nope, not today—accidentally got eight hours of sleep last night), or the chronic summer rain in Texas (nope, I like the rain), or the glass ceiling (nope, my career is advancing ahead of schedule), but none of these contribute to the feeling of dread I feel every morning when I walk toward the front door of the office.

I know it's not just me. I see the auto pilot look in other peoples' eyes as I pass them in the hall. Our high school intern listens to TV shows on her iPod while filing. I catch glimpses of the person that exists beyond the corporate world, but that's it at best. I'm no better than any of them. Often at the end of the day I have minimal recollection of what I've done because I went on automatic mode.

You can only go so many days without feeling inspired before you want to scream at the top of your lungs THERE IS MORE TO ME THAN BEING A CUBICLE MONKEY!!

What do I do on these days when I feel my shoulders slouching in submission?

I go into the restroom and from the safety of a stall, I bury my head in my hands.

Sometimes it only takes one or two breaths to return to the necessary state of complacency to return to my desk, but on most days it's not so simple. This morning, for example: I hid in the comfort of the restroom for twenty minutes with a pen and paper in hand. I always keep a couple slips of carefully folded pieces of paper on me at all times, whether inside my left knee-high boot, pants pocket, sock, or bra if nowhere else (last resort, it gets pokey and itchy). I smoothed one out on my thigh and started writing notes for this very post. Sometimes I write at random or sketch out a little something that will grow into something bigger once I get home, but the point is that the act of writing is my something special. I steal precious slivers of time like this every day, because I have to keep my mind on something that gives me hope.

I don't want my life to be filled with ordinary days. I want something that makes me excited about jumping out of bed in the morning and disappointed to have to go to sleep at night. It happens with my writing, but the writing is still something that happens around my real job.

What about once I manage to make a living from writing? Won't that become dull too?

No. Not when I feel such a strong compulsion to write that I do it in the fucking restroom at work. And that makes me believe that I will not be spending the rest of my life escaping from my cubicle.

One day, motherfuckers. I'll fill my days with doing what I love, and that's anything but ordinary.

The Condom Aisle Is Heckling Me

Tonight I went by a drug store to pick up some things. Sadly, none of them were condoms. I'm at a seminar this weekend—for *work*. You think I'm going to bang any of those fugly-ass guys? NUH-UH. (But if I did, I'm covered—I've got three condoms in my purse and two in my work bag. And a paper bag to put over his head)

Okay, well there was this one cute guy but he was a bit smallish for my taste (I worry I may break anyone who is my size or smaller). Nice body though. Beautiful smile. Cute butt. Asked a good question during Q&A. Nice arms. Not that I paid much attention.

Oh yeah, *drug store*. I was in a drug store, and for some non-condom-related reason I was in the aisle with all the condoms. Look at all the pretty boxes! Black! Purple! Green! Navy Blue! I like all the colors, *awww* so pretty!

Too fucking bad I didn't NEED any condoms. I think they could tell. The boxes of condoms were heckling me. I could hear them talking to each other. They didn't even bother to whisper.

Lubricated Trojans: That girl hasn't gotten laid in ages! See how she looks at us all sad?

Extended Pleasure Trojans: Oh my god, I am sooooo embarrassed for her.

Lifestyles Snugger Fit: I am totally pointing and laughing at her. –points and laughs–

Durex Warming Pleasure: I bet she doesn't bother shaving her legs!

Lifestyles Extra Strength: Or her bikini line! EWWWW!!!

Trojan Value Pack of 36 condoms: Wow, how can she live every day without sex? Think of all the MILLIONS OF PEOPLE out there having sex EVERY DAY like it's no big deal! Isn't she about to *die*? From EMBARRASSEMENT?!

Lifestyles Variety Pack: What happened to her days of being a swingin' single? Didn't she used to get laid *all the time* by hot guys? What the hell?

Piña colada flavored condoms: I bet she smells. She's got nice tits, so she must smell *bad* to keep all the guys away.

Elexa Ultra Sensitive: MAYBE SHE'S JUST REALLY BUSY. SHE HAS A LIFE, YOU KNOW. SHE HAS A CAREER, NAY, *TWO* CAREERS TO WORRY ABOUT, SHITFUCK. NO ONE LIKES PIÑA COLADA, SO WHAT THE FUCK DO YOU KNOW?

Lifestyles Ribbed Pleasure: But she could still get some wangin' and bangin' every now and then. De-stress, you know?

Bottle of Astroglide: I bet her bottle of lube is collecting dust on the nightstand.

Durex Her Sensation: Bet her vibrator collection isn't! HA HA.

Trojan MAGNUM: Aww, the poor girl needs a real MAN to take care of her. *Ahem.*

Trojan MAGNUM XL: She looks hardcore, dude. I think she needs ALL THE MAN SHE CAN GET. *Ahem AHEM.*

Generic drugstore brand condoms: Count me in! GIGGITY. *Allllright.*

153 lbs., alcohol units 2, Oreos 62, calories approx. 9000 (v.g.)

One of my favorite silly indulgences is Bridget Jones's Diary, *in both book and video format. Hey, don't judge. I know more than one of you out there has* Varsity Blues *in VHS, DVD, .avi, and mini-disc format, so shove it up your bumhole. Any-sodding-hoo. This post is written in the style of Bridget, the proud queen of singledom herself (um, if you ignore the crying).*

8:05 a.m. Wake up late. Way late.
8:06 a.m. Don't care.
8:20 a.m. Drag ass of bed, pretend to care about making self-presentable for a bunch of corporate fuckwits.
8:32 a.m. Eat chocolate cake for breakfast while get daily dose of snark and consider calling in sick on grounds that I'm really fucking sick of work.
8:52 a.m. V. late. Leave for office. Drive barefoot until find spare set of shoes in back seat. Think about inner poise. Oh bollocks, shirt buttoned wrong.
9:16 a.m. Arrive at office. Grumble to boss about car. Although car is a half-functioning rat-bastard, car is in no way responsible for tardiness (I blame the cake. Too good to put down. Definitely worth the tummyache.) Congratulate self for arriving less than thirty minutes late (v.g.).
9:23 a.m. Strut to break room for coffee, once again think about inner poise.
9:27 a.m. Begin normal work day, except now am actually very busy at work and therefore have to cram the same amount of daydreaming/sexual objectifying in much less down time. Very inconsiderate of management. Thankful that management is very attractive, albeit married.
4:22 p.m. Receive letter from Perfectly Normal Friend. Enclosed is an Oreos advertisement torn from a magazine. This is why we're friends.
5:47 p.m. Braindead from maintaining an exhausting daydreaming schedule (complete with lots of fantasies of dirty whore sex in the conference room) while doing actual work. Wish had mp3 player with video. Now would be good time to watch episode of *Sex and the City* while "working", the one where Samantha buys "1001 sex positions" for $1.50. Bought own copy from a guy on the street when

lived in NYC. Consider getting it framed.

6:15 p.m. Leave office. Good riddance, mothafuckas!!

6:50 p.m. Back home. Strip. *Yech*, office cooties.

7:10 p.m. Make stir-fry vegetables. Very healthy. Am fine example of health, youthful independence, and responsibility (v.g.).

7:30 p.m. Dinner blew. Eat a row of Oreo cookies. Watch stomach expand. Eat more to forget the pain.

7:40 p.m. Watch DVR. Love DVR. So much kinder than TiVo. Eat more Oreos in celebration of awesomeness of living in age of digital recording devices.

7:42 p.m. Fart. Suffocate in own regret.

9:00 p.m. Brew coffee in preparation for second shift of work (aka management training program). Pout. Think back to less sucky days of college, recall that studying is way more fun when inebriated. Consider adding Kahlua to coffee. Kahlua *is* coffee. -ish.

9:15 p.m. Bury nose in mammoth corporate-issued training manual. Second presentation is in a week. Panic stirring.

9:18 p.m. Studying sucks big donkey balls. Remember how used to draw hearts in text book with initials of favorite boy inside. Now feel urge to draw lewd caricatures in margins with ass tattoos that say SUCK THIS.

11:41 p.m. Discover huge pimple when look in mirror. Cleanse, exfoliate, tone, spot-treat, and finally settle with a firm talking-to. That should scare it away by morning.

11:56 p.m. Take a little nap. Feels like a little piece of heaven. Dream of a consenting Cute Client.

12:05 a.m. Masturbate, "just for fifteen minutes."

1:15 a.m. Oops. Rationalize that all the orgasms are good for my complexion and general disposition as a member of society (perhaps less frequent use of The Finger while driving, as well as less hissing). An excellent step toward developing inner poise. V.g., will reward self with Oreos in the morning.

1:30 a.m. Still going. Have developed a cramp in left leg and crick in back. Work through it. Endurance is key to developing inner fucking poise.

2:00 a.m. Blog. Try to be clever while still swooning from orgasm-fog, decide don't care and write this post any way. Pissed that attempt to develop some semblance of inner poise gave me a charley horse.

3:10 a.m. Glare at pimple in bathroom mirror. Clearly it is not heeding my warning. Hmmph.

3:13 a.m. Fall asleep in wet spot.

Double Drama

Saturday was my friend Barbie's absolutely gorgeous wedding. Although I was very excited for her, I was nervous as fuck about Handsome Nerd. Would he be weird? Embarrassed? Cold? Apologetic for disappearing after one date? (He'd better be, the idiot). Ah fucking *hell*.

In anticipation of the first contact with Handsome Nerd in months, I dressed to kill with a little black dress, stilettos, and an itty-bitty black, lacy g-string (I swear, guys can sense when you're wearing these and not just because there's no panty line. I can't decide whether it's the devilish grin or very faint smell of partially-exposed pussy that gives it away).

It worked. Or rather, I worked it like a bad case of blue balls depended on it.

As soon as I sat down in the church pew with my friends Dr. and Mr. Smarty Pants, I saw Handsome Nerd peering around the open door leading to the groom's suite. My heart skipped a beat and my pussy fluttered. I told both to shut the hell up—we're in a *church*, for fuck's sake.

I think he saw me at the same time I saw him because he went from a relaxed lean to standing up straight and looking anywhere but in my general direction. I groaned. Dr. Smarty Pants looked over and saw Handsome Nerd. "Idiot," she muttered with a head shake. Dr. Smarty Pants has grabbed my ass on more than one occasion, she knows what there is to be had.

Once the ceremony started I did my best to ignore Handsome Nerd, but it was impossible because he was the best man and standing right freaking there at the front, the fuckhole. The only time he really disappeared from my mind was after the ceremony ended and we stood in line to give our congratulations to the bride and groom and their parents. Since we had sat down in the last row with all the other heathens, that meant we were first in line and then stood off to the side where I had a nice view of everyone in attendance. It was time for the *I'd fuck him* game.

I took a survey of all the cute single guys at the ceremony who would most likely also be attending the reception after. The single criterion left very few contenders: most guys came with girlfriends and wives, which is really very rude of them when I'm in hunting mode and IT'S BEEN THREE MONTHS. They automatically went to the Fuck No category. That left only a handful of guys who came alone or with someone resembling a mother/sister instead of a girlfriend to have a shot in hell of qualifying for my Fuck Yes Fuck Me NOW category.

I narrowed the hot/single contenders to four. The first one was Barbie's twin brother, who she specifically told me was off limits. Damnit. She didn't tell me he would be so *pretty*. No matter, no touchie. The second was a classic Tall, Dark, And Handsome sort of guy, but he had a bit of the angry thing going on. Not sure if it was in the bad boy way or asshole way. The third was tall, slim, and had beautiful eyes, but I couldn't tell if the girl with him was a girlfriend or another one of their bajillion classmates in attendance. Must inspect further before touching. The last guy who caught my eye was a tad goofy looking but had a great smile and no hint of a girlfriend, sister, or any female-looking specimen on his arm.

Most of us went back to the hotel for an hour or so until the reception began in the banquet hall downstairs. I was one of the first to arrive because I was hungry and ready for booze. Eventually the room filled and the wedding party (including Handsome Nerd) arrived. Their table was next to ours so I had a clear shot of the back of his head for the rest of the night. The back of his head was very distracting, and not just because he'd gotten his hair cut short. The back of his stupid head was so distracting that I was the last one to finish eating each of the wonderful courses brought out to us (normally I gobble everything down and then start eating food off my friends' plates). My stomach was churning so hard I couldn't finish my cheesecake. That's serious.

Since Barbie and Ken are awesome, they had a fully stocked open bar. Everyone, myself and Handsome Nerd included, enjoyed this to the fullest. Every time he went and stood behind me at the bar I felt the tiny hairs on my back reach out toward him, *just because I'm ignoring you it doesn't mean I don't want you to come talk to me! COME TALK TO ME, YOU IDIOT!!* The little hairs on my back must not have been loud enough, because even though I kept catching him looking at me, he never came over to my table.

Once dinner ended and people started getting up to dance, I saw my chance (with just the right level of in/sobriety) to take the empty chair next to Handsome Nerd. As I got up to walk over, another girl sat down next to him.

What?! Why is she talking to him?! GO AWAY! HOW IS HE SUPPOSED TO BE PINING FOR ME IF YOU AND YOUR PRETTY SHINY HAIR ARE IN THE WAY? MOOOOOOVE!

I sulked. I drank another glass of wine. I wondered if maybe I should have forgone underwear altogether.

Barbie came by to say hello. As I hugged her she whispered in my ear, "There's a guy here who works in your industry. My sister said he's very single and very interested in you."

"What, really? Who!!" I squealed. Please be one of the cute ones please be one of the cute ones or at least not one of the ones who make me wish there were a government-sanctioned *No Fuglies May Procreate* policy.

"The guy sitting between my brother and my sister."

I looked. YES! It's contender #4! We have targeted our prey, viewers of National Pornographic. Let's watch the hunt, shall we?

Barbie and I were discussing the ceremony when her sister walked past and Barbie grabbed her long enough to whisper something and get a snort and a wink out of her. All right, prey and huntress have been made aware of each other. I wonder if the poor boy knows that he has been engaged in the *Sex and the City* generation's version of "The Most Dangerous Game." It's a good thing I came armed with the double guns.

I went to the bar for a fresh glass of wine before heading over to the table where my prey sat waiting. Perfect. I stood behind the empty chair next to him.

"Excuse me, but I was told that there's some poor bastard over here who is in [my profession]? Is that you?" I looked at contender #4. He looked up at me with big, brown eyes and a bright smile.

"That would be me. Hi, I'm Another Nice Guy. Would you like to sit down?"

I joined him at his table. We drank wine, picked at the remains of the bread basket, and got to know each other. We started by talking shop, then school, then family. He lived here in town but frequently visited friends in other parts of Texas.

People began to fill the dance floor. When one particularly sappy/classic wedding song came on, I commented on how crap like this makes one really self-conscious about not having a plus-one who is obligated to dance with you.

"Well, why don't we dance then?" Another Nice Guy asked. Aw, clever boy can pick up on the excruciatingly obvious hints. He has passed the first test.

We went to the dance floor with all the other couples (and at this time I so did not notice that Handsome Nerd was sitting by himself at his table). He gently placed his right hand on my waist and took my right hand in his and held it up old-school style. It was sweet. But I don't want sweet, I want a freak like me. Let's get some "Rock yo' hips" going, eh DJ dude? Help a girl out! I need to be smoochin' within the hour to stay on track to my hotel room.

After the song ended a peppier one came on and he showed me his White Man Overbite dance, complete with some shoulder slides accented by the fact that he was still wearing his suit jacket. I only pointed and laughed a little because there were at least half a dozen guys who were way more embarrassing than Another Nice Guy.

A song later I excused myself for more wine, which I had left on the table. I saw that Handsome Nerd was still alone at his side of the table. I went in.

"Heeeeey there, Handsome Nerd. I liked your toast. It was very sweet." He looked up at me. There was no surprise, horror, or embarrassment. Do I dare say he looked happy to see me?

I sat down and we chatted for a bit about normal things. Eventually I worked up the courage to ask him, *"what the hell was your problem back then, anyway?"* Handsome Nerd looked hard at me, perhaps sizing up how angry I would be at his response? No worries, I have wine and you have a rum and coke! We are good to go! NOW TALK, YOU IDIOT.

Handsome Nerd looked down at his drink and then back at me. Damn, those eyes are killer when he actually looks at you. *No, Vix! Look away!* Remember eyes are a window to the soul and his soul is still stuck IN THE PIT OF DESPAIR.

"I know I screwed up. I've felt bad about it since then."

My mouth dropped. I covered by taking a big gulp from my wine glass. Can we get that on tape? I can't believe a guy who fucked up is actually *admitting* to fucking up. I'm completely confused. Where is the guy speak I'm used to?

"I know that that was *not* the way to handle it, but I have had so much going on that it was all just too much for me to handle. I wasn't weird just around you, but with all my friends too."

He stared into his glass. I stared at him in awe. Wait, is he saying this because he thinks it's what I want to hear? No, he doesn't know how to play the game at that level, even if he did, I don't think he'd have the patience for it.

Handsome Nerd said more, but the specifics have escaped me. Unfortunately, the shock of, "I know I screwed up" completely threw me for the rest of his apology.

I put my hand on his arm. I didn't say, *it's okay*, because it was not okay that he ran off just as my heart was opening up a tiny itsy bit to the idea that there are really cool guys out there, or that he left me with a dripping wet pussy. But I did want him to know that I didn't hate him for it.

He didn't look at me or my hand, but he looked up and got that special smile that is unique to Handsome Nerd. The one that makes it so very incredibly hard to write him off as an idiot who isn't worth my time.

"Hey, Vix, I got you some more wine."

Oh, fuck. It's Another Nice Guy. It's Another Nice Guy sitting down next to me and Handsome Nerd in the middle of our first conversation in nearly eight months. It's Another Nice Guy on my left and Handsome Nerd on my right. THIS

IS NOT HOW IT'S SUPPOSED TO GO. How the fucking fucking FUCK do I get out of this?!

"Oh, hi, uh, thanks" I accepted the glass and hoped neither of them noticed my ears turning red.

"Hey there . . ." Another Nice Guy extended his hand across me to Handsome Nerd.

"I'm sorry. Another Nice Guy, this is Handsome Nerd. He's the best man. Handsome Nerd, this is Another Nice Guy, a friend of the family." And this is me being really, really uncomfortable. I do not know how to act when I'm between two guys I'm interested in if it is anything other than a Chinese fingercuff situation.

So I stood up and left. I said something about breaking the seal and hauled ass away from there. I grabbed Dr. Smarty Pants by the arm and demanded, "Restroom. Now."

She followed me in and I gave her a quick summary. She laughed. "Looks like you got your drama all right." Then she gave my ass a little squeeze and I felt better. Then we stayed in the restroom for another twenty minutes talking with our other friends as they came and went. I was hoping that by the time I returned Another Nice Guy and Handsome Nerd would be at opposite corners of the room.

When I did return, I found Another Nice Guy on the dance floor with his other friends, doing what I hope were impressions of the rejects from that TV show *So You Think You Can Dance*. I joined them for one song then asked Another Nice Guy if he wanted to go into the courtyard to talk for a while. I may have checked to confirm that Handsome Nerd saw us leave together. With fresh glasses of red wine. Red is the color of looove after all. And by "love" of course I really mean "dirty whore sex."

The courtyard was beautiful, which unfortunately meant it was full of other people. Damnit. Not exactly the romantic "kiss me, you idiot" atmosphere I was going for. I led Another Nice Guy to a bench far away.

The conversation was awkward. It hadn't been before. I don't think it had anything to do with me ditching Another Nice Guy to fend for himself with a guy who can testify that, *yes, Vix really does have a clit piercing and booooy does she like it, but you don't know that yet do you buddy? By the way she likes it if you bite her neck really hard. FYI.* I think that was completely lost on Another Nice Guy, and Handsome Nerd is too nice to utter a word to him about our brief history (a brief history which contained one of the all-time hottest make-out sessions I have ever experienced, but that is irrelevant information).

Perhaps it was because it was becoming clear that we had "a thing" going on? Another Nice Guy was sweet, smart, funny . . . not *hysterical* funny like Handsome Nerd, but definitely funnier than the average schmuck on the street. He was getting nervous.

I should probably mention that Another Nice Guy's freaking *mother* was there. When she walked by he introduced us to each other. As she shook my hand she very slowly and deliberately sized me up, complete with a pause at the hemline of my little black dress. I wasn't going to say, "Funny you noticed that, I think that's what got your son's attention too," but it did make me snicker to myself, because I'm classy like that.

After about twenty minutes of awkward chatting (and a few lingering glances at my crossed legs), I excused myself under the pretense of having ignored my friends all evening. Not true. For the first two hours of dinner, I barely left the table, and they all knew I was going out on the hunt. Are you kidding? All my friends there were coupled off and therefore cheering me on to report back with salacious tales of sexual conquest.

I left because I needed to be alone to clear my head. Which meant yet another glass of wine. Somehow, I was well on the side of sobriety throughout the evening. I think it had something to do with the huge steak (steak!) that was served at dinner.

Handsome Nerd was dancing with Barbie. I wonder if he's saying anything about me . . . oh, stop being so self-centered. The song ended. I went to the bar for my wine. When I turned around I saw that Another Nice Guy was dancing with Barbie. OH MY GOD. The goddess of irony is out in full tonight, the dirty bitch. I wanted drama and here she is giving me a double serving of the shit. I sat at my table and chatted with a friend.

A few minutes later a beaming and slightly inebriated Barbie found me. She pulled me onto the dance floor where we danced cheek-to-cheek so she could whisper in my ear, "Who is it going to be? Handsome Nerd or Another Nice Guy? You only get to choose one!"

It took me a minute. I was surprised at myself. Barbie saw the puzzled look register on my face.

"I want Handsome Nerd, but I know better than that. I'm going to say Another Nice Guy because he's so nice and sweet and NOT AN IDIOT. And something about him makes me think he's good at eating pussy."

She nodded solemnly. "Wait, you just danced with both of them—did Handsome Nerd or Another Nice Guy say anything about me??"

Barbie didn't say a word. She just patted me on the back and shooed me away so I could go get myself a nice, big nympho-sized serving of man meat. Time to zero in on my prey of choice.

I returned to the courtyard where I found Another Nice Guy by the fountain. The garden had cleared out a bit so we were almost entirely alone. Exxxcellent. He grinned as I walked toward him (and juiced it up with a little extra hip swing). This time I sat closer to him, which I hoped would encourage him to kiss me. I was the one who introduced myself, he can be the one to take the next step.

Fifteen minutes later I had scooted two inches closer and done the accidentally-on-purpose dress strap slip-off the shoulder bit and *he hadn't done a damn thing*. I think my prey doesn't know he's being pursued, but his mother sure does. Or, if he does, maybe he's scared out of his wits, pissed himself, and now is held hostage in his seat by his piss-filled pants. Hmm.

Patience has never been a quality I possess. In fact my impatience contributes greatly to my charm, I've been told. Time to get things going.

As Another Nice Guy was in the middle of speaking (about what, I have no idea. I hadn't been paying attention for ages), I leaned over, gave him the Sex Eyes, and kissed him. Instantly my hands went up to cup his neck and take him in. The kiss was soft, gentle, nice. Very nice, but nothing that made me soak my panties. When I pulled back Another Nice Guy was frozen in place in complete shock. His hands were still at his side.

Um.

Okay, buddy, there's surprise and then there's complete shock. This ain't what I want to see when I'm trying to get in your pants. Where is the passion? The submission? The *hunger*? HELLO, McFLY!!

A big grin crept on his face. Okay, there's something. I see you don't find me repulsive, that is a start. A bad start, but a start. Another Nice Guy pulled back and looked me up and down. He opened his mouth but didn't say anything.

Hmm. I want a do-over.

I kissed him again. A little harder, with the tongue probing a tiny bit in hopes of inspiring his to come out and play. Not a muscle in his body moved. What the fuck, chief? DO YOU SEE WHAT I'M *WEARING?!* TOUCH ME IF YOU KNOW WHAT'S GOOD FOR YOU. He didn't.

Fine. I picked up his arm, placed it around my waist, and pushed his hand toward my ass. This provoked a chuckle on his part. He broke the kiss and leaned back in his chair. I waited. He still had that deer-in-the-headlights look. Which is so NOT SEXY. We are still a long way from X-rated, sweetie, which is where I'd like to be by 2 a.m.

"I think I'm going to have to get your number."

My number? How about MY PANTIES, you stupid, stupid boy. Dude, the Man Club is about to revoke your penis privileges if you keep being a dumbfuck.

"I was hoping for a lot more than a phone number tonight."

His eyes bulged. (Yes, only his eyes. I checked.)

"Oh, reeeeally?" he got that I-think-I'm-being-sexy-but-really-I-look-like-a-goober grin on his face.

Sigh.

I started talking about how much I hate Texas. His pinky stroked the underside of my wrist. I think he was trying to hold my hand. ARE YOU FUCKING KIDDING ME?! A GIRL WHO IS TRYING TO JUMP YOUR BONES HAS NO INTEREST IN HOLDING YOUR GODDAMN HAND. If I had schmoopie on the brain instead of cock, then I would have gladly held his hand. I am not heartless, I am a hand-holder. *In another life*, one that is full of laundry for two, fighting over who used the last of the toilet paper, and reminding your boyfriend to send his mother a birthday card. But, I am not thinking about "we" bullshit. All I can think about is the two condoms in my purse and The Pussy growing steadily heated with frustration.

We talked for a few more minutes, but in all honesty I wasn't paying the slightest attention to what we talked about. The scent of Another Nice Guy's cologne lingered in my nose and in my mind. It was very sweet, almost powdery. It was so subtle that I only realized he was wearing cologne at all when I was kissing him. *What does that make me think of*, I kept wondering. It's so . . . so what?

It smells like *pansy*. It smells like a guy who won't kiss you, who won't touch you when you kiss him, who introduces you to his mother, who won't cum on your tits during sex because, "it's degrading," who has never had casual sex let alone a one-night stand, and who assumes that all he's getting that night is a phone number, not multiple orgasms.

The Pussy threw up her hands in disgust. WHERE DID YOU FIND THIS GUY?? He all but had on a T-shirt that said, "Will you be my cuddlebum?"

To play devil's advocate for a minute: maybe I was generalizing. He's made it obvious he's into me, even if he moves slow as hell. Why not give him a chance to prove that he's up for it? Maybe he's had lots of casual sex and was up for a romp in the sack and I should have given him a chance. Why walk away from someone willing? But no. I don't have the patience for that bullshit anymore. Some other girl can give him a chance.

If I did anything more with Another Nice Guy, I realized it would only be to make Handsome Nerd jealous. That is a stupid junior-high reason to do anything with a guy. Nuh uh, I couldn't.

My stomach churned. I needed to leave, like *right now*.

"Please excuse me, Another Nice Guy. I *really* need more booze." And with that I walked away. Quickly.

Once inside I realized the open bar had closed down and the DJ was packing up. I stole a glass of wine off our table that may have been mine and wandered off in search of a friend to bitch to about how guys have a talent for cockblocking themselves.

None of my friends were in sight. One of the bride's relatives asked me if I had signed the guest book yet. I had not, so I went into the next room to sign.

I flipped through the photo book where other guests had left such sweet messages. I turned to the very last page where I saw one of my favorite photos of them. *To Barbie and Ken, you give cynics like me hope that a couple can live happily ever after. I love you both.* Just as I signed my name, I felt someone come up next to me.

"Heyyyyy, Vix, what are ya doin'?" It was a very drunk Handsome Nerd leaning on the table next to me with a big, fat smile on his face.

"Signing the guest book."

"I should do that, too!" I handed him the pen and the book. He tried to write on the tablecloth instead. Babycakes is drunkety drunk drunk.

Hmm. This situation begs to be taken advantage of.

"Soooo, Handsome Nerd. Tell me—what was the real reason you never called me back when all I wanted was to mess around?"

He drunkenly hovered closer to me and stared intently at the table. Probably so he wouldn't fall over. I waited. He looked at me with impressive focus for someone so tipsy.

"Because I know that if I have feelings for someone and we mess around, I can't let it go at just that. I know how I am, and I can't do that."

Damn. The guy makes a good point. I was probably lying to myself back then. How can I expect to keep it impersonal with someone who makes me laugh so hard I have to beg him to stop because my face hurts too much?

"I know I'm going to regret saying this, and I know I'm only saying this because I'm drunk and I'm counting on not remembering any of this in the morning, but it really was about all my weird stuff. I kinda told you about it back then, and I hardly tell anyone about [genuinely sucky situation] because I don't know how to talk about it."

"So you're a jackass to me and your friends instead?"

Handsome Nerd frowned and then half-shrugged in agreement. "Yeah, I guess so. But I don't know how to talk about it, so I don't. I don't know what to do, it's like I'm just *stuck*."

I studied him. The bastard is telling the truth, isn't he? It really was all his shit and had nothing to do with me. And he really did (does?) like me. I didn't know how to respond.

Handsome Nerd kept talking. He was talking so much and with such energy that it made me wonder if he had said *any* of this to someone else. Some of what he said started striking chords and so I told him about how I went through depression for a really long time. I explained that it totally sucked ass, and all I could see was the suckiness, but, once I was out of it, I realized how it made me so much stronger . . . depression wasn't all bad.

I apologized lest he think I sounded like a preachy asshole, but his head was cocked in way that made me think he really was taking it in, albeit drunkenly. Then he thought it was his turn to be embarrassed, because he kept saying, "I know I'm going to regret saying all this tomorrow because I'm drunk but then I'll probably be happy I did."

We must have talked for twenty or thirty minutes. At one point I saw Another Nice Guy walk past the open doorway, his head craned for a better look. Fuck. Ugh, I would deal with him later. One drama at a time.

"For the record, you gave up some fine pussy," I told Handsome Nerd.

He closed his eyes and nodded.

"And I do mean *damn* fine pussy."

He scrunched his eyes tight. "I know. I regret that every day, and I will continue to regret it tonight, tomorrow night, the night after that, the night after that . . ."

"Just checking."

We laughed. I wished I knew what he was thinking. I wondered if there were a chance that one day he'd get through his personal shit and I'd get over my relationship issues and if we would actually make things work between us. What if one day Handsome Nerd could be my frog?

The chemistry, it was undeniable. It still is. I have never felt anything like that—and I'm not just talking about the bedroom. I wondered if he was thinking the same thing. As we stood at the table next to each other—oblivious that for the last ten minutes people had been cleaning up the room—I wondered about all the things that may still have a chance.

If I want anything to happen tonight, now is the time to say or do something. What if he's waiting for me to make a move? He wants it too, you know it! Oh, come on, Vix, do something, anything!!!

I bit my lip. I reached up and kissed him on the cheek. "Everything will be okay one day, sweetie. Life is a bitch, but it has a way of working itself out eventually."

And I walked away.

Once out in the noisy hallway of the hotel I was shaken back to the other boy problem. Aw, fuck, what was I going to do about Another Nice Guy? I definitely couldn't mess around with him, especially not now. I couldn't stay here a second longer than necessary.

I would have left right then but I felt like I owed it to Another Nice Guy to give him some sort of face-to-face explanation for changing my mind so suddenly, and preferably one that didn't require saying he kissed like he was stuck inside a full-body cast.

He wasn't in the banquet hall. He wasn't in the side room. He wasn't in the hallway. The door to the courtyard was locked. Daaaaaaamnitttttttttttt, I just want to go back to my hotel room and be miserable in peace!! LET ME LEAVE.

I found Barbie's sister and asked her about Another Nice Guy. She said she thought he drove his mother home but it wasn't far away, and he might be coming back for a party in one of the rooms. I shook my head. Now what, I can't just *leave*. I pulled out one of my business cards (which I intentionally did not write my cell phone number on) and handed it to her. "Would you give this to him? Thanks." [It's three days later. He hasn't called, and I don't care.] She asked me if I was sure I didn't want to stay.

Oh, sweetie, I am SO sure I don't want to stay. In fact, I am leaving right the fuck now.

Once safely inside the elevator, I leaned back against the railing and closed my eyes. What a crazy-ass motherfucking night. I felt miserable for having turned down two things that could have proved themselves to be fun or at least an ego-boost. It was safe to assume I'd be double lonely when I woke up in the morning in a queen-sized bed.

I felt a little proud about the ending to my night. A couple years ago I would have made very different decisions which may or may not have been tainted with regret afterward. I've finally learned that sometimes the best thing you can do for yourself is to go home alone.

Choosing To Be Single, In Sickness And In Health

Attending a friend's wedding a couple weeks ago made me very aware of being single. During the ceremony I sat between two couples. Dateless, I sat between two couples. Both of whom were newlyweds and therefore very *schmoopie!-schmoopie!!* with each other.

At the reception afterward, I sat at a table with four other couples. Four couples and me, without a plus-one. It didn't make me feel guilty or lonely, but it definitely made me feel, ick, *something*.

I think it's marriage cooties.

I've never been sure about the whole marriage thing. I think I was born without the bride gene. I'm hesitant to talk about that though because I know there will be the disapproving stares of all my aunts boring into my cold and empty soul. I'm supposed to be engaged by now, or at the very least have a promising long-term significant other good enough to copulate with as soon as he saves the two months' salary for a ring that would be more to impress my family than me.

I'm sure it's not just my family who pressures anyone over the age of twenty-two to get married. For years all my aunts were convinced I would be the last one of the nieces to marry because I'm so sullen/bitter/odd/dark and –gasp– I don't go to church on Sundays!! That's right I don't because that's when I LIKE TO MASTURBATE.

In spite of my sad little troll of a heart, there is still a tiny bit of hope deep inside. Watching my friends Barbie and Ken get married definitely warmed me up to marriage. I like the idea of finding my counterpart, someone who gets both my dark and goofy sides of humor and thinks I'm dorky (but in an endearing way) when I blow a joke. I try to keep realistic expectations about dating. I'm not going for Mr. Perfect who drives a Porshe and speaks four languages. I'm looking for a frog, not Prince Charming.

What if I never meet that guy? I already met Mr. Perfect, a.k.a. Aussie. Nice, good-looking, smart, upwardly mobile, supportive. We dated for a couple years and talked about marriage. I thought he was the one, but that little voice inside kept trying to get me to ask myself why I never had anything to say. Finally it got through to me that Mr. Perfect is not the same person as Mr. Perfect-For-Me.

The funny thing is that it seems people are more forgiving of middle-aged single women who've never been married because they can't find anyone versus a middle-aged woman who chooses to be single. *What nonsense! She must be a lesbian! She just hasn't met the right man!* Why is it easier to forgive a woman who couldn't find herself a husband than it is to accept a woman who finds happiness in "me, myself, and I"? Isn't that better than settling for less than you want or saying yes to the first guy who asks? It seems that singledom is seen in relation to coupledom, *i.e.* as the absence of a significant other.

How about seeing singledom as it really is? Being yourself, being on your own. It's not a death sentence like some (including my gaggle of aunts) would have you believe. Why is it so hard to remember that being single can be kind of fantastic?

I have always liked the single me more than the coupled me. I'm stronger, more independent, more opinionated, and have all that time that would be spent doing twice as much laundry/cooking doing something that is good for the soul. In my case it's writing for hours every night, playing sports, reading book after book, and doing whatever else I want that makes me happy. It's really quite simple: I like who I am when I'm single. I feel like I'm being all of me instead of just part of me.

Of course, there are times when I feel lonely and wish I could have a boyfriend for, like, a week. However, the majority of the time I love being on my own, doing my own thing. It makes it easier to figure out and become the person I want to be instead of the person someone else thinks I should be. In an ideal relationship there is none of this "should" crap, but in all three long-term relationships I have had I always felt like my boyfriend was either nudging me in a direction I didn't want to go or pulling me away from the path I wanted to explore. I don't want that to happen again, because then I become someone I don't recognize. I'd much rather be alone and happy with who I am than in a relationship where I have to grey out fundamental parts of my identity.

What if I choose to stay single for the rest of my life? I'm choosing to be single right now, and I plan on staying single for quite a while. It's only now that I have a much clearer vision of the strong woman I want to become because there is no one tainting it with all those fucking *should*s.

Cunt

Before you shriek in terror at C-U-Next-Tuesday and turn the page in a hurry, hear me out.

I dig cunt. The word, the sisterhood of fuck-me feminism, slipping my fingers inside, and all those other things *cunt* embodies—I feel it inside and out.

Cunt is not something I will ever be ashamed of. Many people try to take it away from me with disapproving finger-shaking or a snarl of contempt. Fuck that bullshit. It's not about what they think. It's about me, and, let me tell you sweetie, I love my cunt.

The word itself is a hard slamming of consonants against each other. There is nothing soft about the word at all—but it doesn't need to be. Every other synonym is either sweet, delicate, or downright sterile: vagina, vulva, punani, muff, goodies, down there. Of the lot of slang terms, I typically use pussy because it makes my eyes roll the least. A few times I've thrown out cunt while fucking someone and that usually makes the guy stop cold exactly when I want him to be ramming me hot and hard. Oh, come *on*, buddy. What the fuck? Why does this still catch people off-guard?

Because nice girls don't say cunt, let alone have one.

So why do I have to talk about cunt, why not pussy or vagina or secret love garden? Because cunt is so much more than a body part, especially if that body part smells like a meadow. Cunt is a statement.

People have been reclaiming cunt since the 70s. I want to know what's taking so goddamn long that I still have to be careful not to throw cunt into everyday conversation unless the person I'm with knows me well enough to understand that I mean "rock on, babe."

According to *The Woman's Encyclopedia of Myths and Secrets*, the origin of cunt didn't have the foul connotation that it does today: "Derivative of the Oriental Great Goddess of Cunti, or Kunda, the Yoni of the Uni-verse. From the same root came country, kin, and kind." Yoni translates as "divine passage" and "womb," although it also refers to the female anatomy used in giving birth with a tone of great respect. Although there seems to be a lot of dispute over the origin of cunt, what I'm getting at is that it wasn't always uttered with a sneer.

I know a lot of people grew up with cunt being the ultimate bad word, the one you rarely heard so that when someone spat it out it left you momentarily frozen. In my case, I did not come across the word until I was fifteen (read it in a book, asked my father what cunt was, *whoopsies*). It was too late. The contempt and mean-spiritedness of it was forever lost on me. It was like hearing someone call me a "loud-mouthed bitch of a suitcase." Didn't take. Fortunately, that makes it much easier to reclaim cunt as a word that belongs in my Happy Place, along with Angelina Jolie, a bed the size of Rhode Island, and speakers big enough to mount.

What is cunt?

It's *fuck me harder, no I said FUCK ME HARDER*. It's burying my face in the smell of sex. It's enjoying my sexuality without caring about whispers of *slut* or *whore*. It's standing up against every asshole out there who thinks I should stay in my place.

Most importantly, it's pride in who and what I am. If that means I'm a cunt, then I will stand tall and proud.

I'm Mary Fucking Sunshine, Thanks For Asking

Somehow I ended up in the perky department at work. Oddly enough all these perky coworkers are men. The partner I work for is the perkiest of them all, which on Monday mornings like today, can make the not-so-inner bitch fight to come out. The first time he sees me every day he asks me how I'm doing. "Fine" is never enough for this man—he wants a whole paragraph. Nothing but sarcastic answers laced with vinegar fill my head. This means that I actually take time in the mornings to think about what I'm going to say when he asks me so that something respectable comes out of my mouth.

One of these days, I'm worried that my sarcasm filter is going to be overflowing to the point that a piece of poorly-disguised snark manages to slip out. It almost happened today. These were some of the gems that surely would have gotten me fired, or at least put in isolation:

- I'm Mary Fucking Sunshine today, and how are you?
- Over the weekend I found out I don't have crotch rot!
- Don't speak to me.
- DAH OH MY GOD, TURN THE HAPPY PILLS DOWN A NOTCH!
- Golly gee whiz and willickers, I am so FREAKING DELIGHTED it's Monday morning!
- How am I? I'm bright-eyed and bushy-tailed, ready to tackle whatever comes my way!
- I managed to arrive at the office with pants on. I am AWESOME.
- –bursts into tears–
- I ate a one-pound bag of M&Ms last night. My therapist told me to call him the next time I do that, so I will be needing a couple hours off this afternoon.
- When I woke up I was cuddling my vibrator. Again.

- Not so good. –shifts uncomfortably– Ever since I came in this morning I've had a bad case of the runs. –turns and runs right out the door, giggling all the way to the car–

Yes my boss is very sweet and yes, I would rather work for someone who's too nice than too mean, but . . . I think he's one of those people who fills personal emails with exclamation points and smiley faces. That is not very becoming on a man, especially one who has enough power to squish my career into something the size of a dead bug.

I miss my old boss. When he was in a good mood, he was fun. When he was pissy, he didn't try to hide it— I respect that. I hate feeling like I have to plant a big fat fucking smile on my face for eight hours a day. As if having to wear a bra under all these conservative clothes weren't punishment enough. THEY WERE MEANT TO BE FREEEEE!

I Love Being Single *But*

I love being single, I really do. Please don't think that I'm saying this because I'm trying to convince myself it's true, like some sniffly, middle-aged woman who has never had a boyfriend and has resigned herself to a life of loneliness, nor am I saying this as someone who has been dumped one too many times and hisses every time a guy walks by. I only hiss at specific guys, jeez.

I am saying this because *I love being single*. It's just . . . I only feel this way about 90% of the time. That other 10% has a way of really biting me in the ass.

Why is it so hard to completely enjoy being single? I mean, hell, I *chose* to be single. Yet, every once in a while, I see the way my girlfriends talk about their husbands and I can't help but want someone in my life who makes me feel that way. For a week. Maybe two. Also, I would have to catch up on all the sex I should have been having all this time.

When I was writing the outline for this post, I made a list of pros and cons of being single. I filled up the entire pro-single column, meanwhile there was only one item written on the con side: "Snugglebunny." (Oh, shut *up* I'm sick of snuggling with my dog). Once I moved to the con side it took me twice as long to complete the list as for the pro-single column.

Doesn't take Dr. Phil to figure that one out. Just don't tell my mother. She'll revoke her offer to give me cash if I elope, then I'll never be able to marry a gay guy for the cash prize.

There are many treasured moments that I can enjoy every day because I'm on my own: popping pimples in the bathroom in peace, not doing dishes for a week and a half, taking up all the DVR hard drive space with my favorite crap TV shows, eating ice cream at the kitchen counter in my underwear and maybe dancing a little bit to *The Office* theme song.

The career thing is a huge deal. I've said it before and I'll say it again: neither my real career nor my writing career would be going half as well if I didn't have all this time to do my own thing. Hell, as I type this it's four in the morning and I have to be awake in a couple hours. Why am I always up so late? Working on advancing both those careers. Before midnight is office training stuff, after midnight is best creative time for writing. If I had a boyfriend do you think he'd let me get away with this routine every night? I know he definitely wouldn't like to see me writing about hot sex with other people, that's for sure. (Selfish bastard. Think of the blog!)

But.

There's a line from a great movie called *Amy's O* where the lead character says something like, "I'm alone, but I'm not lonely." As if the quotation weren't enough to think about, there's this crucial tidbit about the movie: at first it is convincing that she stands behind her statement, however, by the end of the movie it's obvious as hell that she's lonely. At the end the guy she had been dating comes back into her life, she tears up, *yada yada yada* the ending kind of pissed me off because he kissed her into fulfillment.

Remembering this movie makes me wonder, am I genuinely happy being alone? If I were to meet Mr. Perfect-For-Me tomorrow, would I suddenly realize that I've been miserably lonely this whole time and was living in self-imposed blissful ignorance? Am I on the verge of rolling my eyes at myself?

Then my better sense comes out for a fresh round of bitchslapping and says, I don't need a guy. 90% of the time I don't even *want* a guy. PHOOIE on guys. Boobies are more fun anyway.

That last little bit of me, the part that misses sappy *schmoopie* talk and butterfly kisses, has me questioning whether I'm only 10% lonely. Has it been increasing? Are the scales tipping from one side to the other? Sweet merciful crap, what if the *lonely* overtakes the *happy being alone*? What then?

Or maybe it's just that I miss a regular source of sex. Yeah. I think that's it. Being horny and unsatisfied makes me say all sorts of stupid shit.

How to Talk Dirty

I like to talk dirty during sex. That's why sex is *fun*. You don't have to act like a lady like every other hour of the day. Let loose with the occasional, "I love your big hard cock." If you've already got your hand down a guy's pants, I think that means you can stop pretending you're a good girl. That means it's time for you to talk dirty:

Come on. Unleash your inner dirty whore.

Okay, I know a lot of the things I'm going to tell you to say will sound lame. Of course they sound lame *here*. The hotness comes when you're naked and you're whispering these things in his ear. Short sentences and short words are good. No babbling. No "lovemaking" or "vagina" fluffiness allowed. This post is for beginners, so keep in mind it barely touches on "talking dirty like a porn star." I don't want to scare anybody off with rim-job talk.

A quick note: I'm writing this post for the female readers because they ask me about it much more often than guys do, but most of what I'm saying works well for guys too. Just don't forget to change out the body parts where appropriate. I once told a boyfriend, "I love having your pussy inside my big cock." I can't believe he didn't stop fucking me right there. If I were him I would have, after I stopped pointing and laughing, that is.

If the instructions here require a tittily bit too much thinking, you can flip to the end where I've written out a cheat-sheet of dirty phrases, no assembly required.

Introduction

If this is your first time talking dirty, then it may be easier if you ease yourself into it. You also have to keep in mind that the guy you're with may not be used to the dirty whore sex we are so fond of here in the freak corner of the blogosphere. I've encountered several guys who dropped their mouths and said, "I didn't know girls talked like that." Yeah, we do, babe. Now lie down and take it like a man.

Test the waters

I've met guys who flipped out when I said something as innocent as, "you make me so wet." Most of the time it is just the initial shock that girls aren't always all lady-like. Sometimes it makes a guy really uncomfortable. As much as I want to say, *it's okay, everyone is unique*, what I really mean is, *why bother? NEXT*. Then again, I'm no Nice Girl, so others may be more understanding about an awkward silence after telling a guy, "You're so hot, I want to fuck you all night long." I'm not. I expect my dirty words to be lapped up like my pussy juice should be. Assuming your first attempts at dirty talk are met with a smile and not a door slam, then continue saying these sexy gems as things ramp up.

What you should say

Whatever you damn well please. It's sex. There is no need for "please" or "would you mind terribly . . . ?" It's SEX. Here are guidelines for what to say:

- What you want to do to him
- What you are doing to him right now
- What you are going to do to him next
- What you want him to do to you
- What you fantasize about him doing

This is sex. That means you should use sex terminology. *Lick, suck, fuck. Pussy, cunt. Dick, cock.* You're a big girl. Use big girl words. If these don't flow off your tongue as easily as the wetness flows between your thighs, just give them a chance. After one night of talking dirty, I promise you'll never be able to keep your lips closed around, "I'm going to ride you so hard you'll be begging me to stop."

What you should NOT say

Words you would come across in a romance novel, gynecology exam, or dirty Mad Libs answer. These include: penis, vagina, Miss No-No, Mr. Happy, junior, saucy sausage, spicy tuna handroll, kitty button, or love muffin. Don't believe me? Fine. You tell me how much it would turn you on to hear the following sentence whispered in your ear: *I'm going to pound my spicy tuna handroll deep inside your love box.* Duuuude. That's so sexy it's sex-*ay* with a capital XXX.

What you should say specifically
Simple is fine. No one expects you to be a fucking poet when you've got multiple orgasms on the mind. Follow this basic formula: I want to [verb] your [body part]. For example, I want to . . . suck your fingers/lick your dick (points for rhyming!)/ ride your cock. Mix it up so it's not completely obvious that your taking one from Column A and one from Column B, you can change the beginning part based on the guidelines above of what you want/am/will do to him, or throw in the occasional adjective.

Here is a catalogue of words that you can use to form a thousand combinations of sexy by following the simple formula: I [verb] to [verb] your [adjective][body part]:

verb 1: want to, love, would love to, can't wait to, have been fantasizing about, beg you
verb 2: lick, finger, rub, grind against, suck, fuck, ride, mount, pound, bite, kiss, tease, slap, spank
adjective (male): hard, rock-hard, big, huge, long, thick, throbbing, strong, HARD
adjective (female): wet, hot, smooth, honey, sexy, round, hard, soft, sweet, WET
body part (male): dick, cock, balls, sack, tongue, mouth, lips, neck, fingers, hand, stomach, bicep, back, thighs, shoulders, muscles
body part (female): tits, pussy, cunt, clit, lips, hips, ass, tongue, lips, neck, fingers, hand, stomach, thighs

A few examples using the above formula: I want to rub your rock-hard cock. I love fingering your wet pussy. I can't wait to grind against your sexy hips.

I'm begging to suck your big throbbing dick. Mix and match as appropriate until your mouth is busy being inappropriate.

There is also the approach of instructions cleverly-disguised as dirty talk, *i.e.* "now put your finger on my clit," "suck my tits," "I want you to bite me harder." Or the command-talk can be a hot lead-in to light S&M ("Lie down so I can do whatever the fuck I want to you"), but that's another post.

Note that there was no mention of *feet* in the above formula. I am fine with a finger up my ass, but I will never again suck on a guy's sweaty big toe because it is WEIRD. *Ew ew ew ew ewwwwwwWWWWW.* –scrapes retroactive toe cooties off tongue–

Don't sound like a sex robot

For fuck's sake, say it because you mean it. Don't say "I love licking your balls" if you don't. Enthusiasm is half of what makes dirty talk so damn hot. The eyes and body should be following whatever your mouth is saying. Otherwise it's obvious you're saying these things just because you think you should be, not because you want to.

If there is nothing else you take away from my blog, please understand that one of the many reasons sex is so awesome is because it's one of the few places in life you can indulge in all the things you want to do, assuming you have a partner who's a decent match. Sex is supposed to be *fun,* not a chore. So, let's make it fun, shall we?

The dirty talk doesn't need to be a running commentary of every single thing that happens. That's annoying and it's like you're reciting dialogue from porn. As far as intervals between each time you say something . . . that's something you have to judge on your own. Depending on the guy/heat/action/situation it may be good to say something nasty every fifteen seconds, one minute, or five minutes. It's not something you should keep track of, just do whatever goes with the flow. Your call.

If you can't remember anything else I've said: Quote sexy songs
. . . still got the freak in me. I'm a slave for you. Loosen up my buttons, baby. I'm bossy . . . oh lemme slow it down so ya can catch the flow. Give it up and let me have my way. I wanna give you a taste of the sugar below my waist. And, of course: *I want to fuck you like an animal*. Classic, orgasmic, never fails to induce a moan.

A cheat sheet of things you can say to help you feel inspired to come up with your own special bits of nasty-nasty:

I can't wait to ride you

I'm going to fuck you so hard you'll think you died and went to heaven

How am I supposed to suck you off if you still have all your clothes on?

You bring out the freak in me

I want you to cum on my tits

You're so fucking hot

I thought about you when I got off earlier today

I love getting nasty with you

You know how to make me feel so good

Your cock feels so good inside me

What are you waiting for

I've been waiting for this all day

You like reverse cowgirl? Because I do.

I'm going to blow your mind

Get between my legs NOW

Give me some of that big cock of yours

Bend me over

Bite me

Bite me harder

I said BITE ME HARDER

I'm going to ride you all night long

I'm not done, babe

Put your fingers in my pussy

I think about you every time I masturbate

I'm going to show you how good you make me feel

You make me want to do things I've never done before

Fingerfuck me

    Okay that list was like twice as long as I intended. Forgive me. If I'm not getting laid, I at least want to do what I can to help other people get laid. A*hem*, Karma. You owe me an entire fleet of Navy SEALs by now. You think I'm kidding? That's what it's going to take to satisfy this Texas Platinum Pussy, sweetie.

Look At Me Look At Me oh *shit* THEY'RE LOOKING AT ME!

On Friday a bunch of us went to a bar after work. While driving over it occurred to me that Sexy Venezuelan may be there. I knew Hot Brother would be, and they're friends with a lot of the people on the email list that went around that afternoon.

Just in case Sexy Venezuelan was there, I made sure I looked good. He had not returned my call from Sunday and it was beginning to piss me off. Time to prepare myself: let my hair down, check on The Twins (keep up the good work, girls!), and recite my mantra: *I am not nervous! I am too sexy to be nervous! I am NOT NERVOUS!*

It didn't work.

I was among the last to arrive at the bar because I had to finish up some things for that afternoon's huge meeting. That meant that the bar was packed both inside and out by the time I arrived. Fortunately, I was able to snag the last available spot in the parking lot right by the patio, meaning that everyone there could see me as I approached.

Eep. I am not nervous IamnotnervousIamnotnervous. NO. Stop it. I. am. not. nervous. Get some sexy music going in your head! Ooh la la, *I'm boss-ay!* Okay, here's your chance to strut your stuff! Now GO.

As I walked toward the patio I saw heads turn in response to the loud click of my heels on pavement. *Look at me. Please look at me, I need all the ego-building I can get right now . . . look at me . . .* and don't forget to breathe, dumbass. It's okay, I am cooool. I am so cool, I've come back around to *hot*. I've got on a sexy knee-length pencil skirt and a set of legs so lethal that a guy between them once told me if he had to die, this was how he wanted it to happen.

This may or may not come as a surprise, but most girls love getting noticed (we just don't show it). Assuming the guys doing the checking-out are somewhat attractive, of a reasonable age, and not creepy. Otherwise, don't be too surprised when you stare at a girl my age and she hisses at you just because you were alive back when programming was done on punch cards.

Dozens of eyes turned to take me in. Time to work my strut like I'm going for the jugular. Shoulders back, one foot directly in front of the other for maximum hip-swivel, lead with the tits, and give a lot of attitude. And, of course, I pretended like this was how I always am. That's right, I'm sexy even when I walk the dogs, little bags of poo in hand. I *rock* bags of poo.

On most occasions, guys (at least the smarter ones) wait until a girl passes by to comment, gesture, air-grope, air-hump, etc. Guys who speak another language assume they are exempt from this, but they often forget that there girls may still know what *Mire esta perra!* means. *Pelotudo.*

Not this time. As I walked toward the patio, I saw a guy standing on the left turn, look at me, turn back to his friends, and gesture toward me with his beer bottle. They all turned to look at the same time.

AGHHHH!!! *SHIT!* I wasn't ready for that! I'm not supposed to *see* you check me out, I'm only supposed to *hope* you checked me out! STOP LOOKING AT ME!!!

I lost it. Suddenly my sexy strut dissolved: the nice posture transformed into a stiff torso, the hip rotation went off-balance so that I nearly tripped out of my own shoe, and all grace transformed into a tremble in my hands that nearly had me snap my sunglasses in half. In the span of three footsteps I lost fifteen years of sexiness and self-confidence, all because a couple of cute guys eyed me at the same time. Go figure, I became nervous as hell, because I am a goddamn twelve year-old clomping around in Mommy's heels.

Once I stood with both feet firmly planted on the deck, I looked around for my coworkers. They weren't there. *Shit.* Move, move, *move!* my brain yelled at me, before those cute guys revoke their appreciative glances now that they saw me trip and get flustered! I turned and made a bee-line for the door. As I passed the table of guys, I avoided eye contact and hoped that they at least liked looking at my ass out of consolation for me making a total jackass of myself. Tripping and doing a face-plant on the wooden deck probably would have been better because then at least boys would rush to my rescue and touch me.

Often girls (myself included, as my friend Barbie has informed me on a couple occasions) don't know they're being checked out. As someone who has a tendency to run into corners and bedposts on a good day, I have to say that it's better this way. I can only pull off the sexy thing when no one is looking. Fucking *brilliant*.

I walked inside with only a mild bump of my shoulder against the doorway. My coworkers sat at the first large group of tables inside. The first person I saw was Hot Coworker. Oh, fucking hell. Just the bastard I wanted to see when I'm trying to shake a bad case of dumbass. And there's no Sexy Venezuelan to trill his Rs at me. SOMEONE GET ME A GODDAMN BEER.

I wrote this post for those of you who have said things like, "You can't really be as self-conscious as you make yourself out to be if you're the same girl taking home two guys in one night. Are you holding out on us?" My answer: NO!!!

I would love to be that girl who is so sure of herself that she never stutters when asking a guy for his phone number or looks behind her for some other girl because that cute guy by the pool table couldn't really be motioning at *her*. Seriously? I still can't believe I pulled that off. The entire night I kept expecting one of them to suddenly see through the beer goggles and then take off running out my apartment. This isn't me being modest, this is the ugly nerd from high school still being surprised every time a cute boy talks to her about anything other than math.

Please remember where I'm coming from: the ugly nerd girl with glasses who didn't get her first kiss until she was fifteen—and this after ten years of actively trying. I assumed I was going to be an ugly nerd girl for life, so I made my peace with it and threw myself into books. Imagine my surprise when I woke up one day and realized that I had perky tits and kind of totally rocked the nerd glasses. In spite of that delightful discovery, I've known the ugly nerd girl for far longer than the sexy one standing in the mirror now. I can't help it. After twenty-plus years as a nerd it's hard to see myself as anything else.

I also wrote this post for the nerdy guys out there who are often too nervous to talk to a girl, let alone ask one out. A reality check—we're just as nervous as you are. Don't let the hair twirls and girlish giggles trick you. Those are cover-ups for jittery hands and not being able to put together coherent sentences.

And for fuck's sake, please be a gentleman and help me up off the floor after I fall on my ass because I saw you checking me out.

How To Answer "If You're So Great, Why Are You Still Single?"

As a single person in my upper twenties, it royally pisses me off when some snot-nosed coworker or relative asks me the dreaded question:

> "If you are so [choose all that apply]:
> ____great
> ____funny
> ____sweet
> ____charming
> ____good-looking
> ____successful
> then why are you still single?"

If you are pissed off like me, I'm guessing that the first thing that comes to mind is, "So annoying assholes like you can ask me this question and I have reason to verbally if not physically bitchslap you back to your good sense."

But that's not very nice. Shame on you. Your answer should also be snarky:

1. The last guy I dated was bad in bed, so to make sure that doesn't happen again I make all prospective boyfriends go through an intensive booty-camp. None have made it past the third day of training, and one of them was a Navy SEAL.
2. Hey, you're going through a divorce, right? I've always wanted to get on a cougar.
3. I've been told I have a *smell* situation, and for the life of me I can't figure out where it's coming from.
4. The strap-on always scares them away. What the hell, it's not like I don't promise to use lube!
5. Word got out that my last boyfriend was sacrificed to The Almighty Kegel.

6. –bursts into tears and runs away crying–
7. Excuse me? I'm not single. I'm dating TiVo. Okay FINE we're having problems but he's at the repair center, okay?!
8. Guys say they don't like all my cats. I don't understand, I only have nine. I used to have fourteen, which, I will admit, were too many. But, that's why they had their own room!
9. I'm sorry, my therapist told me I'm not allowed to talk to assholes like you anymore.
10. It freaks out guys when they hear my brain and The Pussy fighting.
11. I'm not ready to date yet. I'm only halfway F2M. Only got the top half ready so far, ya know what I mean? –wink wink–
12. Really?? You think I'm a lovely young woman? DO YOU HAVE A SON YOU CAN SET ME UP WITH? I want to be a baby machine before I turn thirty! BABIESBABIESBABIESBABIESBABIESBABIESBABIES!!!
13. Because I have more balls than they do.
14. I am NOT SINGLE. We're just having communication issues. He's always hanging out with that *girl* and then there's that damn restraining order, neither of which are helping to open our channels of communi*fucking*cation! I even sent him a *cookie bouquet*! A COOKIE BOUQUET MEANS TRUE LOVE, WHY CAN'T HE UNDERSTAND THAT?!
15. I suck them stupid.
16. Most guys can't keep up with my rigorous schedule of TV-watching and fourteen hours of sleep a day. Successful women like me need a guy who can keep up with us, you know?
17. Um, I'm dating *your daughter*. Oh my god, she swore to me that she told you she's gay! THE BITCH LIED. That's it, I want my favorite vibrator back!

Is It Enough To Keep Breathing?

Tonight while cleaning up the apartment, I put on DVR and found the season 3 finale to *Grey's Anatomy*. Even though I've seen the ending several times, it still moves me to sobs. Not tears, *sobs*.

Cristina Yang, a resident who's a total commitment-phobic hard-ass (and coincidentally my favorite person on the show) agrees to marry a wonderful man. At the church, she flips out and he realizes that it is not in her character to get married, so he walks out.

It reminds me of how close I came to losing myself in my previous relationship. Aussie was a great guy—it wasn't his fault that I had started fading away. It was all mine. He didn't know how I was supposed to be, who I once was. The fact that things like a baby shower made me react so strongly has me wondering *why*? I suspect it's not nearly as simple as it seems.

A while ago Aussie asked to meet for a drink and catch-up. At first I brushed him off with apologies of a looming deadline (which was true), but the real truth was that I didn't—couldn't—see him. It has nothing to do with him personally, which was why I didn't understand my reluctance. It is only tonight while writing this that I realized why, that I'm afraid seeing someone who knew such an ugly version of me would somehow bring that person back. Of course, that's crap, but it is enough to keep me from wanting to see Aussie. He represents a life I don't want, at least not right now.

We were never officially engaged, but we often talked about it. He hinted at rings. I hinted back. We talked about how/where we would get married—on the harbor next to the famous Sydney Opera House, since he was from Sydney. I said all the things I was supposed to say. I said few of the things I wanted to say, and eventually I stopped saying anything at all. I didn't write. I didn't cry. Instead, I slept.

I hate to think what my life would have been if I had stayed on that path. Aussie was a good guy, so our marriage wouldn't have been bad, it just would not have been right. Husband, a couple kiddos, a house, an eight-to-five job—it would have been fine. Just fine.

The song that plays during the break-up scene, "Keep Breathing" by Ingrid Michaelson, is what I have been listening to while writing this post. So simple, such soothing repetition, yet so full of emotion. I wish this song had existed a couple years ago—it might have been the slap I needed to wake the fuck up.

> The storm is coming but I don't mind.
> People are dying, I close my blinds.
> All that I know is I'm breathing now.
>
> I want to change the world . . . instead I sleep.
> I want to believe in more than you and me.
>
> But all that I know is I'm breathing.
> All I can do is keep breathing.
> All we can do is keep breathing now.
>
> All that I know is I'm breathing.
> All I can do is keep breathing.
> All we can do is keep breathing now.
>
> All we can do is keep breathing
> All we can do is keep breathing
> All we can do is keep breathing
> All we can do is keep breathing.
> All we can do is keep breathing now.

For so many years I slept through my own life. There was no cancer, no suicide, no personal tragedy that kept me hiding underneath my covers day after day. It was all in my head, which is exactly why it was so hard to shake it. There are entire semesters of my undergraduate years that I can barely remember because I slept through them. Twelve, fourteen, sixteen hours a day in bed. How I passed classes or didn't get fired is a mystery.

Years. I lost years of my life in sleep.

Eventually I started peeking out from under the covers—seeing my relationship, my life for what it was and wasn't—I didn't want to spend the rest of my life like that. It took a long time to lower the covers enough to show my face, to sit up in bed and feel a deep breath fill my lungs, to touch my foot to the ground and stand up. When it finally happened I was surprised to find such strength in my muscles. It had been so long since I'd stood on my own that I assumed I would sink to the ground as soon as I tried. Although it was the most difficult step I've ever had to make, it was also the one that changed everything.

Seeing how happy I am now, it pains me to think how far away I could have been from here if I had stayed. Every day for the rest of my life, I will think back to the day I made that first shaky step and smile knowing it was worth the anguish.

I don't give a fuck how lame it makes me look to say the things I have in this post. I've been crying nearly the entire time it has taken to write this. A moment ago the sobs shook my body so hard that they stirred something deep down in my gut. With each heave of my ribcage I felt the resolve growing inside. It coursed through my body with such force that it felt like my chest thickened with each heave. Then the crying subsided and I felt the determination settle in my spine, in the straight set of my jaw. *I felt it.* It's the strength that can only come from the darkest and most precious of places.

On the typical day of working late at the office, studying all evening for my real job, and then writing until three in the morning, I often wonder if it's worth it. When I meet douchebag after dumbass after dipshit, I wonder if they're worth it. When I think about how much I miss New York City and how far away it feels all the way down here in Texas, I wonder if I'm stupid for hoping to make my way back there one day. And what about Mr. Perfect-For-Me? If I'm such a cynic, why do I still find myself hoping that eventually I'll fall in love? Is it worth wondering how many more times it will take before I find someone I know I wouldn't leave one day?

I don't know what I would be doing if I didn't think it were worth it— because it is not enough to keep breathing, not for me.

163 lbs., alcohol units ~~2~~ 4, bowls of Cinnamon Toast Crunch 3, calories acknowledged 7

9:14 a.m. Arrive at office.

9:15 a.m. Wonder if have been seen, *i.e.* if too late to run back out and call in sick from car in parking lot.

9:47 a.m. Pants are tight. Bollocks. According to scale at gym, have gained ten pounds in last two months. Would blame boss for making me abuse love of comfort food, but ass still looks better than hers despite ten extra pounds concentrated in mid-section. Karma must be starting at my boss's ass. Rejoice.

10:10 a.m. Poke stack of papers on desk with ballpoint pen. Consider faking a nervous break-down to get out of work. Wouldn't have to fake very much.

10:11 a.m. Stack of papers fell over, nearly got killed under the weight of menial tasks.

10:15 a.m. Examine finger for blood from (invisible?) paper cut. Wonder how much blood it would take to be sent home from office. Start poking hand with envelope opener. Oh, bloody hell, must have skin as impregnable as that of Superman.

10:16 a.m. Wonder who would be if were a superhero. Maybe Super-Peon? Super-Peon, defender of cubicle monkeys everywhere!

11:15 a.m. Boss is using That Tone with me. Resist urge to bitchslap her five ways from Sunday. Should receive an Inner Poise award, complete with gift certificate for a massage and mani/pedi.

2:56 p.m. Haven't been to gym in week and a half. Must go to gym tonight to tone inner poise. Must have goals and determination to reach state of peace with self, like all the books on TV say. Books are very smart, *ipso facto* those who read books are very smart and that much closer to state of excellence and envy of fake-friends. Excellent.

4:44 p.m. Wonder when it's too soon to start listening to Christmas music made by assorted sell-out pop artists. No, Mariah, all I want for Christmas is *you*.

6:38 p.m. Leave office, work bag freshly stocked with assorted pens, Post-it pads, highlighters, and a new bottle of Tylenol thanks to the office supply closet.

7:09 p.m. Undress, free self from uniform of Responsible Adult. Put on knee socks and Coyote Ugly tanktop. Work cooties gone now. V.g.

7:11 p.m. Stare at belly in bathroom mirror. Poke belly for evaluation of jigglyness. Only have jiggle rating of 3, v.g. Can skip gym for one more day. V. tired from dodging boss's finger of accusation all day.

7:17 p.m. Cook broccoli and snow peas for dinner. Skipping gym, make up by eating healthy. Excellent.

7:21 p.m. Eat healthy, not v.g. Eat bowl of Cinnamon Toast Crunch. V.g. Eat two more bowls. V.v. g. Surprisingly good with wine. Not really, but don't care. Wine + cinnamon sugary goodness = my happy place.

7:42 p.m. Dog has been staring at my arse for much longer than usual. Can feel the dog judging. Perhaps should go to gym after all, right after finish this glass of wine.

8:03 p.m. Play movie *The Devil Wears Prada* while attempt to organize tall stack of papers on writing desk. Wonder if all papers in daily life are conspiring to bury me alive one day.

8:08 p.m. Conclude yes. Leave stacks of papers alone.

8:19 p.m. Turn off size six Anne Hathaway. Put on more realistically sized Bridget Jones. I too choose vodka and Chaka Khan.

8:50 p.m. Wonder what the conversation would be between Bridget and Dwight, with the occasional voice-over by Carrie.

8:52 p.m. Should watch less TV. Should go to gym. There is TV at gym.

8:54 p.m. But seriously, imagine! I couldn't help but wonder . . . shouldn't he be loved just as he is, bears, beets, Battlestar Galactica and all? "It has been a lifetime struggle, a never-ending fight, I say to you and you will understand that it is a privilege to fight the war of relationships and 'happily ever after' as single men and women. WE ARE WARRIORS!" [applause]

9:01 p.m. It's not too late to go to the gym. Really should go to gym if for no other reason than to run off work-induced stress. Weights nice too. Like making loud noises.

9:04 p.m. Half the wine is gone, might as well finish the bottle. Hate to leave perfectly good bottle of $5.99 wine chilling in fridge when wine would obviously prefer to be in my tummy.

9:35 p.m. Still not too late to go to gym.

9:40 p.m. Stare at feet lying on top of ottoman. Stare at glass of wine. Stare at running shoes. Stare at feet. They'll move any second now, just know it.

9:58 p.m. Can feel arse growing. Must be long-awaited inner poise beginning to develop. Congratulate self with another glass of wine.

10:20 p.m. To hell with it. Sitting on my big fat inner fucking poise. Very cushy, quite lovely. V.g.

I Have Tits Too, You Know

The last few weeks it seems like all I do is work, work, and then work some more. How intellectually titillating. *Rub my brain harder, oooh, just like that! Stimulate me! Yes, yes, keep going!!*

My brain is going on over-drive, which is not wise when The Pussy is running on empty. When I work all day, work all evening, then dream about work all night—I start to feel unappreciated as a piece of ass.

No girl should ever have to feel that way.

It's a fine balance one looks for in her life, feeling equally appreciated intellectually, emotionally, and sexually. The day job and night writing have the intellectual realm more than covered, friends keep me emotionally stable-esque, leaving sexuality far behind in the "special needs" group.

"What about those guys who hit on you at the party?" you may ask. You mean The Douchebag, Clueless Guy, and the "girlfriend? what girlfriend?" guy? The ones who made three cheers for thighs? Yes, what *fine* specimens of the twentysomething male demographic. How dare you remind me. NEXT.

Now don't get all huffy and throw feminism at me with something about how today's women are strong, independent, and empowered based on their minds alone. Yada yada YES WE KNOW. Wee, power, let's burn something. I love my mind, it's one hell of a sexy bitch who brings home a paycheck every two weeks—but sometimes I want to scream *there is more to me than my brain! I HAVE TITS TOO, YOU KNOW!!!*

Forgive me. It's been two months. I think my boobs are shrinking due to lack of recognition.

Most of the time I love being all professional-looking on the outside and then pierced, tattooed, and horny as fuck on the inside—but most of the time there's some sort of pay-out for that. What fun are having secrets when no one in your daily life bothers to wonder if you have any?

This isn't about needing to see myself through someone else's eyes or feeling validated in my sexuality. I know I don't need that, but I still want someone to look. Meanwhile I feel like I'm the only one walking through the office or filling my car at the gas station who is aware of the fact that I have an ass. Sometimes it's just nice to be noticed, especially when you're so caught up in your own head that you can't remember the last time you shaved your legs, let alone had someone to touch them.

All I want is the occasional appreciative eye—from a guy at the grocery store (who is non-douchey, not stupid, mostly functional and half attractive), a cute office temp, a super-hot, sexually confused girl at the coffee shop. They don't even have to say anything! It's better not to say anything because then they don't ruin my happy memory with stupid *talking*. Don't talk. Just look at me like you know there's a nympho hidden underneath these slacks.

I need the blood to pump somewhere other than my brain. I need to go to sleep at night fantasizing about a guy I met who damn near made me cum with his eye contact alone, not thinking about the stack of papers waiting for me at my desk in the morning. Papers don't remind me that I have a body. They just give me paper cuts.

There's more to me than my brain. I swear. If I flash you then you'll believe me, right?

More Than A Blowjob Queen

Some days I'm feeling sexy and so I write about blowjobs or threesomes. Other days I'm feeling funny so I write about dating or the skeeze-bags who want to buy my underwear. On a really good day I hit the snark just right and out comes pure bitch-gold. Then there are the times like tonight when I find myself ankle-deep in shit water in my bathroom.

As if standing in shit weren't bad enough, it was my own shit. MY SHIT IS NOT SUPPOSED TO TURN ON ME.

It was poo time. I got my magazine, dropped my jeans, and was having a lovely time. *Flush*, pull up jeans, wash hands, walk out with a smile on my face. Then I heard that dreadful sound of rushing water that can only mean one thing: aw *fuck*. I ran to the bathroom. The toilet was overflowing with brown water. POOP IS EVERYWHERE! *EWWWWWWWWWWWWWWWWWWWWW!*

What's my first impulse? *Save the* Cosmopolitan*!* [I know, I KNOW, okay?! Shit water is covering my fancy white tile and I save the fucking *Cosmo* magazine with "Hair That Gets You What You Want" printed on the cover. There is no need to point and laugh. I mean, *fuck*, I spent twenty minutes standing in shit water, is that not embarrassment enough?]

Water hits my toes, then the bottom of my jeans. My eyes dart from toilet to feet to floor. Why won't the fucking thing stop?! It's never done this before! THE TOILET PASSED THE POO TEST MONTHS AGO, OTHERWISE I WOULDN'T HAVE RENTED AN INFERIOR BATHROOM! WHY IS IT DOING THIS TO ME NOW??? WHY AT MIDNIGHT ON A FUCKING SUNDAY NIGHT?! WHAT HAVE I DONE TO ANGER THE TOILET GODS?! IT'S NOT MY FAULT! I ATE A FUCKING SALAD, YOU ASSHOLES!!

Frantically I pulled up the legs of my jeans to my knees, flung the bath towel off the shower rod onto the floor, and pulled off the top of the toilet tank.

It's times like this I really wish I had a boyfriend. Boys like icky things and potty jokes. They are one with poo. Where, oh, where is my imaginary boyfriend? *Hey sweetie, why don't you fix this and I'll go make us some flan? BJ later! Love ya, okay kisses!!*

The water wouldn't stop overflowing. OH MY FUCKING GOD THIS IS ICKY, ICKY, *ICKY!* GOOD LORD ALMIGHTY MAKE IT STOP!!!!

I ran into the living room where I had left yesterday's pool towel [it's Texas. It's mid-October and it's still ninety degrees. This is normal.] The water had nearly made it to the carpet in the hallway. With a triumphant flourish I threw down the huge towel as a barricade to keep the water inside the bathroom. It worked! The water was backing up in the bathroom! And now I'm standing—I AM STANDING IN SHIT WATER. I perched one foot on the bathtub and raised up on the tip-toes of the other. WHY HASN'T THE WATER STOPPED YET?! I pulled up the floaty ball thing because it is the only thing I know to do to fix a toilet other than duct taping the whole fucking thing closed and praying the water pressure doesn't create a geyser of shit water in my neighbor's bathroom. I waited a few seconds. All is quiet except for the slow drip of water from the toilet to the pool on the floor. I let go of the ball floaty thing. The miniature Niagara Falls of shit water starts again.

FUUUUUUUUUUUUUUUUUUUUUUUUUUUUCK.

I pull it up again. I am standing on one foot in shit water with the floaty thing in my hand. I have no idea what to do. The phone is too far away for me to use my free toes to dial my father. I am fucked.

NO. I AM A SMART, INDEPENDENT WOMAN! I DO NOT NEED A MAN!! (At least not for this.) I AM A FEMINIST! I OWN POWER TOOLS! I CAN FIX SHIT! I WILL FIX THE SHIT SITUATION ON MY OWN!! *GRRR*, MOTHAFUCKAS, GRR!

I run out of the bathroom and grab a couple more towels from the dirty laundry. Two go directly in front of the toilet to hold back the worst of the water. The third one goes directly in front of the one protecting the carpet.

The big scrubby brush I use for cleaning the tub is lying on the floor. In shit water. It has a handle. A handle covered in shit water. I grab it and maneuver the handle to tuck under the metal arm while the larger part rests on the porcelain. After a couple tries I get it to hold so that the floaty thing is still and water stops flowing.

Silence.

By this time I am ankle-deep in shit water. I wish I were exaggerating. I would love to be exaggerating about this, but it was so bad that four of my ten little piggies are still crying in horror of the memory.

Once the water stopped, there was a dam of towels holding back three inches of shit water.

Fuck. Fuck fuck fuck fuuuuuuuuuuuuuuuuuuuuck. THIS IS NOT HOW MY RELAXING SUNDAY NIGHT WAS SUPPOSED TO GO.

I spent the next hour cleaning the bathroom and unclogging the toilet. To top off the fun, the cleaning products I use are kept by the toilet. That meant they were victims of Shitfest '07 and required extensive cleaning before they themselves could be used. It took a total of seven towels, an entire roll of paper towels (the good ones! This is why you don't buy the generic crap, *Mother*), two loads of laundry, innumerable and frightfully creative expletives, a 25-minute shower, and a chug from the bottle of wine in the fridge.

So that story was nice and cute (in a totally disgusting let's-never-speak-of-this-again sort of way) but there's more to this post than the simple shit water situation.

Every once in a while, I feel the need to remind readers that there is more to me than sex. When I see that nearly 75% of my daily readers find me from Google searches for "how to give a blowjob" or "nympho," it gets depressing. I may write about sex and I may love writing about sex, but I cannot always write about sex. I'm fucking human. I go four and a half months without getting laid. I get caught up in work I have to do for my "real" job. I cry. I have shitty days, and on those shitty days, I don't give a fuck about sex. All I want to do is get in the shower and scrub the scent of shit water off my skin.

Many days I am damn proud to be Google's #2 blowjob queen, but sometimes I want to scream *there is is more to me than sex*. Not that I have a right to be angry—what is to be expected when I call myself the Over-Educated Nympho and write detailed posts about blowjobs, sex, and threesomes? It's fun and I enjoy it, but I'm not like that all the time.

Do I ever think about ending OEN? Not at all. I can't. I'm not all sex, but I'm not all serious either. Sometimes, I look at my blog and wonder how so many different voices come out of one person (sweet merciful crap, I had an aunt with schizophrenia). Sometimes, I wonder if I should quit OEN and call myself something else that wouldn't be such a let-down to those who come in search of nothing but dirty whore sex and find themselves face-to-face with this side of me. Then I remind myself that this is how I am. Moody as hell, horny as fuck, and everything in between. I don't know any other way to be.

[P.S. It was after I posted this that several helpful readers informed me there's a water valve at the base of the toilet that I could have easily shut off, if only my father had told me of this sometime in my nearly 30 years on the planet.]

My First Time Sparkled

After receiving a delightfully large year-end bonus, I decided that I was going to buy one fun thing (not that getting the brakes on my car fixed isn't a barrel full of jollies. (W*eee, look at me stop suddenly and safely!)*, I also don't think buying more work clothes to replace the shirts with food stains and pants with coffee stains is exciting, but more a professional requirement so I don't out myself as a dumbass playing grown-up for all this time).

On Friday, I decided that I was going to walk into a nice jewelry store and buy myself whatever the fuck I wanted.

When the idea to buy a diamond necklace first came to me, I dismissed it as being stupid and frivolous. *Put the extra money in savings! You would only like the necklace for a month and then when you're sixty and living off Easy Mac you will wish you had put it in your IRA instead! Be sensible! For fuck's sake, at least buy new tires.*

I couldn't get it out of my head. The bonus check was substantial enough to have some fun with and still have plenty left over to use responsibly. Besides that, I wanted a little something special for myself—something *I* gave myself. Sure, I already own some nice things, but all of them have been either gifts from boyfriends or "on loan" from my mother. They're not special in the way that something can only be special when buying it for yourself, which is why diamond promise rings from boyfriends have never dazzled me. I assumed I was undazzleable. I would be one of the few chicks ever to get married who refused a diamond ring in lieu of something simple. What's the big deal over a stupid diamond? *Wee* it sparkles, so the fuck what?

Now I get it. And let me tell you, it doesn't have a damn thing to do with a boyfriend.

I wanted my first diamond-shopping experience to be perfect. Is this not an experience I'll remember for the rest of my life? I wanted nothing but magic. The weather was beautiful, although unseasonal (eighty degrees in December in Texas), I had managed to avoid my evil boss for most of the day, and I was full of smiles and booty-shakes.

When I walked in, several sales people approached me, but I waved most of them off. One was a crotchety-looking old man who would clearly prefer to be doing inventory than interacting with others, one was a vile middle-aged woman who looked like she should be smoking three packs of cigarettes while bitching about her last three ex-husbands, and the last was a nice-looking guy slightly older than myself. *Ah yes, my darling diamond boy, you will do just fine for my first time!*

When he started pulling out pieces for me, I noticed a tattoo on his wrist peeking out from his shirt-sleeve. Later, I saw a Celtic tattoo at the base of his neck that had been hidden by his collar. Ah, crisply ironed by day, freaky by night. Yes, exactly the guy I want to remember for my first diamond-shopping experience.

After he showed me the pieces I pointed out in the cases, I chose a white-gold necklace with a pendant made of three small diamonds hanging above one another. Simple, classic, and perfect. It was exactly what I wanted.

I must have been giddy while I was looking at the jewelry because the sales guy eyed me curiously and asked if I was shopping for myself. I beamed yes. He warmed up and told me about his own first time with a sheepish, but proud smile.

After the guy rang it up, he started putting the necklace in a dark, velvet box. *No!* I squealed. *I want to wear it out.* He dropped the necklace into my open hand. With anxious hands, I undid the tiny clasp and struggled to fasten it around my neck. At that moment I knew that I would never forget the feeling of the necklace laying on my bare skin for the first time.

Something so simple—a small diamond necklace I bought myself—means so much more than if someone else had bought me the same thing, or something five times bigger. I don't give a fuck how many carats it is. That's not the point. It's not about the money or even the diamond necklace.

It's special because it sparkles just for me.

Waking Up Next To Hairy Man-Ass

The other night, I watched the movie *Knocked Up*. After the lovely Katherine Heigl sleeps with Fugly Dude, she wakes up in the morning to his pale, fat ass in her bed. Youtube it. Yeah. I know that hairy man-ass moment all too well.

There have been many hairy man-asses in my day. This was why I stopped bringing guys back to my place. Nothing sighs *casual sex* like finding a freakishly long pubic hair on the bar of soap in your shower. I trim. Ain't no way that shit is mine. Who does it belong to? Mr. Harry Man-Ass.

The last time I was single was when I was in college. Cute and horny guys were a dime a dozen. They came knocking on my door, beeping on IM, and calling on my phone. The condoms tucked away in my purse didn't stay there for months at a time like they do now. I'm sure the latex melted and congealed to the inside of the packaging months ago. If I got one of those in every color and hot-glued them to a cucumber I could sell it as an installation piece from an up-and-cumming artist.

Now I don't get nearly as much action as I did back then. I've been with six people since the break-up a year and a half ago. Six? Really, that's it? Damn, does that mean my virginity is going to grow back any day now? It sucked plenty the first time around.

The months between fucks keep growing longer. Now each day that passes is a new record. Currently I'm at four and a half sex-less months. I'm getting like *really* mean.

Last time I was single I was not so picky about who I fucked. Between that and the weekly parties it is not surprise that I got laid so often. *A guy is a guy, a dick's a dick*. Back then, I chased anyone who caught and held my attention. The outcome was always a crap shoot: is he going to be good? Bad? Terrible? Downright embarrassing? Or so amazing that to this day I still get instant wet between the legs when I think about him?

Of course, there are plenty I remember fondly, but there are plenty whose names I don't remember. I promise you however, that I remember something about every single one of them. If not the image of his naked, hairy ass burned into my brain, then it's something equally sexy.

One guy opened my beer bottle for me by pulling the cap off with his teeth and then spitting it out on the floor. Stepping on one of those serrated bad boys in the morning was the perfect way to finish off an otherwise lousy night (and that was the only thing that got finished off). Once, when I asked for a drink, the guy gave me a glass of water that tasted of cigarette butts. The one time I ever brought home a drunk guy he ran through the apartment looking for orange juice ("electrolytes!") with his woody bouncing up and down, much to the horror of my Baptist roommate. One guy came out of the bathroom demanding to know why I had so many bottles of prescription pills in my medicine cabinet. All these stories make the ones who vow their undying love for you after the first blowjob not seem so bad.

Although I have many amusing stories from that time in my life, there are just as many stories that leave a bad taste in my mouth. Do I regret any of them? Yeah, a couple. I also regret maxing out my credit card when I was twenty-three and not breaking up with any of my ex-boyfriends sooner. Those are things I would actually take back. [And may I just say, I REALLY regret not starting this blog years earlier, although it probably wouldn't have the bite or wit that it does from having started at a later/pissier age.] But this long strand of guys I remember mostly as hairy asses in the faint glow of a bedroom lamp? Not worth the five seconds of regret, not when so many other moments shine so bright that I shudder when I think of them.

The thing is, now that I've what, matured? Counted more bad fucks than good ones? Realized that after casual sex guys *do* like to cuddle regardless of what *I* want, which is for them to get the hell out? I don't want to ever again wake up next to hairy man-ass. I want to wake up with a hard-on pressed against me, and if I can't have that, then I will continue waking up alone with my own hand between my legs.

You Know You Need to Get Laid When

1. With great horror you realize that you could grow a huge icky fly-eating mole right on the middle of your stomach and it would have absolutely no impact on your sex life.
2. The old man at work who calls you "Lady Longlegs" is beginning to not look so bad. Maybe even a little cute in a hairy-eared gremlin kind of way.
3. You catch yourself singing "Little Lady Awesomepants" to the tune of "London Bridge is Falling Down."
4. The cute college intern refuses to come near you after you sniffed him one too many times.
5. Watching your dogs licking each other makes you really jealous. And maybe just a tittily bit turned on. The bitches. THIS IS WHY YOU GOT FIXED.
6. You know that your fiftysomething parents are getting way more action than you are and you kind of hope Dad breaks his hip. (Oh, that's not nice.) Fine. *Fractures* his hip.
7. You press your ear to the shared wall every night, desperately hoping that by being within a twenty-foot radius of someone who is getting laid will bring you some sort of cosmic boning.
8. You find yourself reminiscing about the good ol' days of high school sex with your boyfriend who couldn't spell orgasm let alone give you one.
9. You actively avoid the condom aisle because last time you were there it heckled you.
10. Every time you leave your hand alone for more than thirty seconds it wanders down to your crotch.
11. Every time you wake up in the morning your hand has wandered down to your crotch.
12. Every time you're in front of a mirror, you stare at your crotch screaming, "WHAT DID I EVER DO TO YOU?!"

13. You stop trimming your pubes and remember just how German your ancestry is.
14. You masturbate so much that you sprain your wrist, your other wrist, four fingers, and use up every battery in a twenty-pack. In one week. Okay, five days. Oh, shut up.
15. Your dogs pant as you change clothes and you feel a little bit sexier.
16. You wonder if this is some sort of divine Catholic punishment for having sex before marriage. Then you think about going to a church to confess your sins because you heard the new priest is a nice piece of eye candy and if you're already going to hell you really want to go to hell.
17. Getting your nipple pierced sounds like a fantastic idea because that means someone else will touch it for the first time in five months. If you tip him maybe he'll keep touching it.
18. You open the birth control packet in the morning and all the pretty pink pills have rearranged themselves to spell out "HA HA."

Who's On Track?

Today one of my coworkers told me she's four weeks pregnant. She's my age.

In theory, I know that twenty-seven is a perfectly reasonable age to have a baby, but I look at myself and think, oh holy FUCK there's no way I'm mature enough to have a child. Don't let the bank account and vibrator collection fool you, I am a twelve year-old tottering around in heels.

I wouldn't exactly say I'm good friends with Pregnant Coworker, but we talk and email at the office enough that I'm one of the few people she's told so far. We both started the management training program at roughly the same time, and have stuck together because we're the two youngest people involved, as well as being two of the few females in the program. Although she's done more of the units, she has to make up two of her presentations due to unsatisfactory evaluations. Theoretically, that leaves us dead even on our desperate scamper up the corporate ladder.

Or at least we *were* dead even. What is going to happen now that she's on the baby track? It takes a year to complete the training program and we both still have a long ways to go. Pregnant Coworker has a new house to finish remodeling before the baby comes, in addition to being swamped at the office. I wanted to ask her if she planned to bust her ass and finish the program before the baby comes along, but I didn't for fear of sounding like I was judging her if she didn't give me the answer I expected.

Even though there's a good chance I'll pull ahead of her career-wise over the next two years, why do I feel like such a kid? She's married, owns a house, and is glowing with her first pregnancy. I . . . have two dogs. And TiVo. That doesn't exactly scream, "I am woman, hear me roar." It's more like, "I'm a girl! *Weeeeeeeeeeee!*"

Within the period of only two years all my friends went from being single to being engaged/married and buying houses. I went from having a boyfriend to having an Oreo consumption problem and the obnoxious habit of cursing like a Brit.

Although I am perfectly happy with the current state of my life—I still see marriage as a four-letter word and the thought of babies makes me fish the bottom of my purse for a spare Xanax—I feel like I'm missing something. Not a boyfriend, oh, hell no (okay, maybe every once in a while, or when it's been FOUR FUCKLESS MONTHS), but . . . But what?

Am I going to wake up one day ten years from now and wish I had jumped on the marriage/Mommy track at the age of twenty-seven? Am I so hellbent on the career track that I'm blind to any other path?

Please don't misunderstand me, because I am damn proud of where I am in my life. I worked hard to get here and stay here. Living on my own, taking care of myself, advancing in my day job and busting my ass at my writing—it's exactly what I want. At Thanksgiving and again at Christmas I was granted the sweet affirmation from The MOM that out of all the cousins my age, I am advancing the fastest (take THAT Ivy Leaguers and Ms. JD/MBA).

This is in large part due to the fact that I AM single and have the luxury of spending my time any way I please. My cousins/competition are getting married, buying houses, and having babies just like Pregnant Coworker. I'm not, and that was a conscious choice. There is no doubt in my mind that I would not be this far career-wise if I were still dating Aussie. All the hours of studying and overtime for my job, on top of another couple hours of writing every night—he wouldn't have put up with it.

Now my hours are mine and mine alone. Although I'm making the most of them, I still feel like I'm being left behind.

It's My Cooch, Not a Venus Fly Trap

Many of my girl friends and female readers have told me that their man doesn't like going down on them. *Why the* fuck *not*, I ask politely. Cooch is awesome. I've gone bush-diving and I'm down for another round or three any day.

I've always known that it was common for girls to find the penis icky—it grows, it shrinks, it waves hello, it shoots things in your eye, it may wear a turtleneck. What is all this bullshit? Pussy is way better than dick.

I'm going to be honest. That's a deal-breaker for me. But don't take my opinion too seriously, because I'm kind of a huge bitch when there's something like an orgasm on the line.

On one hand, I want to try to be understanding to the guys out there who think cooch is less than appetizing, and I will try my very best here to play devil's advocate, but . . . well . . . I . . . I just have to say it: sweetie, *it's pussy*. Pussy is nothing short of pure awesomeness, and you should be so lucky to have a girl opening her legs and lips for you. RESPECT THE AWESOMENESS OF THE PUSSY.

To the female audience out there who doesn't care that your guy doesn't eat you out because then it means you don't have to suck on his icky thingy: congratulations to the happy couple. That means one more guy who keeps his tongue to himself is off the market and out of what little there is of my hair. You may freely proceed to less orgasm-centered posts on my blog.

To the members of the male audience who try even though you don't have a damn clue what you're doing: I applaud you for trying. Pussy can be an indecipherable and downright confusing thing to approach.

Okay, now I'll be understanding. I will address the common excuses and issues I've heard about not wanting to go down on a girl.

It smells funny. No, it smells like pussy. It's not supposed to smell like rainbows and sunshine, it's supposed to smell like *pussy*. (Don't guys ever watch "The Vagina Monologues" in college?) There's nothing like pussy, and it's hotter than Hell.

It looks funny. Hey man, don't point fingers when you have your own goofy stuff going on. Yeah, pussy may look like a Georgia O'Keeffe painting, but it doesn't exactly look like it's going to beat you up and take your wallet either. Just like breasts, hips, and eyes, pussy looks very different from girl to girl. Part of the fun of being with someone new is enjoying all the curves that make her like no one else, all the way down to what her pussy looks like when you spread the lips open for the first time. It's supposed to be like a flower blossoming and opening up for you or some such poeticness. Whatever. For the love of all things Star Wars, get between her legs and take a good look at what you see waiting for you, because you never know when you'll be going months without seeing it again.

It tastes funny. Yeah, exactly. It tastes *like pussy.*

It feels funny. Okay, this is getting old. Pussy has a taste, smell, look and texture all its own. There's nothing like it, and that's one of the bajillion things that makes pussy rule so fucking hard. If you don't understand that then I think your pussy privileges should be revoked.

No, seriously. It smells funny. The smell of pussy can change a lot throughout the day, especially if she has been sweating from the summer heat or exercise. Some guys like the raw smell of pussy sweat (don't knock it 'till you've tried it), but many don't. No biggie, ask her to shower or better yet get in the shower together. *Weee*, slippery sex and spooge on the ceramic tile!

Is there a way to make it taste better? The taste of pussy juice is directly affected by what she eats and drinks that day. Same thing for guys. This is unfortunate for the world of hook-ups, because they often occur after a night of drinking. It pains me to say this, but the foulest mouthful of cum I've ever had was after the guy had been drinking beer all night long. Coffee isn't too good either (my own culprit), but it's easy to change all that by altering the food and drink a couple hours before you expect to get some. Anything sweet–maple syrup, apple juice, pineapple juice, fruit, or anything healthy like vegetables (and wheatgrass shots, according to *Sex and the City*) improve taste. For girls we have the option of avoiding taste altogether by deep-throating, but our partners don't have that convenience.

The texture inside is gross. So eat out instead of eating in, jackass. Many girls are happy with clitoral action alone, especially if you happen to luck out with a girl who has her clit hood pierced. Lick her clit while you finger her. Although, allow me to say: the hottest time a guy (who happened to be an ex-stripper, wannabe history-professor from Spain, and the all-time best neighbor I could have ever asked for while living in New York City) ate me out was so hot because he *lapped me up* like he wanted every last drop of sweet pussy juice he could reach.

It's too hairy. I respect the whole *au naturale* thing (also known as the "I wasn't expecting to get laid today" thing), but I am more concerned about the pubic floss situation. Pubic floss is so not hot, it slows things down (always at a crucial time, of course), and it covers up all the pretty things that make pussy pussy. Ask her if she'd consider shaving or trimming. A lot of girls are down with this, but not all, so broach carefully. Hint: "I'd eat you out more if you shaved your damn crotch" is not considered "broaching carefully." You might as well be saying "I slept with your twenty-dollar whore of a sister and she gave me chlamydia again." Try, "Hey, why don't we trim for each other? I'm always wanted to try it."

Will a girl break up with me if I don't go down on her? Uhh . . . I'm not a good person to ask. Because I would. Then again it's safe for me to say this because 1) I've never dated a guy who wouldn't eat me out and have therefore never had to make that call, 2) I've never fucked a guy who wouldn't eat me out (not that I threw him out when he wouldn't, I've just never personally encountered a guy who wouldn't. Ever. Which is why this whole thing leaves me befuddled). 3) I place a lot of emphasis on sex in a relationship. More emphasis than is healthy, some might say, to which I respond: if I agree to fuck you and only you, you'd better do a damn good job of getting me off every possible way you know how and then some. 4) I mentioned that I'm not a good person to ask, right? The Pussy speaketh, and She wanteth some tongueth.

What if I'm really bad at it? What, like *not* trying will make you better? Get your face down there and start practicing. Yeah, you know what? Your first time you're probably going to suck. But your second time you'll be better, and the third time you'll be better than that—it helps a lot if you're with a girl you're comfortable with because then you can ask her what she likes and how she likes it. Hopefully, she's in tune with herself enough to be able to answer.

I don't know what I'm doing down there. First, don't call it "down there." Not hot. Second, there's this really spiffy thing called the internet where you can look up anything you want to learn about. Read, read, read! Maybe one day girls will call you the Pussy Whisperer. It also helps if you watch porn because then you can see what's what. Porn certainly isn't the best place to study technique, but it's not a bad start if you have no clue.

I've tried eating pussy before, but the girls always tell me I'm bad. Now I'm afraid to try on anyone else. Please re-read previous paragraph. First of all, enthusiasm counts for a lot. If I'm with a guy and he's not getting off from eating me out, then I'm never going to call him again, no matter how good his technique may be. Second, you have to have some confidence in yourself even if your history makes you self-conscious. Fake it 'till you make it. Just aim for that first moan. Ask her what she likes, what she wants, and keep doing it until you get that moan. [Note to female readers: DO NOT FAKE ORGASMS. YOU ARE HELPING NO ONE. All you have to do is tell him, "Touch here, lick this, harder, faster." It's not that hard. Don't let me hear you've been faking or I will come find you and beat you senseless with a 10" rubber dong.]

Vagina scares me. All new things are scary, including awesome things like Thai food. Man up.

Vagina really scares me. Most pussy plays nice. The scary ones are usually preceded by black lipstick or spiked collars.

No, seriously, vagina really scares me. I'm going to assume you've moved past the "what if I'm gay?" problem, but, just in case, I'll address it quickly: in this post, do you fantasize about being the one on your knees or the guy having his cock sucked? If this isn't the source of your anxiety, then I wonder if you had a really scary first experience? I've known guys who refused to let a girl's mouth anywhere near his dick because his first girlfriend accidentally bit it (YOWCH) or threw up on it. But pussy doesn't bite. Maybe you got female ejaculate in your eye? If that was the case, then that's something you should spend the rest of your life bragging about, okay, chief? If you're still scared and nothing above hits a nerve, then it's something beyond the scope of this blog post.

For the female readers:

When you finally get him to eat you out: Show him lots and lots of encouragement. Even if he sucks, be encouraging. This will hopefully increase your chances of getting him between your legs again so you can start slowly introducing him to what you like without having it sound like criticism.

What to tell him if he puts up a fight: "Sweetie, I'm not asking to let me fuck you with a strap-on, I just want you to spend some quality time down between my legs every once in a while."

How do I get him to eat me out? PG-13 version: Ask nicely. Don't nag, don't be condescending. Tell him you think it's hot when he licks your pussy and it makes you wet instantaneously. Bonus points: tell him you you think it would make him more interested in sex.

How do I get him to eat me out? R-rated version: This is the response you won't hear on Oprah. Only say this if you mean it. Milk your bi-curiosity and tell him that sometimes you think about eating out a girl when you're masturbating because pussy is so hot. Elaborate. Give him sex eyes and work your feminine wiles until you have his head between your legs. Use porn (regular or female-friendly) if necessary.

If that, uh, doesn't work and he breaks up with you for having gay inclinations—well what the hell are you listening to me for? I haven't been laid in months. I walk around humping lamp posts.

Because I Love Cock

I love cock. I know that is a common sentence on this blog, which is part of the reason I was happy to accept when the queen Fellatrix asked me to join as the Friday contributor. I love cock, and I want to do everything I can to help others enjoy cock as much as I do.

I love cock. I love cock. I love cock. I could say that all day long. There have been many occasions when I have said that all night long, including tonight. As I write this it is five in the morning and I still have the faint taste of cum on my lips. I have to be at work in less than four hours and I don't care, because I love cock.

I remember the first time I ever sucked a dick. It was the first time I had ever seen a guy naked. I was fifteen and after careful planning one summer day I had managed to get a boy and an empty house at the same time. Although I don't remember the guy that well, the color of his hair, the feel of his body, the way he kissed, I remember every last detail about sucking cock for the first time.

As soon as he dropped his pants, I reached out and held his hard dick in my hand. It grew more. I rubbed my hand up and down, fascinated. It was even better than I had hoped. Since I still had a bit of a good girl mentality at that age, I had not yet seen porn. I had no idea what I was doing, but I didn't care because I had a cock in my hand and it was all for me.

Without thinking I dropped to my knees and took his cock in my mouth. The hunger for the taste of a guy's cock was something that had been inside me all along, before I even knew what it was. As soon as I felt him in my mouth, I knew that I was entering a new world. It promised nothing but discovery and excitement. It felt right in a way that I had never felt something before.

I still feel that way now, years later, when I've seen and sucked many dicks. The hunger has remained, if not grown. The more I get, the more I want. My body reminds me of that over and over when I find my hips slowly rocking and a moan coming from deep inside my throat. Because I love cock.

I love cock. I love everything about it. The shape, the texture, the taste, the smell, the way it reacts when I squeeze, lick, suck, and fuck—I can't get enough. Because I love cock.

162 lbs (5 pending), Thin Mints 127, calories zero b/c don't count on N.S.A.D., v.g.

8:01 a.m. Wake up late. Stay in bed.

8:15 a.m. Wake up again. Stay in bed.

8:31 a.m. Wake up again. Sigh heavily.

8:32 a.m. Get up. Fling body across bed in final gasp of heartbreak over departure.

9:18 a.m. Arrive at office. Sigh heavily.

9:21 a.m. Realize it is sodding Valentine's Day. Roses and balloons and happiness in abundance.

9:23 am. Accidentally pop nearest heart-shaped balloon with a freshly sharpened pencil.

9:30 a.m. Sit down to get to serious business.

9:33 a.m. Get up for coffee. Must be fully aware in anticipation of evil-doings in the name of anti-Cupid, who must have been the perviest little boy around, always walking about with willy in hand.

9:37 a.m. Lots of calorie-filled yumminess out on table in break room. Look around for witnesses, then shovel all chocolates into empty coffee mug and walk back to desk with hand on top. Brilliance.

9:45 a.m. A Valentine has magically appeared on keyboard. Hoorah! Must be from cute guy in Human Resources. *I have lots of special human resources to offer you, My Yummy Valentine.*

9:47 a.m. Bollocks. Not from cute guy. From boss (sweet boss, but *married* sweet boss, who is of no use to me). Pin card up because has cartoon of Spiderman on it. Peter Parker/Spiderman is totally sexy-nerdy. *With great power comes great orgasmibility.*

9:49 a.m. Dream about being in *Spiderman 4*. Would be way cuter than Mary Jane, plus provide better back-up in arch-enemy encounters. Spidey may have the guns, but I've got twins of mass-distraction that can take down any villain.

9:50 a.m. Spreadsheets. Supposed to be updating spreadsheets.

10:05 a.m. Can't concentrate on spreadsheets with all these silly bouquets of flowers being delivered left and right. Have developed sudden allergy to 1-800-

Flowers. *Achoo, achoo!*

10:10 a.m. Enter number 5318008 in spreadsheet. Snicker.

10:11 a.m. In moment of clarity realize this may be why still single.

10:12 a.m. . . . because of unmatchable Awesomeness!!!! High-five self in head. Shake boobies in borderline office-appropriate manner.

1:45 p.m. Cookie Mom Coworker comes in with a dolly full of Girl Scout cookie boxes. Immediately jump to attention and selflessly offer young strong arms to help bring in rest of cookies.

1:46 p.m. That was last round of cookies to be brought inside. Excellent timing. Look like selfless individual without doing any actual work, meanwhile ensure a minimal wait in the afternoon's cookie deliveries throughout huge office.

2:24 p.m. Where are fucking Girl Scout cookies? Does buying six boxes of Thin Mints and a half-sincere offer to help do *nothing* for my level of priority?

2:28 p.m. Pop another balloon. "I heart you" in pink sparkles. Should be thanked by society for ridding world of such a monstrosity.

2:44 p.m. No cookies in sight. Pout.

2:47 p.m. Go scavenging for cookies. Valentine's Day is the most sweet-intensive holiday in county, so where is all the fucking candy?!

2:49 p.m. Swipe some Sweet-Tarts from administrative department.

2:52 p.m. Mail room only had icky chalky candy hearts. Bleh. Steal stamps instead.

2:57 p.m. No candy in reception, but huge vase of orchids. Steal orchid.

3:00 p.m. Investigate executive area. Daring move, but highest returns. Homemade chocolate chip cookies with pink M&Ms. Shove one in mouth and make a run for it.

3:02 p.m. Human Resources. No food, no cards, no flowers. All men. Bastards. Steal highlighters.

3:04 p.m. Second floor break area. Nothing. Steal a coffee mug that says *LMAO*. Appreciate irony.

3:05 p.m. Take a poo in restroom next to break area. Steal tampons.

3:10 p.m. Return to desk. Six boxes of Girl Scout cookies sitting on chair.

YESSS!!!!!

3:11 p.m. Young Annoying Coworker comes by to complain about fifty-dollar bouquet had to buy for fiancée. Follows by complaining about seventy-minute drive to office.

3:12 p.m. Counter with insincere "at least you have someone to buy flowers for" and look sad. Cackle quietly inside when he hands over two beers from his "Beers of the World" basket given by fiancée. V.g.

3:14 p.m. Go to Married Coworker's desk. Look sad about not having a special someone. Accept pity-cupcake.

3:21 p.m. Go to department full of women. Look sad. Engaged coworkers dieting, give me their chocolate-covered strawberries and pieces of cookie-bouquet. Pregnant coworkers give me their exotic dark chocolates and candies. Love benefiting from unsuspecting engaged and pregnant women.

3:50 p.m. Fall asleep under desk from sugar high. Successfully hide from boss by building fortress of Girl Scout cookie boxes and assorted stolen items.

4:19 p.m. Go to office of Cookie Mom Coworker. Buy six more boxes of Girl Scout cookies. Bond over our misery-filled memories of being Girl Scouts once. Have proved that Den Mother was wrong about basket-weaving being a highly-respected skill.

6:30 p.m. Leave office with cardboard box full of Thin Mints, candy, cookies, strawberries, and new mug.

7:14 p.m. On couch with a jug of milk and Thin Mints. Refuse to do anything remotely responsible or productive tonight. Arse needs freedom to grow, v.g.

7:58 p.m. Scratch self, play with boobies, and bask in awesomeness.

8:08 p.m. Rejoice in not spending three hours cooking fancy dinner for a boyfriend who won't put out.

9:10 p.m. No boy in sight. Fart without guilt.

11:00 p.m. Rejoice in National Singles Awareness Day. Commence celebratory booty shake of awesomeness.

Part IV

Be yourself. Above all, let who you are, what you are, what you believe, shine through every sentence you write, every piece you finish.

John Jakes

Jazz Man, Meet Awkward. Awkward, Meet Jazz Man

Tonight, I went to the bar where I knew Jazz Man would be playing. We met through Handsome Twosome when I talked about how hard it was to find a reliable fuck buddy.

I arrived late, but Jazz Man was not there. Unusual, considering he is typically on time if not early. I sat alone at the bar and hoped he would arrive soon.

I ordered a drink and waited.

After fifteen minutes I felt someone sit down at the barstool next to mine. There were three empty stools in a line, so the logical choice for a newcomer would have been to take the middle one. The stranger sat next to me. I made no attempt to be friendly and smugly enjoyed being the girl at the bar who was about to be hit on. It's been a while since a complete stranger hit on me, especially a cute one with tattoos.

Slowly, I sipped my drink and watched the band. I kept looking at the door for Jazz Man to come in. When I wasn't doing that, I kept checking my phone for text messages. Meanwhile I sensed the guy at the next bar stool was quietly keeping tabs on me. I had nothing to lose, so I intentionally kept from turning in his direction.

The guy held out his phone. I ignored him.

"Good stuff. I'm recording it."

It took me a second to realize he was actually talking to me—and using this as his line. I looked at his phone and saw a timer running. I looked up at him expectantly.

"I like to record music and play it as my ring tone. These guys are really good. I'm [John], by the way. I recognize you from somewhere."

Seriously? This is the best he can come up with? Oh, like I'm one to talk. I've actually said, on more than one occasion, "Hey I like your pants. Can I touch them?"

"Hey. Vix. Nice to meet you."

We shook hands and started chatting. The guy seemed normal enough, and it was nice to be blatantly hit on for the first time in months. At least the guy didn't do or say anything weird like comment on my thighs. He was definitely hitting on me.

The next time I looked up I saw that Jazz Man had just entered the bar. My face brightened and I waved to him. *Um . . . I know this looks incriminating . . . HE STARTED IT. I SWEAR.* I was giving the Cold-Hearted Bitch act and he drove through it. Kind of admirable, when you think about it.

I waited a little longer before excusing myself with a, "Hey, watch my purse for a minute, would you?" and went over to say hi to Jazz Man. He gave me his usual happy smile and then some of his music friends came over and started talking about industry stuff I didn't understand. I caught Jazz Man's eye and pointed toward my empty seat at the bar.

The new guy I'm sure saw me being very friendly with Jazz Man. It would be hard not to notice. I went back to the bar and prepared myself for awkwardness.

Once I sat down again, the guy continued flirting just as before, if not more so. Meanwhile, I kept the corner of my eye on Jazz Man as he prepared to join the other musicians on stage.

The new guy kept talking. It was only another minute before he took out his cell phone and asked to exchange phone numbers. I hesitated for a split second, then told him my phone number. My real phone number (yes, there are ugly times in my past when I fake-numbered someone to avoid the "um, NO, I think you're icky" conversation, I ADMIT IT). Immediately, he called so his number would be stored on my phone.

Jazz Man finished talking with his friends and came over by me to talk for a few minutes. He was cool, I was cool, the confused guy next to me was cool. Jazz Man went up on stage and worked his jazz magic.

"So . . . that guy . . ." asked the guy next to me.

"Um . . . dating. Casually."

Damnit. Why didn't I think to say I was a lesbian and avoid this whole fucking mess?

"Cool. He's cute."

"Dude, don't be weird," I said. Oh, who am I kidding. THIS IS TEN DEGREES OF WEIRD.

"Okay, I'm going to grab a smoke now and leave. It was very nice to meet you." He shook my hand. He looked like he was going to leave but then he stopped. "Listen, if you decide to call me, I'll answer. If I don't answer, I'll call back because it was really cool talking with you. So . . . call, okay?"

I nodded. I wasn't sure if I meant it or not. Before he had said that, I had no intention of speaking to him ever again. Something about his tone just now made me hesitate to dismiss him so easily.

He left, and I turned my attention to Jazz Man's performance. He was amazing. He *is* amazing. I spent the next hour watching him in awe.

When the band took a break we sat together and talked. When the gig ended, Jazz Man walked me to my car and was just as funny and sweet as he always is. We kissed. We made plans to hang out Thursday night. We kissed one final time good night.

As he walked away, I wondered, *what the fuck am I doing?*

The Cubicle Monkey Escapes

It's a beautiful day. Too pretty to stay inside the office for lunch. I came home at noon for the sole purpose of driving on the highway with the windows down, radio blasting, and feeling my mess of hair whipping around my face.

If anyone saw me peeling out of the parking lot at work, it would be no secret that I need to get the fuck away from there, which is nearly every day. I do this

so regularly I've got it down pat—one hand rolling the window down, the other hand shaking my hair loose from its professional up-do and then twisting the radio dial to find the perfect *SEE YA*, CORPORATE MOTHAFUCKAS song, all while driving with my right knee.

It's the days like today when I wish I lived further away from the office, so I could enjoy the seventy mile-an-hour rush of freedom for just a little longer—especially now that I can experience the full effect properly with sunglasses thanks to Lasik surgery.

–looks at clock– Twelve forty-five. Fuck. Time to go back to the Land of Professional Behavior. Fucking asswipes can suck my left one and choke on it. –slips feet back into stiletto heels and takes final bite of cold lunch–

They may drag the cubicle monkey back to her desk, but they can't keep me from escaping day after day. I'm only getting feistier.

–peels out of apartment parking lot to go back to office–

The Rhythm of Jazz Man

Once Jazz Man lay his long lean body on top of mine, I felt my pussy come alive. The power inside having lain dormant all this time was now burning burning burning burning. My hips started to move to the rhythm of my pussy muscles.

My back arched and I turned to expose my bare neck. His mouth skimmed my lips, teasing, then plucked at the skin over my throat. I let out a long, low lilt.

His hands never left my body. His eyes may have made me feel like a woman, but his hands made me feel like a goddess. They barely left my body the entire night.

His warm tongue drummed against my neck and then I felt a light bite. I moaned. The nibble turned into a real bite. I shuddered. I love having my neck sucked and bitten. It's one of the most delicate areas of the body, and my biggest turn-on. No bite is ever hard enough, not for me.

Wait, I have way too many clothes on. How did he get away with wearing only shorts and I'm fully dressed?! What the hell is this shit? I wiggled out of Jazz Man's arms and pulled my miniskirt off, revealing low-cut lacy panties underneath. Jazz Man's face lit up in a smile. His hands reached out to my naked thighs and slowly moved down the entire length of my legs. On his way back up his hands paused at the edge of my panties and both thumbs teasingly traced the skin just along the inside of the lace.

He did that once, twice more, and then crawled back up and hovered his body above mine just enough so that his hand had free range. A moment later he started biting my neck again, this time grinding his pelvis into mine. I lifted my long legs up in the air to make it easier for Jazz Man to reach every part of me that he wanted. *Glad I painted my toenails for the first time in four months. Wee, look how pretty as my feet wave back and forth in the air!*

He stopped so he could pull off my shirt. Underneath I wore a sheer, lacy, black bra. Jazz Man's eyes drank me in. He grabbed my hips and guided me over onto my stomach. "Time for a look at chapter two," he laughed.

Silence.

Shit. It's my cellulite, isn't it? IT'S BEEN GIRL SCOUT COOKIE SEASON, OKAY?!

"Goodness *gracious*. *WhoooooooooooooWHEE!*"

Oh. That was definitely a happy sound. My big booty gets a big BOOYAH! Which is something people said once upon a time.

I felt his fingertips graze my lower back. His hands became bolder, each cupping one side of my ass. He exhaled. His fingers dug in.

"Okay," he stopped with a laugh. "Now for the part I suck at . . ." His fingers fumbled at my bra strap. I buried my laughter in the mattress. A couple seconds later I felt the clasp release. *Weeee, I'm free!*

I rolled over so I was on my back once again. Immediately, Jazz Man reached over to fondle my breast. My pussy started to flutter again, now in time to the jazz music playing in the background. He leaned over so he could take my nipple in his mouth, his hand on the other. His hands, oh, how I love his hands.

Our eyes met. The smile in Jazz Man's eyes made it clear where he was headed next. His hands rested on my hips before finally—finally—tugging down my lace panties and pulling them off my legs.

IT'S NAKED TIME!

With the biggest grin I'd seen on Jazz Man's face the entire night, he bent down between my legs. Soft at first, he grew harder with each lick of the tongue. At first his hands lay on the inside of my thighs, but he gradually moved them underneath my ass. He dug his fingers in and lifted my pelvis up slightly for a better angle to eat me out from.

I played with my tits, meanwhile doing my best not to grab him by the hair and shove his face deeper into my pussy. Jazz Man took his sweet time, which was wonderful and yet incredibly mean. I wanted to see and feel him buried in pussy juice—droplets on his eyelashes, a sheen on his nose, and the smell on his fingers for days after.

And then Jazz Man did one of my all-time favorite moves. Using his whole tongue, he lapped me up and down, as if he needed every single drop of pussy juice to be on his tongue right fucking now. No one does that unless he is possessed by incredible hunger and devotion to pussy. He did it over and over and over. *Up, down, up, down, up, alllll the way down.*

I wanted some of that. I pulled him up toward me so I could kiss some of that sweet juice off his own tongue. He reeeally liked that. He kissed harder, his tongue digging deep in my mouth. I broke the kiss so that he could watch me lick my lips, now covered in the cunt honey he'd just tasted himself for the first time. *More*, my eyes demanded.

I needed something inside me NOW. I grabbed his fingers and pushed them inside me. He looked a bit surprised, but I had already been more restrained than I thought I was capable of. Time to finger-fuck me.
He didn't move a single muscle.

What the hell? Then I realized that my kegel muscle was going already, flexing, tightening, gripping. It wasn't conscious, it just happened. I have always said the pussy had a mind of its own.

I looked over at Jazz Man. He had a dreamy look in his eyes.

"You feel that, don't you?" I asked. I clenched tighter.

"Uh huh," he said. He stayed motionless, enjoying the changing rhythm of my pussy.

I clenched even tighter. He started moving his fingers in and out, finding the right pace to match my pussy. I let out a happy sigh. A minute later I could tell he was holding back, so I whispered, "Harder." He went harder, but not hard enough. "Harder," I said. I held his hand and ground hard against it. Suddenly, I stopped and pulled his fingers out, so I could suck them dry. I thought Jazz Man was going to cum right there.

He returned his fingers to where they belonged. We kissed deep and hard. He brought me closer and closer until finally my pussy clenched and held for the wave of orgasm. My entire body tensed and then collapsed. Jazz Man waited for me to calm down, then he brought his fingers toward me for a final suck.

Our eyes widened at the same time. Blood.

"What the FUCK?!" I squealed.

GODDAMNSONOFABITCHWHOREMOTHERFUCKER, NO, NO, NO, NO, *NO, NO, NO.*

Jazz Man giggled. I was mortified. And furious. "Seven months without sex and when I finally get some ass I START TO BLEED FROM THE CROTCH?!! WHAT THE FUCK!!!"

Jazz Man burst into laughter at the sight of me pouting. I smacked him.

"STOP IT! IT'S NOT FUNNY!!" He was too busy muffling his laughter in the mattress to answer.

I was beyond mortified. What the *hell*? I'm not supposed to get my period for weeks! This makes no sense! What–

"Oh my God. My virginity grew back! YOU BROKE MY VIRGINITY! THAT'S WHY I'M BLEEDING!"

Jazz Man erupted in a fit of laughter all over again. I gave in and started giggling too. *Stupid virginity*, like it didn't suck enough the first time.

First Mission with The Marine

Last night The Marine and I went on our first date. We met at a Korean barbecue restaurant that he swore was the most authentic Korean he could find in the city. When I walked in and saw that we were the only white people, I knew he was serious.

As soon as The Marine walked in, I noticed his hands. The guy is six foot five inches tall, which makes me look like a fucking pygmy next to him, even in four-inch heels. His hands were large even for his body, which made it hard for me to concentrate on anything he was saying. They were pretty hands considering how many jobs he's had doing manual labor. Long and muscular, those hands needed to be all over me as soon as possible.

Since I wasn't sure what The Marine's expectations were, I made a point of steering our conversation toward past relationships and therefore future relationships. I told him that after my last boyfriend I still wasn't ready for anything serious, just looking for someone cool and fun to spend time with. He reacted when I said that, but I couldn't read what his expression said. Relief? Disappointment? Surprise?

The Marine said, "I hadn't really thought about any of that. I was like, here's a cool chick I want to get to know better. But you know, it's all good."

I felt relief, and then excitement—

The Marine said, "I'm down with having a girl to get close to and hold hands with and take places, but it doesn't have to be any big thing."

"So . . . it's cool that I don't want to be your girlfriend? Keep it casual?"

Could I be so lucky? All the benefits of a boyfriend without any of the relationship crap? Please, please, please, because that would be so awesome.

"Yeah. Casual's good." He gave me an I'm-imagining-you-naked-smile.

Oh HELLS YEAH. I am totally bootyshaking in my head.

We eyed each other over this new understanding. It was the first of many looks we exchanged that said, I've met my match.

After The Marine paid the check, he suggested we go to one of those adult-arcades so we could continue our date. I said I'd follow him in my car. Once in the parking lot, I pulled him toward me by his shirt and wrapped my arms around him. His face showed happy surprise just before we closed our eyes in a long, hungry kiss. He smelled clean, like shaving cream and soap. By the end of the kiss his hands had made their way from my waist down to my hips and ass, which made me hopeful that I wouldn't have to be the aggressive one like usual.

Eventually we broke apart and drove to the game place. In the parking lot there he offered me his hand. I held out mine and we linked fingers. Everything felt so easy, so right with The Marine.

Once inside I paid our arcade fees and bought the first round of drinks. I like being fair on dates, especially since I've heard so many guys feel like girls use them for free meals. Nuh-uh, I pay my share *and* put out. That's fuck-me feminism.

We walked around the arcade games holding hands and drinking beer. It was obvious we were on our first date. We enjoyed every moment as the rare indulgence it is when two people have immediate chemistry.

I already knew The Marine was a smoker, and I had guessed correctly that he was a pothead. BIG pothead. If I were thinking about a serious relationship with The Marine, both of those would be a deal-breaker for me. Since I'm only in it for fun, I can overlook the smokey ickiness. Everything else about him I liked: street-smart, people-smart, chill, fun, and most importantly—old enough (34) to have gotten through his dumbass phase of life.

After checking out all the games, we settled on skeeball. I sucked. He didn't. He got tons of tickets and I barely got any. Silly me, I forgot that I had feminine wiles to my advantage in distracting The Marine from doing so well. I stuck my ass out and accidentally on purpose bumped into him.

"I don't think you're doing it right," he said. "It's more like this." He stuck his ass way out and bent over. I giggled and imitated his stance. He threw a ball and completely missed. I nearly fell over laughing. The Marine smacked me hard on the ass in a futile attempt to stop my giggling. Instead I backed up into him just enough to make him play a horrible last round.

We got more beers and played more games. The Marine told me stories about his friends and all the crazy jobs he's had over the years. He kept asking me about my job and each time I made a face, saying I didn't want to talk about work. I intentionally didn't tell him I write because I'm not sure if I want him to know about that side of me. I keep my writing very private. The Marine is a curious guy, so I knew if I mentioned it, he'd barrage me with questions. What the fuck am I supposed to say? "I write about sex and dating. As a matter of fact, I'm going to write about you as soon as I get home. I hope for your sake you're good in bed, because thousands of people will be reading about it."

Best to avoid that discussion.

As the evening progressed, we grew more bold. We stole kisses in dark corners and grabbed each other's asses as we walked around. It was fun to be silly-sexy. When we sat at the bar he turned to face me so that his long legs were on either side of me, making it easier for me to keep a hand warm on his thigh. I tickled the inside of his leg and whispered that we should get more cozy together in my car.

The place closed and we headed out to the parking lot with a dozen other people. The Marine is ridiculously tall and I'm not shorty, so we needed all the maneuvering room we could manage. We climbed in the front seat and pushed the seats back as far as they could go. At first we sat next to each other and kissed, but that was not the best arrangement for hand access. I climbed my big ol' body (in a small SUV I felt like an Amazon) over so that I was straddling The Marine's lap.

He buried his face in my tits, which were easy to reach thanks to my strategically low-cut top. His hands went up my legs to my ass, nicely displayed in a tight pair of jeans. We kissed and groped and fogged up the windows. It was fantastic. I ground against him the best that I could between the confines of the car and our long limbs.

Eventually my bra came off and then my shirt. The Marine took his time enjoying my breasts with his hands then mouth. Harder, I urged. He sucked harder.

No, bite. He bit down with his teeth. Harder, I whispered in his ear. He looked up at me with wide eyes. "If you like this, that is *awesome*." I laughed and nodded. He bit harder. My whole body sighed.

My hair was coming out of its clip and sweat covered my back. The Marine's huge hands ran up and down my bare back, exploring every curve and muscle. He sucked on my nipple, reminding me that he had said his nipples are pierced. I unbuttoned his shirt partway and slipped my hand inside. My fingertip found the ring and he smiled. I played with it for a few seconds before lowering my mouth to his nipple. I flicked it with my tongue and then sucked on it. He moaned.

It was getting very late. One last thing before we go—

My hand slowly moved from his nipple down his long torso to his cock. I worked around the thick cloth of his pants to get a better grip. He shifted and pressed his hand over mine, *harder*. I felt my way up and down. From what I felt, I was very impressed.

But another time. I wanted to leave him wanting more.

It was very late and we both had work the next day. I told him I needed to get home. The Marine looked at his watch and agreed. With a few more long kisses we said our good be.

As I drove home I thought to myself, it was worth the seven and a half months without sex. After a long drought it's nothing but rain as far as I can see through the steamy windows of my car.

Base Camp One

This evening I went over to The Marine's apartment to "not watch a movie." The Marine was the guy who hit on me at the bar during Jazz Guy's performance. He took me on a great first date to Korean barbecue. Without being cramped into the front seat of a car, we were able to have a lot more fun this tie. Now let me just say—

Wow. The Marine has the biggest cock I have ever seen in my life. When he pulled down his boxers my jaw dropped to the floor.

I must have stared at it for a full five seconds before I could speak. *There's no way— No, it must be the lighting, a shadow, something . . . That can't be right*

. . . But . . . GOOD LORD, IT'S HUGE.

I looked up at The Marine. He looked at me nervously. Now I understand why he had seemed self-conscious before he took his shorts off. God knows how many girls have looked at the girth of his dick and run for the hills. It looked like two dicks had melded into one freakishly wide Superdick.

Cautiously, I reached out with my left hand. Who knows what secret powers the Superdick wields. My fingers wrapped around the shaft but the tips didn't touch. I gulped. The Marine still looked nervous. Well no fucking shit, now I was nervous too.

In all my years of sucking dick, I never met one I couldn't handle. I am the blowjob queen, I am a goddess of cocksucking, and now I understand that all those dicks have prepared me for this moment right here with the Superdick. IT IS MY DUTY AND AN HONOR TO TAKE ON THE SUPERDICK.

I took a deep breath and went down to work. With the utmost concentration I took as much of him in as I could. My hands still had plenty of room on his shaft. GodDAMN. I kept trying. Stretched to its limits, his girth filled my entire mouth. I stopped for a breath and to let my lips relax. *Re-energize, now GO GO GO.* I took him in again. This time I worked in another inch of length, but the girth was an obstacle. I could tell my body was starting to give.

Time for another pep talk: *I have been graced with the presence of the Superdick. I must honor the Superdick. I must not be intimidated by the Superdick. The Superdick would not have presented itself to me if it did not think I could handle the Superdick. I will conquer the Superdick!*

The Marine led the way. I followed each moan and shudder toward the glorious end. The more he encouraged, the more I could take. Soon I heard little gasps escaping from The Marine, then he whispered, "I'm cumming." With great pride I stretched my lips and tongue for his final gasp of orgasm. His whole body shook, but I held on through each wave. A moment later he relaxed and I finally retreated in a heap on the bed.

"Hollllllly SHIT, that was my biggest orgasm ever!"

Hmm? Sorry, can't talk. Mouth broken.

"Wow," he said. "That was AWESOME." He reached out and gave me an appreciative squeeze.

I tried to smile. Nope, smile broken. Instead, I let my eyes tell him how much I loved sucking his cock. Once I figured it out, that is.

No Superdick is too much for this nympho. It will be even better next time! YOU HEAR ME, SUPERDICK?! I'M COMING FOR YOU.

It's going to be a while before I have sex with The Marine. Seriously, I have to prepare. This weekend I need to dig out my biggest dildo and start warming up my pussy for the biggest hunk of man I have ever witnessed. Golly gee whiz, what an unfortunate situation in which to have a tight pussy. I never really considered that a liability, but, well, irony always finds a way to be a bitch. Sorry, my nice tight pussy, but you have to learn to open up and let the love shine in.

The whole thing reminded me of that scene from *Sex and the City* when Samantha dates Mr. Cocky:

Samantha: I'm really going to psych myself up before I try it again.
Carrie: You're going to try it again? Why?

Samantha: Because it's there…

Carrie: Sweetie, it's a penis, not Mount Everest.

Samantha: Well, let me tell you, if it was Mount Everest last night I could only make it to Base Camp One.

I laughed when I first saw that episode. How ridiculous! No dick is too big, especially not for Samantha! Oh, those silly TV writers.

But now? Oh, *fuck* no, I'm not laughing now. How can I when my mouth is full?

Loving Pussy

The other night while I was packing, I watched an episode of *Sex and the City* where one of the characters is completely grossed out when a guy tries to kiss her after going down on her. She tells this to her friends, they all go *ewwww* and discuss proper sexiquette. They even admit to there being a double-standard, because if a guy wouldn't kiss a girl after she blew him, she'd be pissed.

Please allow me to ask, WHAT *THE FUCK?*

I love pussy. Now that I've had sex with a woman I've been on both sides of the orgasm and I know for damn sure I love pussy every way I can get it. I love everything about it—the taste, the smell, the look, the smell, the feel, the smell. What's not to love? Pussy is a wonderful and glorious thing that deserves to be worshipped.

I love pussy, whether my own or someone else's. It gets me hot to smell a hint of pussy when I lower my pants in the restroom. Everything about pussy is so *raw*, so full of sex and lust. Every time I smell pussy it reminds me of someone, of some random time a guy got me off in the car or told me he smelled pussy on his hands all day while at work or got me off so many times I squirted or spent an hour between my legs with what could only be described as complete pussy-worship. How can I not love pussy when these are the associations with it?

Sometimes when I smell pussy and it takes me a million miles away from where I am now (usually the office restroom), I like to rub the tip of my finger between my legs along my bikini line. It has picked up a faint hint of sweat and hungry pussy, which I smell on my finger. Many guys have told me this is one of their favorite parts of the body because it has that smell of natural pussy, the way pussy was meant to smell. No perfume, no deodorant, no body wash, just pussy.

Since many girls don't like touching/smelling/tasting pussy, it gives those of us who love it that much more of an advantage. When clothes first come off (or hell, when they're still on). I like to dip two of my fingers in my pussy, give a little wink as my guy's mouth drops, then pull them out and lick them off. His eyes pop open too if you wiggle your tongue a little between the two fingers (the universal sign for eating out pussy) and then lick off both fingers with long, slow movements up and down of the tongue.

Another move I like is when a guy (or girl) has been finger-fucking me until I'm completely wet, then pulling his (or her) fingers out of my pussy so I can lick off every last drop of cunt honey. After I do that once or twice with someone, they start offering me their fingers every chance they can stand to take them out.

And, of course, I love it when a guy kisses me after eating me out for ages. My taste is all over his face, his lips, his tongue. Sometimes I can see the gleam of juice on his lips, which is almost as sexy as the gleam in his eyes. The first time he is often hesitant to kiss me with a mouthful of *me*, I assume because he's encountered the *SATC* situation above with a few too many girls. Since I know that's what is going through his head, I put both hands behind his head and pull his face into mine. I kiss him hard, search for his tasty tongue with my own, and lick all around his lips so I can pick up every last drop of pussy juice. A coy move after that is when I wipe a tiny bit of juice now on my mouth with the tip of my thumb, lick it off as I hold his gaze and then bite my finger with a look that says nothing but *I love pussy*.

Pussy is the taste of sex, the feel of your body welcoming sex, the smell of sex, and the look of someone wanting your sex. Again, I ask, what's not to love?

You'll Shoot Your Eye Out

Call me a dirty whore, but I love it when a guy cums on my face. I think there is nothing hotter or more animal than a guy hovering above me with a hard cock about to shoot his load. When he cums on my face I lick it all up, and if any goes on my tits, I rub it all over my skin. I've been that way since I gave my first blowjob at fifteen.

As Jazz Man made clear, not many girls feel that way. Last week he gave me a very long and impassioned speech on how much he has wanted to cum on a girl's face but has rarely been accommodated. I politely waited for him to finish talking (the poor guy obviously needed to vent), and then I said, "I'll do my very best to make up for what you've been missing out on."

A few minutes later I was on my knees and well on my way to giving Jazz Man the proper cocksucking he has deserved all this time. I licked and sucked with all the love for cock I have in my body. The whole time I looked up at him with hungry eyes to let him know how turned on I was just thinking about his cum on my lips.

He started whispering "Oh, fuck, fuck, *fuck*," so I knew he was about to cum. His legs stiffened and then he sighed. I tilted my head up to him just in time to catch some cum on my open tongue. Once he finished, I grinned and licked off as much as I could reach with my tongue.

"Whoa," he said. "That was a lot . . ."

"It's okay," I said. "I like it." *Except when it's in my nose. Oh, fuck, it's IN my nose.* "I got some in my nose." I tried not to snort it out. Snorting spooge is not sexy.

He started laughing. "I'm so sorry . . ."

"Oh, fuck, it's IN MY NOSE!" I jumped up and ran for the nearest sink. I can't be sexy when I have spooge dripping from my nostrils. NASAL SPOOGE IS NOT SEXY.

Jazz Man, the considerate bastard that he is, nearly fell over laughing as I ran naked to the bathroom.

I looked in the mirror. There was cum all over my nose and just above my right eye. "OH MY GOD, IT'S EVERYWHERE!!" I splashed my face with soap and water. When I dried off, smudged mascara ran under my eye. GODDAMNIT. First cum up my nose, now I have racoon eyes. Shit.

The entire time I was splashing around in the sink and maybe cursing a little under my breath, Jazz Man was dying with laughter. "Don't laugh, it's not funny!" He howled. "Okay, FINE. Maybe it would be funny if it had happened to someone other than me!"

I came back out and scrunched my nose up at him in fake-anger. We lay down and started talking. A few minutes later I felt my eye starting to sting. I rubbed my eye and figured it was the running mascara. It got worse. Finally I got up and went back to the bathroom.

"OH MY GOD MY EYEBALL IS *PINK*!" I shrieked.

"Oh, um, yeah, I thought it looked a little weird . . ." Jazz Man said innocently.

"IT'S IN MY FUCKING EYE!!" I splashed more soap and water on my face. Jazz Man's laughter filled the apartment yet again. "Ow, IT BURNS, OH MY GOD, *IT BURNS*!"

Dude, that was an expensive eyeball! RESPECT THE LASIKKED EYE. Do you know what I went through to be able to see properly out of that eye?! And now IT STINGS LIKE A MOTHERFUCKER.

A minute later I came out with my right eye squeezed half-shut. Jazz Man stifled laughter. I attempted to glare at him through my good eye.

"I'm so sorry," he said.

"I know, it's not your fault. It's not the first time that's happened." I patted his naked leg and smiled at him. "Aim for the tits next time, okay?" I giggled to let him know I was teasing.

Today's lesson: sex eyes are only sexy as long as there isn't spooge in them. Holy shit, I can't go back to the eye doctor complaining about "inexplicable stinging which only occurs between midnight and four a.m. on Saturday nights."

The smartass would probably give me an eye patch and tell me to close my eyes next time I'm near a loaded cock.

Because I Believe

Last night I had a wedding to attend. Yesterday afternoon, I started writing a post complaining about how I like weddings less each time I go to one. *Yada yada* I fell asleep and woke up just in time to drive to the wedding out in the suburbs.

I knew two people in the entire three-hundred-person wedding, who were the bride (my newest friend, Favorite Coworker) and maid-of-honor, which of course meant they would be too busy to talk much throughout the evening. Although I had invited my friend Sweetie Pie to attend so I wouldn't be lonely, she came down with a nasty cold and had to stay home. Great, I thought to myself as I drove to the church. I didn't want to go to a wedding in the first place, and now I have to go to a wedding where I have no one to talk to for five hours. I hate weddings.

The wedding was a bit on the country side (big hair and Southern accents as far as the ear could hear), which meant I stuck out like a slutty city girl. The pastor had eyed me suspiciously as I walked toward the door. Was it the spaghetti-strap dress or could he tell that a non-believer was entering the house of God? It took all my self-control to keep from rolling my eyes at him and hissing, *Hey, be happy I didn't show up NAKED, asshole.* I hate weddings.

Since I was one of the last people to arrive, having driven all the way from the big city, I sat in the last row. Squirmy children sat in front of me and a very unfriendly middle-aged woman sat next to me. The wedding program promised lots of readings and singing. I sighed. I hate weddings.

The processional music started. We stood up. As the bridesmaids walked past, I scanned for cute single guys in the pews on the groom's side. None. They were single and plain or cute and taken. DAMNIT. Now how am I supposed to entertain myself? I hate weddings.

Then the bride appeared in the doorway. For all the smiles we had exchanged in the short time we've been friends, I had never seen a smile like that on her face. I felt my eyes tearing up. Oh my God, I can't stand showing emotion in public. Or anywhere else. I looked down and stared at my feet. Oooh, what pretty chipped nail polish! I hate weddings.

A minute later we were all listening to family members read passages from the Bible. I played with my cuticles and then spun my ring around my pinky really fast. I hate weddings.

A cousin went to the altar to sing something he chose especially for the couple. I thought about what a waste it was that I was wearing a tiny, white, g-string and no bra under my dress that no one was going to get to see. Note to self: send sext to The Marine when ceremony is over. Damn, this guy singing must have chosen the longest song in the history of boredom. I hate weddings.

The pastor told the ring bearer to present the rings to the bride and groom. At last, we're getting somewhere. The pastor stated the standard vows you hear in every other wedding: *I offer you my solemn vow . . . in sickness and in health . . . to cherish you as long as we both shall live . . .* yada yada yada. I want cake. If I have no one to talk to, no one to flirt with, then there had better be some fanfuckingtastic chocolate cake at the reception. I hate weddings.

Then I noticed that while the groom was holding the bride's hand in his own, he was stroking her skin with his finger. I felt my eyes start to blink faster. I hate weddings.

The groom kept caressing his future wife's hand with his finger. It wasn't the vows, the vows I've heard a thousand times on TV that made me stumble in my attempt to be cold-hearted. It was that single gesture there between the man and the woman, something that can't be rehearsed or faked. I sniffled. I hate weddings.

The groom beamed at the bride. My eyes fluttered and my nose filled with snot. I hate weddings.

The bride beamed back at the groom. Do brides always look this happy? Really? My eyelids blinked rapidly, trying to fight back tears. *I hate weddings.* Together they lit a candle. They looked so incredibly happy. A tear slipped out. *I HATE WEDDINGS.*

Now hand-in-hand, they stood to face us. Tears slowly escaped. I couldn't watch any more. *FOR THE LOVE OF ALL THINGS UNHOLY, I HATE WEDDINGS!*

I hunched down so I could no longer see them standing at the altar, safely hidden behind a very tall man sitting three rows in front of me. A moment later the bride and groom walked past our pew, their smiles of joy impossible to miss. Tears and snot dripped off my face onto my slinky dress. I looked around at the other people next to me. No one else is crying! What the hell?! Am I the only sap in this entire church? What's wrong with you people? HAVE YOU NO HEART?!

As soon as the bride and groom had cleared the doors, I ran out of the church.

Once safely inside my car with the local hip-hop station blasting on the radio, I blew my nose and gathered myself. What is going on? Why do I keep trying to convince myself I'm a cold-hearted bitch when it comes to love, but then I'm the first person to cry at a wedding?

I leaned my head back against my seat and closed my eyes. BOOM BOOM BOOM went the sound of barely decipherable rap over the speakers. Ah, dear sweet reassuring gangsta rap, how I love thee.

Although the weather had looked like rain before the ceremony, it was now as clear and sunny as could be. Fucking son a of a bitch, I thought to myself. If this were a movie, it would be *raining* right now. Stupid real life gets things all wrong. I WANT RAIN, YOU SON OF A BITCH SKY!

So what's the deal?

As much as I lie to myself about hating weddings and shunning serious relationships, one day I know I'll want that for myself. I want to be the one who beams at her someone special, who feels a tingle every time he smiles, who wants *happily ever after* and actually lives it.

I see my own friends fall in love, and I find myself wondering when is it going to happen for me? When will I be ready? What if it's too late? Then I smack myself because that kind of questioning is why so many people settle for someone who isn't right. It almost happened to me. I'm afraid it will happen again if I let my guard down.

As often as I tell myself I'm being silly (and unrealistic and naive and stupid), I still believe in love that lasts forever. I have a heart that's bigger than I know what to do with, which is why most of the time it's easier to pretend I don't have one.

Secretly, I know that one day a guy will see through all my bullshit and leave me no choice but to fall in love with him. I'll fight it, but he'll know I have to because that's the way I am.

If I have to wait twenty years to fall in love, I'll wait. I want to get it right. Until then, I'll believe.

But I'm Straight. -Ish.

When I masturbate, I think about girls. But I'm straight. When I see a hot girl walk past me in a short skirt I wonder what kind of underwear she has on, if any at all. But I'm straight.

When I see a hot girl, I check out her legs, her ass, her tits, her stomach, her eyes, everything. But I'm straight.

Yep, I'm as straight as the vibrator I'm shoving up my pussy when I'm thinking about sucking on some perky tits.

In meetings, I stare at the beautiful new girl and I get so caught up in her pretty smile that I don't realize it when someone is talking to me. But I'm straight. When I see a sexy photo of a girl on the internet, I start to play with my nipples. But I'm straight.

When I'm at the pool with the guy I'm fucking, we are often checking out the same people. But I'm straight.

I've had sex with a girl. Awesome sex. But I'm straight. -ish.

For the most part, I consider myself straight. I just want to have sex with other straight girls. I'm the kind of girl that proper bisexuals disregard because I still favor the heterosexual side of the sexuality spectrum. I may love pussy, but I crave cock. I agree that I'm not a so-called proper bisexual because I only want to fuck girls—I don't want to date them. Which is why it's no big deal that the spank bank of my computer only has photos of girls in it.

But if my mother asks, I'm straight. And a virgin. Aw, hell, why don't you tell her I'm a practicing Catholic, too.

Farting In The Face Of Sex

If I were a gorgeous model or movie star, I'm sure I would never fart. I would also never piss, shit, vomit, or bleed from the crotch because nothing more offensive than a ray of sunshine would ever come out of my body. As a normal person, I am forced to acknowledge not-so-sexy things like cellulite and queefing. Which brings me to confession time.

My name is Vix, and I am haunted by the need to fart during sex.

It started in childhood, with my family. Perhaps the red meat-heavy diets are to blame, or maybe some ethnicities are predisposed to flatulence (we're German—which means we didn't stand a chance in hell. The women in my family however tend to have big asses, so perhaps that was an adaptive trait to muffle the sound/smell. Dear God we probably would have killed each other if we had been born with flat ineffectual asses).

My mother, normally a very classy and worldly woman, was known for her SBDs (a.k.a. Silent but Deadly). Dad preferred to be loud and obnoxious, but was generally able to avoid noxious gases. My brothers and I sat firmly in middle ground, which is actually a worse situation because then you never know what you're going to get. A 7 on the Fart Richter scale one day, unnatural and terrifying in stench the next. We were one big nose-holding family of gurgly bellies.

Enter sexual awakening.

As if the need to fart weren't problematic enough in general, I cannot tell you how many times my efforts during sex have focused on NOT FARTING. Sure, I can put on a sexy face, but really it is concentration on holding it in, or devising an excuse to stand up (*look sexy!*), move away from the bed (*look sexy!*), release (*look sexy and hold your nose!*), wait a moment (*look sexy and GOOD GOD DON'T BREATHE IN*), and walk back to the bed (*look sexy! Hell, if you feel better go for double sexy!*) in what hopefully comes across as an alluring ploy in seduction. Never mind if that seduction hinted at that evening's beef fajita and refried bean plate.

The first time I became aware that farting could be a huge problem during sex was when I was in high school with my first boyfriend. He was going down on me (holy frijoles, I really don't want to think about this let alone admit it anonymously on the internet) and I farted. Just a little. It was more like a tiny little *poot*. Right in my boyfriend's face.

He jumped up in disgust. I tried to play it off like it was no big deal, but of course I was mortified. What could be worse than pooting when your boyfriend's face is *right there*? He refused to go near me for the rest of the night. [Excuse me, I had to take a moment to cover my face with my hands in residual embarrassment. Even my ass is blushing at the memory.]

That horrible incident has followed me from bed to bed, making me very self-conscious if I've had anything more offensive than a bowl of cereal to eat in the last six hours. Forget the ass cellulite or tummy pooch, those so-called "problems" don't SMELL LIKE BURNED BURRITOS.

What brings out the farts? I don't get it. Sometimes there is no correlation to food. Maybe it's all the jostling about during sex, it stirs up the contents of the belly into the most ungodly combination of smells, brewing as if in a witch's cauldron until it finally unleashes itself on some poor unsuspecting fool.

About a month ago, The Marine and I were having sex after eating some especially tasty Chinese food. He was on top pounding away. The more he pounded the more gurgly I felt, but I was able to suppress it. He slowed down and then I heard it. A loud and distinct fart.

It wasn't me. I think.

The Marine froze, mid-thrust, holding each of my ankles in the air with his hands. His eyes looked left, then right, and finally down at me. I could smell the guilt coming from him.

I busted out laughing. Not because of the fart, but because the face The Marine made was one of the funniest things I have seen in all my years of fucking. I'm still giggling.

His face scrunched up in embarrassment. I patted his knee with my hand and said, "Oh good, I thought I was going to do that first!" Seriously, the guy beat me by about thirty seconds. In the Olympic event of Mid-Coital Flatulence, The Marine took home the gold.

His face broke into a goofy smile and he laughed. Once the air cleared we kept going. Duh.

When I was living with Aussie, we had been together long enough that it wasn't a huge deal if a little something eeked out. To the best of my memory there were no [*shudder*] incidents during sex, but there were dozens of times when we were watching TV that I saw Aussie sniffing the air before turning a raised eyebrow toward me. What, like *he* never farted?

"The dog! Oh my God, that is SO DISGUSTING," I would say, then shake my finger at Great Big Pit. If the fart had been really bad, I would stand up from the couch and make a run for it—cursing the dog all the way to safety.

After months of this, Aussie was convinced we needed to take the dog to the vet to get her digestive system checked out. I started eating more fruit and less dairy. The dog seemed to improve.

What No One Tells You About Losing Your Virginity

Lately I have received several emails from readers hoping/planning to lose their virginity soon. Virginity does not get much coverage in this blog for obvious reasons, but that doesn't mean it is not blog-worthy.

For the younger (or less sexually fortunate) readers out there, I'm going to tell you everything that I wish I had known when I was an adolescent eager beaver without easy internet access at my disposal. Damn my parents for keeping the computer in the office next to their bedroom.

The most important thing that no one tells you about losing your virginity is that the first time sucks.
Seriously, it is not fun or magical or even worth turning the TV off for. I remember laying there spread eagle after my first time wondering to myself, *That's it? WHAT THE HELL.* There are many people out there who have had wonderful first times (probably), but I do not know any of them. My first time sucked, and my second time sucked, and my third time sucked. Luckily for me I had a serious boyfriend at the time, so we kept going at it like good little horny Catholics until it became somewhat enjoyable.

After lots and lots of fucking (and a new boyfriend who obviously had better internet access), sex got to be awesome. It takes a while. Imagine that sex is like calculus: only one freak in a million knows how to do it right off the bat. The rest of us have to learn to add, divide, solve, and continue practicing until integrating is no big deal.

What Not to Expect
The female orgasm is a fickle little son of a bitch, and it can take years to find it. It took me a while to be able to orgasm every time. That means that you are clueless if you expect the girl to cum the first time she has sex. A thousand cool points for

you if it happens, but don't expect it. For most girls, clitoral orgasms are easier to achieve than vaginal. Practice, practice, practice. It will cum eventually.

What To Expect

Bodies are beautiful things, yada yada they also make really weird noises. They can be kind of disgusting at times. Queefing, for instance. Did you know the pussy can make noise? By Jove! It does, and it will at the worst time. Or did you know about the sex-farts when a couple is going at it, chest-to-chest, and the sweaty/smacking combination sounds like farts? Then there's the cellulite, the bouncing, the jiggling, the accidental smacking. There are long periods of ugly between the moments of sexy. The people on TV *lie*. But don't let that stop you. The bouncy-bouncy is fun and no guy is thinking about your cellulite when he's fucking you doggy-style. They're more like, "I'M HAVING SEX!! I'M FUCKING A GIRL DOGGY-STYLE! I WANT TO HIGH-FIVE MYSELF LIKE THE TOD!"

Having Sex for The Right Reason

If you answer yes to any of the following questions, then you are thinking about losing your virginity for the wrong reason. I'm not saying you have to do it for love (come on, we all know what it's like to be a horny teenager. It never goes away actually, hence the existence of my own site), but I will say you should do it because you want to. YOU want to. Not because someone else is telling you that you want to.

- Do you want to have sex to get someone to like you?
- Did someone ask you to have sex or else he/she will break up with you?
- Do you want to have sex to be cool?
- Do you want to have sex because there's nothing to watch on TV and your Xbox is broken?
- Do you want to give up your virginity because none of your friends are virgins anymore?

- Is anyone pressuring you to lose your virginity?
- For straight female readers: Is your potential partner a douchebag or a manipulative bitch?
- Are you nervous? Like so-nervous-I'm-going-to-piss-my-pants or about-to-cry-nervous, not *weeeeeeeeeee I'm-gonna-get-laaaaid* nervous?

Who Are You Going To Have Sex With?
It's okay if it's not a boyfriend or girlfriend, but it had better damn well be someone you like and respect. If he is a douchebag—no. Just don't sleep with a douchebag, okay? The world will be a better place if you don't encourage them. Make sure the person is someone nice who will show patience and understanding.

It can be nice to have sex for the first time with someone else who is a virgin, because then you're both nervous/clueless/on equal ground. However, it can also be nice to lose your virginity to someone who has been around the block a few times, because he/she can help lead the way. "Put your leg here," "go slower . . . not so hard . . ." is a big help. Besides that, if they know they are your first, they often want to help make it special (like they wish their own first time had been). Just please don't have sex with some random person you met on Facebook. Unless you're over the age of twenty-five, then just get it done.

Do not have sex if you are drunk.
That is a good rule to keep for yourself regardless of whether you're a virgin or not. Do not have sex if the other person is drunk either. I've never understood that. Okay, I get the whole "my inhibitions are lower so I'm not so nervous about hooking up with someone," but let me ask you this: What kind of fun is getting laid if you were too drunk to remember it? What if you had beer goggles and the person you slept with was ugly? Or an idiot? Or someone you would be too embarrassed to ever admit having sex with? Learn from millions of stupid drunk people before you and do not have sex when either of you are drunk.

I mean, come on. Do you want to look back ten years from now and tell your friends "my first time was with this total asshole who dumped me the next day because he didn't want his other girlfriend to find out about me" or "I lost my virginity to this chick whose screen name was EZhottie6969 because my buddies told me she'd sleep with anyone"? NO, YOU DON'T. Because mean people like me will make fun of you.

Don't Pretend You Aren't
If you're a virgin, don't lie about it. You may feel embarrassed, but everyone has been a virgin. You have no reason to lie about your lack of experience. If your partner has a lot more experience than you, then let him/her know it will be your first time. Assuming your partner is a decent human being, he or she will help guide the way. But don't lie. You can't fake experience like that.

Preparations
Condoms
Don't you dare consider having sex without a condom. If you do, I swear I will materialize out of thin air and smack the dumbass out of you so hard you'll be seeing a little cartoon bird with a hard-on flying around your head for weeks. All it takes is one time to get pregnant, one time to contract an icky sexually transmitted disease like herpes. Don't play the odds, because they are not in your favor. Condoms are also the most effective protection against STDs. This is serious. Do you want crotch rot? Then don't be a dumbfuck. Always use condoms.

If you're embarrassed about buying condoms in public, buy them online. I use Undercovercondoms.com because they have a huge selection and the shipped package is completely generic looking. It shows up as "PCPD, LLC" on the address label and on the credit card bill. I get mine sent to the office. This site also has a wide selection of lubricant, which YOU DO NEED. No matter how wet a girl gets during sex, she may still need lubricant. Spit works in a pinch, but that can be off-putting. I recommend Astroglide. There is an impressive display of lubricants at CVS and I imagine other drug stores would have a similar stock.

In an ideal world, the guy is the one to bring the condoms. Some bring only one (dude, what if it breaks?), smart ones bring a box of three. Idiots don't think to stop for condoms beforehand, or they expect you to have them, even though you're paying for birth control pills already, in an ideal world. In conclusion, you can't rely on the guy to be ready, so always have a box of 12 stashed somewhere near your bed. Better to be overstocked than pregnant. Case in point: I have never had to get an abortion, and I plan on keeping it that way.

Birth Control Pills

For girls considering having sex, you should get on birth control. It comes in many forms although I have always found the pill to be the easiest. *But why do I have to get on birth control if I promise to use a condom?* Because condoms break. It has happened to every one of my friends, and it has happened to me several times. There are dozens of pills available in generic that it's easy to find one for a $10 copay. If you're worried about your parents finding out, you can go to Planned Parenthood on your own. Their purpose is to make it easier for everyone to practice safe sex. They also give out free condoms by the handful. Keep one or two stashed in your purse, and grab a couple for your friends who are too embarrassed to buy any. Keep in mind that birth control pills do NOT protect against sexually transmitted diseases in any way. They are exclusively for protecting against pregnancy. And improving acne.

OH SHIT: Emergency Contraception

If the condom breaks and you don't have a back-up method of contraception, then get your ass over to Planned Parenthood for emergency contraception a.k.a. the morning after pill a.k.a. Plan B. Don't let the name fool you, it's effective if you start up to five days after sex, although most effective if started within three. It costs under $70, which is way cheaper and less scary than an abortion. I knew someone who bought the morning after pill and kept it in her medicine cabinet in case she or a friend ever needed it. All this stuff may sound incredibly not fun, but I promise it is a lot harder to get laid if you have crotch rot or a baby bump.

Finally Having Sex

Keep it simple. Don't go for reverse-cowgirl your first time. Stick with missionary (the default position = guy on top) because you don't want to risk kicking the guy in the head or falling off the bed. You're doing good if Tab A makes it into Slot B in three tries or less. Once you get the mechanics down, explore other positions. Don't show off when it's obvious you don't know shit. And, sweetie, no matter how ready you think you'll be, you won't know as much as you think. But that's okay. It's part of the experience and builds character and yada yada you need to start somewhere.

Some advice from the spread-eagle troops in the trenches: It may feel stupid the first few times, but missionary is much easier if the girl sticks her legs straight up in the air and keeps them there. She can grab onto her legs to keep them up/spread open. It will feel less weird if the girl is wearing some sexy shoes, has painted toenails, etc. And for fuck's sake *shave your legs*. No guy wants a paper cut from touching a girl's calve.

It Hurts, It Bleeds, It's Not Pretty

For many girls the first time can hurt. Maybe a little, sometimes a lot. No need to worry, there are ways to make sure it won't hurt much. My first time was no big deal because my boyfriend had been fingering me for months beforehand. The first time he fingered me hard I bled a little, and that was it. Besides my boyfriend helping to loosen up my pussy, I had been using a tampon for years. The first time I used one I damn near fainted, but I'm glad I got used to things being up there because it made things much easier later on. If you're worried about bleeding, lay a dark towel out beforehand.

Within half an hour of finishing sex, go pee. It helps lessen your chance of getting a urinary tract infection, a.k.a. a bladder infection which is not the ideal memento to get out of the experience. If things are very itchy and uncomfortable, that means you got a UTI. Drinking lots of cranberry juice is a good home remedy (just make sure it says 100% juice on the label, otherwise you can drink all the cranberry cocktail in the store and not get anywhere), and if that doesn't do it then you probably need to go to the doctor for antibiotics. The lesson here: Pee after sex. It's much easier than all that other crap.

Before the actual sex, make sure your pussy has been loosened up a little. It will be much easier for entry if you are already relaxed and wet. If you're tight or dry, then it will hurt. Keep lubricant on hand to eliminate friction. Don't go straight for the sex. That is a truly terrible habit to get into. Foreplay is fun and can last hours longer than the sex. Yay foreplay!!! If you've never used a vibrator, get one now to loosen yourself up so the penetration doesn't hurt so much.

Just So You Know
Girls talk. Guys talk. Both can say filthy things that the other would be mortified to hear. Assume the other person told their closest friends, and hopefully they have the class to stop there. If you think he/she doesn't, then you may want to hold out for someone you know won't start a rumor about you. All it takes is one rumor to turn you into the school or office slut, regardless of its inaccuracy.

Final Reminder
Sex is supposed to be fun. Eventually. If the idea of losing your virginity isn't fun or exciting, then reconsider why you're thinking about having sex in the first place. And remember, practice, practice, practice. Then read about the awesomeness that is the almighty kegel.

Other Resources

Planned Parenthood is one of the best resources out there for birth control, abortions, STD tests, information, and a bajillion other things.
www.plannedparenthood.org

Our Bodies, Ourselves is an awesome book that should be given to every girl on her twelfth birthday.
www.ourbodiesourselves.org

Wondering About Him

I know I'll meet Mr. Perfect-For-Me one day. I may be a cynic and a little bit of a bitch when it comes to dating, but I'm a sucker for love.

Sometimes I find myself wondering about him when I see a cute couple walk by or when I'm holding hands with my favorite brown-eyed distraction. I'm not ready to meet Mr. Perfect-For-Me yet, but I like to think about what he'll be like.

Who is he? What is he like? Where is he right now? What is he doing with his life? Is he searching for the same things I am? What will it take for us to find each other? When will I be ready to meet him and not run screaming the other way?

I often wonder what he'll be like. Hopefully, he will have some of the things I imagine in my ideal mate: warm eyes with laugh lines at the corners, a hearty laugh like my father's, a love of storytelling, beautiful hands. Forget the "tall, dark, and handsome" bit, or the modern version of "tall, hot, and sexy." As much as I joke around about guys with hairy asses, I know that love comes in any shape it damn well wants to be in, man boobs or not. All that's fine, as long as I'm in love.

When am I going to meet him? When will I be ready? What do I have left to figure out in my own life before I'm prepared to share it with someone else?

There's an old cover of *The New Yorker* I have up on the wall here above my desk. For a long time I didn't know why I kept it, but I think I finally understand. In the illustration, a girl sits by herself on the subway reading. As she looks up from her book, she sees a guy reading the exact same one in a passing subway car, and their eyes meet.

Reading has always been one of my favorite things to do since I was a child. My parents spent many evenings trying to tear me away from a book because I was so caught up in the world in my hands that I was missing out on my own life. "Why don't you go play with your friends?" they'd ask, or "Why don't you play soccer with your brother in the backyard?" All I wanted to do was read.

I'm not quite as bad any more, but that's because the time is offset with writing now. Friends call me up to hang out, coworkers invite me to happy hours and I say I'm can't. They don't question me, and I don't explain. Instead I stay up many nights writing and staring at the wall in frustration.

What I'm getting at is I want someone who gets my world. It's a bizarre little world full of grey. Although I have a few friends who understand my world enough to talk about it occasionally, there isn't anyone who *gets* it, who gets me the way I want to be understood. What will it take for that to happen one day? What if we're both so busy in our own little worlds that we miss each other entirely?

Since it would be easy to let that depress me, I try not to think about it. Sometimes I wonder if I'm stupid for being hopeful. Other times I tell myself that I should believe there is someone out there for me. All night I have been staring at the illustration on the wall and wondering if he is out there wondering about me too.

Why We Got The King-Size Bed

It was the first full day of our sexcation in Puerta Vallarta, Mexico, and that evening I wanted to go drink and check out the live band playing in the hotel pavilion. The Marine grumbled that he needed some sleep. No problem, we didn't get in until late the night before. We lay down on the king-size bed for a much-needed nap.

I woke up an hour later feeling frisky as hell. We had not yet had sex on our vacation, first because of the delayed flight and then that morning as soon as I saw the sun was shining I took off running for the pool. I nudged The Marine to wake up. He didn't move. I put my hand on his shoulder and sweetly said, "It's time to get up." He didn't move. I slid my hand over his crotch and started massaging.

He didn't move. "Marine?" I asked louder. My hand massaged harder. At least one part of his body was beginning to wake up.

"I'm sleeping," he mumbled.

Okay, fine. He's tired. But, jeez, I was tired too. Supposedly, I was even more sleep-deprived than he was because I had been up late every night that week working on my presentation at work. I don't know, something about BEING IN MEXICO ON VACATION kept me energized. I got up and changed into a sexy little sundress, then casually walked around in front of him in hopes that he would feel inspired to GET THE FUCK UP.

The Marine's response was to begin snoring. My sundress felt a little insulted.

I decided to read and try waking him up again in an hour. I lay on the bed and read, being sure to make lots of loud noises to encourage The Marine to wake up. He snored louder.

An hour later I snuggled up behind The Marine. He didn't move. I put my arm on his side. Nothing. I rubbed his hip and crotch with my hand. Nothing.

As I patted The Marine softly on the shoulder, I whispered in his ear, "Time to wake up and go out."

"LEAVE ME ALONE!" he snapped. It was the first time he had ever snapped at me.

My eyes narrowed into little slits. Did he just *snap* at me? IN PUERTA VALLARTA?!! How *dare* he snap at me like that.

I lay stunned on the bed for a moment. Then I got up, took off the insulted sundress, and put on a fuck-you T-shirt. No boobie show for The Marine. I climbed back into bed under the covers and pulled out my book. Hmm, it's kind of dark. I flipped on the bedside lamp. Ooooh, nice and bright!

I turned on my side and accidentally on purpose kicked The Marine a little. He didn't move. I accidentally kicked him again, harder this time. He grunted.

My stomach began to feel funny. Uh oh, I felt a fart coming on. Normally I would find a discreet and non-offensive way to let it out, but The Marine had pissed me off. WE ARE ON SEXCATION IN MEXICO. WHAT IS THE FUCKING POINT OF SEXCATION IF THERE IS *NO SEX*?

I looked over my shoulder. My ass was pointed directly at The Marine, sleeping soundly like a little cranky angel.

I farted. It was silent but deadly. HAHA, TAKE THAT! I JUST GAVE YOU A DUTCH OVEN, ASSHOLE!

I looked over my shoulder again. The Marine's nose was not anywhere near being under the covers. *Shit.* What's the point of a Dutch oven if no one is there to die in it?

In a huff, I turned onto my back and lifted the covers to shake out the smell. *ACHHKKK.* It hit me full-on in the face. Shit *I did not think this through*, I thought to myself as I covered my nose with my hands in a futile attempt at protection.

With the covers placed down safely around my waist, I turned onto my side and kicked The Marine one more time. It was a hard one because it knocked one of his legs out of position. "*HA HA*," goes Nelson.

An hour and a half, two walks around the hotel and several chapters in my book later, The Marine woke up. I was fuming. Not only did I not get laid—in

Mexico—but we missed the live Mexican band I had wanted to see. Sure, I went out and looked around on my own, but some things are way more fun when with someone else. LIKE SEX.

I felt The Marine turn to face me in bed. I was focused on pretending that I was reading.

His hand rested on my hip. I hissed at him.

"I'm sorry I slept all night, babe." I ignored him. "I didn't feel very good." Really? Maybe it was all the kicking.

He attempted to spoon me. I was not having it. TONIGHT I AM A BUTTER KNIFE, A-HOLE. NO SPOONS FOR YOU. I continued fake-reading until he fell asleep.

I read a little longer until I was tired, then I turned off the lamp and snuggled under the covers. Keep in mind this was a king-size hotel bed, so we had a lot of mattress to work with. The Marine had started the evening well on his side, with me only a crotch-grab away.

As the night progressed, I moved farther and farther away from him. With a king-size bed there is a huge expanse of avoidance to be utilized.

Once he woke up and attempted to snuggle, he invaded my half of the bed. That's MY HALF. It is only for people WHO WANT TO HAVE SEX WHILE ON VACATION. YOU SIR ARE NOT WELCOME ON MY HALF. Thus the kicking continued throughout the night. The Marine continued to pursue my snuggles across the vastness of the bed, to no avail.

SNUGGLES COME AFTER *SEX*, ASSHOLE.

Slipping By

When we were flying back from Mexico last week, I sat by the window and read a book I had borrowed from Favorite Coworker. As I flipped to a new page I found a note tucked inside the pages. *You're going to be my wife!! I love you XOXO.* It must have been from Favorite Coworker's new husband when they were engaged.

I touched the note with the tip of my finger and smiled. It warmed my frigid heart.

With the book still open in my lap I peered out the window of the airplane. I have always loved the window seat on flights, especially on long trips when you can watch the land change in color and terrain. The Marine had scoffed when it became apparent that I had assumed he would let me have the window seat on all four of our flights. On the outside I graciously offered to take turns, but on the inside I pouted. The little girl in me didn't want to share.

I watched the land slowly slip by thousands of feet below us. I stared out the window with the same wonderment I have had every time I have been in an airplane since I was a child. It amazed me that we were up here in a tiny little aircraft zipping across thousands of miles of land as if it were no big deal. The view is probably something I will never see again. I will take many more trips in my life, and the views will always be different. Sometimes I will see mountains, other times hills or plains or a huge lake or nothing but miles of ocean in every direction. The colors of the earth will change and I will get to see it from miles above. It is remarkable that people are able to experience this across the world every single day, and today I am lucky enough to be one of them.

As I turned my attention back to the book, my thoughts returned to the note I had found. I studied the curves of the lettering, the slant of the words across the torn piece of paper. My eyes teared up, because I want that. I want someone who will write sweet little things like that for me one day, and when I discover one, I will smile because I will know that I got it right.

I looked over at The Marine next to me. His hard jawline, his clever eyes, his crooked smile, those pale green eyes that never asked anything of me. With every part of my being, I felt a simple, *No*.

Sure, he's nice and sweet and fun to fuck, but no. Just no. There may be affection, but there is no love or future here.

I turned my head back to the window. The land passed beneath us slowly. I wondered if we were still in Mexico or had crossed the Texas border yet. Everything looked so much prettier from this distance. I wished I could stay there forever, but you can only watch life slip by for so long.

One day I'll get there. I sighed and turned the page in my book.

Recommended Reading

Authors listed without titles means that I don't have a favorite

Memoirs & Blogs
Jen Lancaster
Suzanne Finnamore
The Liar's Club by Mary Karr
Mary by Mary Karr
Dry by Augusten Burroughs

Fiction
Bad Behavior by Mary Gaitskill
Beautiful Bodies by Laura Shaine Cunningham
Dancing After Hours by Andre Dubus
This is Not Chick Lit edited by Elizabeth Merrick
Middlesex by Jeffrey Eugenides
Lust by Susan Minot
Justin Cronin
Alice Munro
Antonya Nelson
Anna Quindlen

Nonfiction
The Bitch in the House edited by Cathi Hanauer

Poetry
Sylvia Plath, Complete Works
The Gold Cell by Sharon Olds
Rose by Li-Young Lee
A Working Girl Can't Win by Deborah Garrison

Play
The Vagina Monologues by Eve Ensler

Photography
Miss Aniela: Multiplicity by Miss Aniela
Lady: Lisa Lyon by Robert Mapplethorpe
Dessous by Gilles Neret

Art
Love for Sale: The Words and Pictures of Barbara Kruger by Kate Linker
Georgia O'Keeffe: American and Modern by Charles C. Eldredge

Feminism & Sexuality
Sex and the City, complete TV series available on Amazon Prime for free
The Ethical Slut by Dossie Easton and Janet Hardy
Nymphomania by Carol Groneman
Woman: An Intimate Geography by Natalie Angier
Women and Desire: Beyond Wanting to be Wanted by Polly Young-Eisendrath
The Technology of Orgasm: "Hysteria," The Vibrator, and Women's Sexual Satisfaction by Rachel P. Maines
Talk Dirty to Me: An Intimate Philosophy of Sex by Sallie Tisdale

Sex
The Good Girls' Guide to Bad Girl Sex by Barbara Keesling, Ph.D.
Expanded Orgasm by Patricia Taylor, Ph.D.

Depression
I'm sure there are more recently published books, but these are the ones that helped me.
Darkness Visible by William Styron
Undoing Depression by Richard O'Connor, Ph.D.
Breaking the Patterns of Depression by Michael D. Yapko, Ph.D.
Get it Done When You're Depressed by Julie A. Fast and John D. Preston, Psy.D, ABPP

ADD/ADHD
Thom Hartmann's Complete Guide to ADHD by Thom Hartmann
The Gift of Adult ADD by Lara Honos-Webb, Ph.D.
Driven to Distraction by Edward M. Hallowell, M.D., and John J. Ratey, M.D.

Getting Out
What Color is Your Parachute? By Richard N. Bolles

Because Everyone Should Own a Copy
Oh, the Places You'll Go! by Dr. Seuss

Afterword

I'd do it all again. Every last mistake, I would do it again. How else do you learn and gain life experience and acquire hilarious stories to share with your friends? It was all worth it, every last fuck. It made me who I am today, and I don't know if you know this, but I'm kind of a badass.

I'd do it all again.

Vix

October 27, 2018

Excerpt from Next Book

TITTYSPRINKLES

Smitten

After finally discovering the new, cute IT Guy was single, and after waiting a few more days to feel him out, I talked to him today. Actually, first contact was over email. How many times have I said that I come across much better in written form than face-to-face? You can delete the dumbass side of your personality in an email much more easily than pulling the foot out of your mouth.

And like a good Hollywood movie, our relationship started just before a weather crisis. Hurricane Ike was two days out, and the entire city of Houston was hunkering down in preparation.

It started with an email. IT Guy sent out a generic email to the entire company about preparing the server for backup before the hurricane hits. The clever little biscuit that I am, I thought to myself, Alas! The perfect opportunity to display my wit and charisma to IT Guy! Must proceed with *Operation: Charm Pants Off* immediately!

It took several minutes to construct the perfect three-sentence email response with which to bait him. How to stand out as being funny and clever, yet sexy and endearing, and somehow make this an appropriate reply to a generic information technology email? Like I said, I toiled for *several* minutes, which included deleting only two pieces of dumbassery.

I waited. Meanwhile I pretended to work: Picking up papers and putting them down in different places on the desk, shuffling things around, furrowing my brow in concentration while I anxiously awaited a reply.

Shortly after, an email from IT Guy popped up. Squealing at a workplace-appropriate level, I clicked it open and scanned the response. He was biting. He was funny. Like *smart*-funny, not frat-boy-funny or poop-funny. YESSSS!

The emails began. Quickly he found an indirect way to ask if I were in a *we* situation. Nope! No one! Technically! The Marine was on his way out already. I beamed with delight at how well things were going.

Except we still haven't actually spoken to each other after half an hour of emailing. I can't be sure that he knows what face belongs to the emails. Time to suck it up and introduce myself properly. As soon as I stood up, I felt king-kong size butterflies in my stomach.

With each step I heard a big Chinese gong in my head: Stop while you're ahead! What if he thinks you're funny-looking? Don't get your hopes up, you stupid girl!

By the time I reached the IT department, it felt like my stomach was going into self-destruct mode.

I walked up to IT Guy's cubicle. The back of his head is so cute.

"Hey, I'm Vix." Please think I'm hot.

He turned his chair around toward me and started laughing. He was all smiles. Good. I'm in. Right?

We talked for fifteen minutes. It was fifteen minutes of pure awesomeness. The memory of those fifteen minutes glows in my mind like a ray of non-cheeky sunshine. Under the watchful eyes of partners walking by, I reluctantly went back to work. Although I also wanted to stop talking before I said something so back-asswards stupid that there was no hope of redemption before I got to see him naked.

And we were off. IT Guy matched me email for email for the rest of the afternoon. Every joke, no matter how odd, was too much for him to volley. I was amazed. Not only was the content smart and funny, he wrote emails properly. That includes capitalizing words that are supposed to be capitalized, spelling out words the way they are meant to be spelled, and using fancy things like commas and paragraphs. The guy gave good email. As if that weren't awesome enough, he is just sexually suggestive enough to be playful without being too forward.

With great finesse, IT Guy dropped hints at the many ways we could spend time together outside work. If it weren't for the hurricane mess shutting down half the county, we probably would have gone to happy hour after work today. Once we figured out how close we live to each other, he suggested that I come over to wait out the storm with him and his friends. At first I thought that sounded a little bit much, but the only vibes I got from him were warm, fuzzy ones.

When the office closed early, I went to say good-bye and we ended up talking for another hour. Then for a few more minutes by my desk when I was logging off. And again in the parking lot. The chemistry was so thick you could reach out and touch it. I'm not just referring to the sexual pull, but the meshing of personalities. In such a short amount of time, it feels like he gets me as much as my closest girlfriends do.

IT Guy reminds me of a mix between Jim from *The Office* and my brother. Chill, easy to talk to, funny as hell, and impossible not to like. Great personality and cute enough that I want to bite him like a soft, buttery pretzel. I could see myself with IT Guy. Like introducing him to all three of my friends and breathing out the "B" word without gagging.

How can I feel so drawn to IT Guy when I've known him for such a short amount of time? The chemistry was undeniable, but how much can you tell in half a day of emailing, texting, and talking? Am I itching to see what I want to see?

What if he turns out to be a stalker who likes to watch me sleep through my bedroom window? What if it turns out he's a huge let-down? What if I scare him off? Besides having a strong personality, there's the sexual history, the sexual present (The Marine who has been all hugs-and-snuggles lately is staying at my place during the hurricane. Wow, this makes things about five times more complicated), and assuming IT Guy can hold up through all that, telling him that I'm a sex blogger after hours?

It takes a special kind of friend to wade through a waist-high secret life, but it takes an extra special guy to be willing to commit to someone with many documented reasons for why he should proceed with caution. There is a lot of room for me to fuck things up as we get to know each other.

I haven't felt this way about someone in a long time. Ever, actually. My chemistry with Aussie was half this and took twice as long. Could IT Guy be too good to be true? Can I freeze time at this point right here, the point before the first date when everything still has the potential to be more wonderful than I ever imagined? I like it here. Where every text message is flirtatious, and every phone call is an hour-long banter session.

How can this be happening? If I were someone reading this post, I'd cock my head to one side and wonder if the blogger were making this up. How can someone say, "Okay, I think I'm ready to enter a relationship" and then BOOM, less than a month later there's a hilarious guy with a beautiful smile and an ice cream obsession that rivals mine? I thought things like that only happened in five-dollar chick flicks.

Who knew I would say something like this so soon? I'm concerned that I'm not more scared this is happening. Am I getting my hopes up for someone who turns out to be a total tool? What if he has a small dick? What if I let him in and he breaks me in half? Am I really ready to see where this leads?

And yet in spite of all my what ifs, I'm anything but scared. Our first date is Monday night.

Made in United States
Orlando, FL
10 January 2024